The Clinician's Guide to Alaryngeal Speech Therapy

D1120888

The Clinician's Guide to Alaryngeal Speech Therapy

Minnie S. Graham, Ph.D.
Department of Special Education,
Communicative Disorders Program,
San Francisco State University

Foreword by
Philip C. Doyle, Ph.D., CCC-SLP
Associate Professor, Department of
Communication Sciences and Disorders,
Vocal Production Laboratory,
The University of Western Ontario,
London, Ontario, Canada

Butterworth–Heinemann
Boston   Oxford   Johannesburg   Melbourne   New Delhi   Singapore

Copyright © 1997 by Butterworth–Heinemann

℞ A member of the Reed Elsevier group

All rights reserved.

No part of this publication may be reproduced, stored in a retrieval system, or transmitted in any form or by any means, electronic, mechanical, photocopying, recording, or otherwise, without the prior written permission of the publisher.

Every effort has been made to ensure that the drug dosage schedules within this text are accurate and conform to standards accepted at time of publication. However, as treatment recommendations vary in the light of continuing research and clinical experience, the reader is advised to verify drug dosage schedules herein with information found on product information sheets. This is especially true in cases of new or infrequently used drugs.

Recognizing the importance of preserving what has been written, Butterworth–Heinemann prints its books on acid-free paper whenever possible.

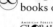 Butterworth–Heinemann supports the efforts of American Forests and the Global ReLeaf Program in its campaign for the betterment of trees, forests, and our environment.

Library of Congress Cataloging-in-Publication Data

Graham, Minnie S.
    The clinician's guide to alaryngeal speech therapy / Minnie S. Graham.
        p.   cm.
    Includes bibliographical references and index.
    ISBN 0-7506-9862-4 (alk. paper)
    1. Speech therapy. 2. Laryngectomees--Rehabilitation. I. Title.
    [DNLM: 1. Speech, Alaryngeal. 2. Speech Therapy.
    3. Laryngectomy. WV 540 G741c 1997]
    RC423.G674 1997
    616.85'506--dc21
    DNLM/DLC
    for Library of Congress   97-21510
                                                                      CIP

British Library Cataloguing-in-Publication Data
A catalogue record for this book is available from the British Library.

The publisher offers special discounts on bulk orders of this book.
For information, please contact:
Manager of Special Sales
Butterworth–Heinemann
313 Washington Street
Newton, MA 02158-1626
Tel: 617-928-2500
Fax: 617-928-2620

For information on all Butterworth–Heinemann publications available, contact our World Wide Web home page at: http://www.bh.com

10 9 8 7 6 5 4 3 2 1

Printed in the United States of America

To my husband and our son for their consistent and enthusiastic support throughout this venture. In appreciation of their patience and understanding, I lovingly dedicate my work to them.

Contents

Foreword

Those of us who teach speech after laryngectomy accept the fact that we are not indispensable. We see ourselves as sharing information gained directly from previous experience and indirectly from the writings of others. For some laryngectomees we need do little beyond providing that information. For some laryngectomees we need to do more.*

Reminiscent of the suggestion made by Dr. James Shanks nearly 20 years ago, *The Clinician's Guide to Alaryngeal Speech Therapy*, by Dr. Minnie Graham, offers a contemporary resource for the primary parties at the unique clinical roundtable of alaryngeal speech rehabilitation. Dr. Graham has prepared her guide to not only meet the direct needs of speech-language pathologists, but also to meet the needs of a very special group of individuals with whom these clinicians work. Although the connection between clinician and patient seems obvious, written works in most areas of communication disorder often address only the specific problem of interest rather than the problem *and* the patient. Although it is common for clinician-oriented texts and guides to provide approaches and materials for treatment, the general background and rationale underlying such approaches, tasks, or materials are frequently omitted. This guide is a clinical resource that has successfully merged both requirements.

The most successful clinicians are almost certainly those who reflect on their own experiences—both successes and failures—and carefully consider the contributions of others found in both the scientific and clinical literature in making clinical decisions. The likelihood of clinical success is improved when the clinician carefully evaluates the rationale behind his or her choice of any given clinical task or protocol he or she asks the patient to perform. Success in the clinical domain finds its foundation in defining the problem, choosing a treatment plan based on a sound rationale, and more often than not, being comfortable enough in one's abilities to "tweak" the task when difficulties are encountered. When success is observed, this information must be shared with others so that other laryngectomees will benefit. The presentation of Dr. Graham's experience serves that purpose.

---

*From JC Shanks. Essentials for Alaryngeal Speech: Psychology and Physiology. In RL Keith, FL Darley (eds), Laryngectomy Rehabilitation. San Diego: College-Hill Press, 1979;469.

An additional advantage of *The Clinician's Guide to Alaryngeal Speech Therapy* is the manner in which it addresses the topic of laryngectomy—one that will permit both new and experienced clinicians to consider the process of speech rehabilitation after treatment for laryngeal cancer and the ultimate impact it has on any given patient's life. The information provided by Dr. Graham is appropriate for those patients who "need little" and for those with whom we "need to do more." Similarly, Dr. Graham's guide provides a point of departure for the clinician who is uninitiated into the clinical voyage with laryngectomees, as well as a continuation point for those clinicians who have previously undertaken this journey. This guide will be long used by students and professionals.

As we move into the twenty-first century, the traditionally accepted profile of the laryngeal cancer patient will no doubt change dramatically. Epidemiologic data suggest that an increasing number of women will be diagnosed with laryngeal malignancy and that the age of both men and women at time of diagnosis may be younger. Concomitantly, the likelihood that these individuals will live longer after diagnosis and treatment of disease is increasingly evident. These and other changes in patient and prognostic demographics demonstrate a clear need for more comprehensive approaches to speech rehabilitation after laryngectomy. *The Clinician's Guide to Alaryngeal Speech Therapy* meets this need. The strength of this work centers on its well-organized, thematic, and cohesive presentation, including an extensive array of speech stimuli. Dr. Graham's expertise is reflected admirably as she provides the critical link between the clinician and the patient. This guide provides the most comprehensive collection of practice stimuli currently available for alaryngeal speech training.

The timeliness of Dr. Graham's book is important for one additional reason. If one asks new clinicians what background preparation they have with regard to alaryngeal speech rehabilitation, the most likely answer will suggest that their preparation is limited. To my knowledge, very few programs in communication sciences and disorders in North America provide any detailed, formal course work in laryngectomy and alaryngeal voice and speech rehabilitation. In many instances, classroom exposure to laryngectomy comprises one or two lectures. Thus, although enhancement of the "voice" curriculum in many educational programs has been observed throughout North America and abroad during the past 15 years, the component of academic curricula that addresses clinical care of laryngectomees has been omitted entirely or severely restricted. The current scenario is in stark contrast to the curricula of old, in which alaryngeal speech rehabilitation was often a prominent component of many academic programs. This criticism of the current trend is not presented to suggest that we return to the old curricular practices, but rather, to acknowledge that educational exposure and clinical training in the area of alaryngeal speech therapy is likely inadequate in many venues. Because this important clinical area is now often overlooked, newer clinicians are facing an increasing awareness of the limitations of their clinical preparation.

In summary, *The Clinician's Guide to Alaryngeal Speech Therapy* is a concise yet comprehensive resource that will guide clinicians through the often arduous clinical process with the laryngectomee. This guide will serve both the clinician and the patient as they move through the rehabilitation process together. Dr. Graham has provided a resource that offers the potential for better patient care and an enhanced likelihood of a favorable rehabilitation outcome.

Philip C. Doyle

Preface

Seventeen years ago, I accepted part-time employment with two other speech-language pathologists (SLPs) to conduct a laryngectomee group supported by San Francisco Community College and later sponsored by San Francisco State University. This book is the culmination of 17 years of challenging and inspiring interactions with these remarkable laryngectomees and their families as we explored alaryngeal speech rehabilitation together.

The Clinician's Guide to Alaryngeal Speech Therapy is written in a practical, clinically oriented style for the SLP who is interested in working effectively with the laryngectomee and family. At the risk of labeling this text a "how-to" book, I have attempted to organize the material in a sequential manner so that the clinician can follow the laryngectomee step by step through the rehabilitation process. The design of the text will appeal to the SLP who has limited experience providing alaryngeal speech therapy; the chapters progress from the time the individual and family are informed of the cancer until the conclusion of therapeutic intervention. The experienced clinician will appreciate the extensive practice activities as well as the ready-to-use forms that appear throughout the text and in the appendixes.

In Chapter 1, a description of the development of laryngeal cancer, the causes, and the most common symptoms of laryngeal cancer are provided. The reader is supplied with current facts and figures about the incidence of laryngeal cancer in the United States. The procedures involved in the medical evaluation are explained as are the available treatment options if the tumor is cancerous. The importance of preoperative counseling of the individual and family by the SLP is emphasized.

Many speech clinicians meet the laryngectomee for the first time in the hospital. Chapter 2 presents the anatomic and physiologic changes that occur as a result of laryngectomy. The intake interview is designed to obtain and provide information, express and explore feelings, problem solve, and plan for future action. Instructions are provided for conducting the oral examination using universal precautions developed by the Centers for Disease Control. The primary goal of postoperative counseling is to establish a communication system for the laryngectomee as soon as possible.

The selection of a communication system by the laryngectomee calls into consideration a number of factors. The advantages and disadvantages of oral communication options, including the artificial larynx, esophageal speech methods, and tracheoesophageal speech, are discussed in Chapter 3. A systematic approach to therapy facilitates the acquisition of intelligible speech by providing an objective method for analyzing and modifying the laryngectomee's behaviors. In Chapter 4, a hierarchical approach to teaching alaryngeal speech is explained.

The information and guidelines presented in Chapters 5–7 are specific to teaching the laryngectomee one or more methods of oral communication. Chapter 5 is dedicated to teaching the use of the artificial larynx. Five target behaviors are identified: finding the best placement, coordinating the "on" control with speaking, improving articulatory precision, using appropriate rate and phrasing, and attending to nonverbal behaviors. Solutions to problems commonly encountered by the artificial larynx user are offered. An activity hierarchy guides the speech clinician and laryngectomee through a series of exercises designed to develop proficient use of the artificial larynx. Six levels of production are identified, from short phrases to spontaneous conversation. At each level of production, the laryngectomee progresses through three phases of difficulty: initial, intermediate, and advanced.

There are two primary methods for moving air from the oral cavity into the esophagus to achieve esophageal speech: the injection and inhalation methods. In Chapter 6, a rationale for following a hierarchical approach to esophageal speech training is presented, along with a review of the literature on this topic. Specific techniques for teaching the injection method for obstruents, the injection method for sonorants and vowels, and the inhalation method are described in this chapter. Goals tailored to meet the distinctive needs of each method are accompanied by discussions of potential problems and their resolution. Esophageal speech training uses a systematic approach: Within three phases of difficulty, activities are determined by the number of goals, the phonetic context, and the level of production. By definition, *proficient esophageal speech* means the laryngectomee successfully combines the use of both injection and inhalation methods to produce spontaneous speech. Chapter 6 concludes with a special section, *Proficient Esophageal Speech*, which offers the advanced esophageal speaker a number of activities using advanced goals: articulatory precision, rate, phrasing, intonation and stress, and loudness.

Chapter 7 discusses tracheoesophageal speech. The clinician is informed about the function of the prosthesis and the contents of the prosthesis user's kit. Teaching tracheoesophageal speech encompasses five primary goals: attention to valving, articulation, rate, phrasing, and nonverbal behaviors. In step-by-step fashion, the activity hierarchies take the clinician and laryngectomee from the short-phrase level to spontaneous conversation. The chapter includes troubleshooting procedures specifically related to care and maintenance of the tracheoesophageal tract and prosthesis.

In the early stages of teaching any of the oral communication techniques, one-on-one therapy is an essential part of the learning process. In Chapter 8, however, the SLP will find a framework for a combination of individual and group therapy of special importance in alaryngeal speech rehabilitation. The group environment serves different functions in a variety of ways—incorporating educational, speech activities, social interaction, and support-counseling themes. Meeting in a group affords the laryngectomee the opportunity to benefit from communal knowledge about anatomic and physiologic changes, medical conditions and procedures, diet, and personal hygiene. Speech activities for the enhancement and generalization of functional communication skills are provided. Within the social interaction theme, the focus is on peer feedback and pragmatics. Counseling allows the laryngectomee to address psychological issues, such as fears of aging, death, and recurrence of cancer, and physical, sensory, behavioral, psychological, and social losses.

Accountability is an important issue in the field of speech-language pathology. In Chapter 9, the clinician is introduced to the procedures for evaluating the alaryngeal speech of the laryngectomee-in-training as well as guidelines for goal setting, lesson planning, writing therapy logs, and report writing.

In Chapter 10, closure of the therapeutic relationship is discussed. Therapy may be terminated for a number of reasons—the laryngectomee may achieve functional communication, move away, seek the services of another speech clinician, join another laryngectomee group, withdraw voluntarily or be terminated by the clinician, or expire. The chapter concludes with a challenge to the SLP to strive for proficiency in alaryngeal speech rehabilitation.

An extensive guide to suppliers of alaryngeal speech products and services appears in Appendix A. A relaxation exercise and oral-facial exercises are found in Appendixes B and C, respectively. The stimuli lists in Appendixes D–G are arranged according to the alaryngeal speech methods discussed in Chapters 5–7. Stimuli derived from an unrestricted phonetic context are found in Appendix D. The lists are arranged according to level of production—beginning with two- to four-syllable phrases and sentences and ending with spontaneous and extended conversation. These stimuli lists are designed for practice by individuals learning artificial larynx speech, combined methods of esophageal speech, and tracheoesophageal speech. For the laryngectomee who needs specific articulation practice, consonant contrast drills for consonants in the initial and final positions in words are shown in Appendix E. Stimuli for teaching the injection method for obstruents in esophageal speech (Appendix F) are arranged in a hierarchy beginning with unvoiced obstruents and concluding with five- to six-syllable phrases and sentences using both unvoiced and voiced obstruents. The practice stimuli in Appendix G are used by the laryngectomee who is learning either the injection method for sonorants and vowels or the inhalation method in esophageal speech.

Stimuli for the evaluation of alaryngeal speech—artificial larynx speech, the injection method for obstruents, the injection method for sonorants and vowels, the inhalation method, combined methods of esophageal speech, and tracheoesophageal speech—appear in Appendix H. Instructions for their use are given in Chapter 9.

MSG

Acknowledgments

This book was made possible by the experiences I have had with laryngectomees and their families during the past 17 years. These wonderful people continue to teach my students and me how to provide effective alaryngeal speech therapy. I stand in admiration of their ability to turn affliction to advantage, vulnerability to strength. A special thank you to Rudy Cook, Seiichi Harada, Jim Harren, Joe Lorenzo, Margaret McGlew, and Mark Wester for their desire to educate others about alaryngeal speech rehabilitation by appearing in this text.

For their dedication and for the knowledge shared so generously by the professionals who care for laryngectomees—physicians, nurses, social workers, audiologists, and fellow speech-language pathologists—I am indebted. The American Cancer Society provided a wealth of laryngectomee rehabilitation literature. Thanks to Bivona Medical Technologies, Griffin Laboratories, and InHealth Technologies for their assistance in providing a number of photographs and illustrations found in this text.

More than 100 graduate students in speech-language pathology have provided therapy in the alaryngeal speech clinic at San Francisco State University. These bright young people have contributed significantly to my understanding of laryngectomee rehabilitation. Four extraordinary individuals—Arlene Arceo, Denise George, Ann Papale, and John Thompson—in their quest for knowledge, challenged and inspired me to write this book.

Finally, I wish to thank Barbara Murphy, Senior Medical Editor at Butterworth–Heinemann, for her enthusiasm as well as encouragement during the writing of the manuscript. Jana Friedman, Assistant Editor at Butterworth–Heinemann, provided expert technical assistance that brought this manuscript to production. The copyediting advice offered by Dana Tackett, Production Editor at Silverchair Science + Communications, was truly singular.

The Clinician's Guide to Alaryngeal Speech Therapy

1

Laryngeal Cancer: An Overview

DESCRIPTION AND DEVELOPMENT

Cancer of the larynx is a disease in which squamous cells undergo an abnormal change and begin a process of uncontrolled growth and spread [1–3]. These cells grow into masses of tissue, called tumors, in the laryngeal area [3]. The danger of cancer, a malignant tumor, is that it invades and destroys normal tissue and organs [3]. The primary site, or location, of the tumor is an important variable. In the beginning stages of laryngeal cancer, cancerous cells may be found at the level of the glottis (vocal folds); the supraglottis (area above the glottis, including the epiglottis, false vocal cords, ventricles, aryepiglottic folds, and arytenoids); or the subglottis (below the vocal folds) [3, 4]. In this stage, the cancer is said to be *localized*. Over time, the tumor may invade neighboring organs or tissue by direct extension of growth. This spread is termed *regional* when the cancer cells are confined to one area of the body—for example, the lymph nodes in the neck region [3]. In some individuals, the cancer cells invade tissues of the pharynx, epiglottis, esophagus, base of the tongue, and mandible [3]. If left untreated, some of the cancer cells detach from the tumor and enter the lymph or blood systems to be carried to distant parts of the body. This movement from a primary to a secondary site is termed *metastasis* [3].

PRIMARY CAUSE

Heavy smoking and alcohol abuse are characteristics of the histories of individuals diagnosed with laryngeal cancer [1, 2, 4–7]; approximately 80% of all laryngectomees used tobacco before their diagnosis of cancer (a *laryngectomy* is the surgical procedure to remove part or all of the larynx; a *laryngectomee* is the person who has undergone the operation) [8]. King et al. [9] reported an even higher incidence of smoking history among laryngectomees—from 92.5% to 99.5%. Further, they found that a "significant portion" of the laryngectomees had "serious problems with alcohol." Casper and Colton [4], among others [6, 10], state that there is "a synergistic effect between smoking and alcohol intake that increases the level of risk for laryngeal cancer." These two agents are suspected of causing a malignant change in the cellular lining of the

1

larynx. Wynder et al. [11] proposed that an individual who smokes 35 or more cigarettes per day is seven times more likely than a nonsmoking individual to develop laryngeal cancer. Further, they predicted that when this cigarette habit is combined with a daily intake of more than 7 oz of alcohol, the risk increases to 22 times that of the individual who neither smokes nor drinks.

OTHER CAUSES

The link between smoking and alcohol abuse and the development of laryngeal cancer is well supported [1, 2, 4, 5, 9–11]. In addition, other environmental factors as well as hereditary conditions have been cited in the development of cancer [4, 10]. Cancer may result from the interaction of inherited predisposition, immune deficiencies, or hormones with external agents such as chemicals, radiation, and viruses [1, 2, 10]. Rohe [6] suggested that for a relatively small number of individuals, "laryngeal cancer is believed to be secondary to occupational exposure to toxic substances, such as in the metal, lumber, railroad, and farming industries." Due to the widespread occurrence of and possible combinations of exposure to these environmental factors, identifying a specific source as a cause of cancer is a challenge [12].

INCIDENCE

Cancer is the second leading cause of death in the United States, superseded only by heart disease. California leads the nation in the number of new cancer cases each year and cancer mortality; Florida and New York rank second and third, respectively [1]. The American Cancer Society [1] predicted that 174,000 Americans would lose their lives to cancer related to tobacco use in 1997. An additional 19,000 cancer deaths related to alcohol abuse, often in combination with tobacco use, were forecasted. The tragedy of these statistics is that *100% of the cancers caused by alcohol abuse and tobacco use are preventable* [1].

Tens of thousands of men and women have undergone surgery for laryngeal cancer. There are more than 50,000 laryngectomees living in the United States [2]. More men than women experience laryngeal cancer; the ratio is approximately 4 to 1 [1, 2, 6, 11]. Between 1970 and 1993, the incidence of laryngeal cancer decreased by 11% in men, yet increased by 67% in women [1]. Data reported in *Cancer Facts and Figures—1997* [1] estimated 10,900 new cases of laryngeal cancer in the United States for the year 1997 (8,900 men and 2,000 women). Further, 4,230 individuals were projected to die in 1997 as a result of laryngeal cancer (3,300 men and 930 women).

The average age of individuals diagnosed with laryngeal cancer is 60 years [2, 6]. Colton and Casper [4] report 85% of all cases of laryngeal cancer occur between the ages of 50 years and 70 years; Rohe [6] suggests the percentage is closer to 64%.

The percentage of black Americans, both male and female, with laryngeal cancer is greater than the percentage of white Americans [1, 4, 5]. Black

American men have the highest incidence of laryngeal cancer of any other reported group, with 12.1 cases per 100,000 population compared with 8.3 for white men [5].

A summary of these statistics regarding laryngeal cancer is presented in Table 1.1.

SYMPTOMS

The symptoms of laryngeal cancer vary based on the size and location of the tumor [3]. The most common location of early-stage laryngeal cancer is on the true vocal folds. These glottic cancers are responsible for approximately 75% of all laryngeal cancers and frequently result in lowered pitch and hoarse vocal quality [2–4, 8, 13]. A supraglottic tumor often creates the sensation of a lump in the throat and may interfere with swallowing [2–4]. Pain may be experienced when the tumor is located in the pharynx, epiglottic region, or the entrance to the larynx [4]. As the tumor enlarges, there may be a visualized growth on the neck [3]. Coughing, shortness of breath, and audible breathing can occur when the tumor restricts the airway [3, 4]. If the tumor presses on the sensory portion of the vagus nerve, which connects the laryngeal and auditory areas, the person perceives the pain as an earache [2].

One or a combination of the following symptoms may be reported by an individual during preoperative contact with the physician:

- Persistent and progressive hoarseness
- Persistent sore throat
- Change in vocal pitch (usually becomes lower)
- Difficulty swallowing (dysphagia)
- Shortness of breath (dyspnea) and audible breathing (stridor)
- Feeling a lump in the throat
- Chronic coughing
- Pain on breathing or swallowing (odynophagia)
- Coughing up blood (hemoptysis)
- Visualized growth on the neck
- Earache
- Weight loss
- Foul breath (halitosis)
- Swelling or tenderness in the neck
- Lumps at the base of the tongue

MEDICAL EXAMINATION

The otolaryngologist is an ear, nose, and throat (ENT) specialist and is the most qualified physician to make the diagnosis of laryngeal cancer and prescribe treatment [3, 4]. The preoperative office visit begins with a medical history, a

Table 1.1 Laryngeal cancer statistics

Ranking of California, Florida, and New York as the states with the greatest number of new cancer cases and cancer mortality	First, second, third, respectively
Number of predicted deaths in United States in 1997	
Tobacco-related cancers	174,000
Alcohol-related cancers	19,000
Percentage of preventable deaths from alcohol- and tobacco-related cancers	100%
Percentage of laryngectomees who smoked before laryngeal cancer	80.0–99.5%
Number of times an individual is more likely to develop laryngeal cancer (compared with nonsmoking individuals and individuals who neither smoke nor drink)	
35 cigarettes/day habit	7 times more likely
35 cigarettes/day + 7 oz of alcohol/day habit	22 times more likely
Number of laryngectomees living in the United States	50,000
Ratio of men to women with laryngeal cancer	4:1
Percentage of change in incidence of laryngeal cancer between 1970 and 1993	
Decrease for men	11%
Increase for women	67%
Estimated new cases of laryngeal cancer in the United States for 1997	10,900
Number of men	8,900
Number of women	2,000
Projected number of deaths from laryngeal cancer in 1997	4,230
Men	3,300
Women	930
Average age of person diagnosed with laryngeal cancer	60 yrs
Percentage of cases of laryngeal cancer occurring within the fifth to seventh decades of life	85%
Cases per 100,000 of laryngeal cancer	
Black American males	12.1
White American males	8.3
Black American females	1.9
White American females	1.3
Successful treatment rate for laryngeal cancer when detected and treated in early stages of development	95%
Percentage survival rate for laryngeal cancer	
White Americans	68%
Black Americans	52%

Source: Data from references 1, 2, 4, 5, 6, 8, 9, 11, and 24.

physical examination of the external structures of the head and neck, and an oral assessment.

During the examination, the otolaryngologist is committed to making the best possible estimate of the extent of the disease before treatment. The assessment of the primary tumor requires visual inspection as well as palpation, if possible. The physician examines the laryngeal structures using one or more of the following procedures [3, 4]:

1. *Indirect laryngoscopy.* The ENT specialist views the vocal folds and surrounding areas using a small laryngeal mirror positioned in the back of the patient's mouth. This procedure is painless; however, the physician may use a topical anesthetic to reduce gagging. Indirect laryngoscopy allows the physician a preliminary examination of the laryngeal structures.

2. *Fiberoptic evaluation.* Complete examination of the laryngeal structures requires the passage of a flexible, lighted tube (fiberoptic endoscope) through the nasal cavity into the laryngeal area. To reduce discomfort, a topical anesthetic is used. Because the tube is placed through the nose instead of the mouth, gagging is reduced or eliminated. The procedure is performed in the physician's office or hospital.

3. *Direct laryngoscopy with biopsy.* If a malignancy is suspected, the patient is placed under general anesthesia, and a laryngoscope is inserted through the oral cavity into the pharyngeal area. Tissue samples are collected for microscopic laboratory analysis (biopsy) [8]. The majority of laryngeal cancers are squamous cell carcinomas and result in a thickening of the epithelium.

4. *X-rays, computed tomography (CT) scan, magnetic resonance imaging (MRI) scan.* For some individuals, the physician orders additional examination of the laryngeal structures to include x-rays or a CT or MRI scan. These tests allow the physician to view the soft structures of the larynx to determine the
   a. Exact site, extent, and type of primary tumor
   b. Presence or absence of regional lymph node metastasis
   c. Presence or absence of distant metastases (e.g., lungs, abdomen).

Using the clinical term *staging*, the ENT specialist indicates the severity of the lesion according to the tumor-node-metastasis (TNM) classification system (Table 1.2) for malignant laryngeal tumors [14]. T describes the site of the primary tumor, N denotes the presence or absence of lymph node involvement, and M indicates whether the lesion has progressed to other parts of the body (metastasis) [14]. Numbers are paired with the indicators: The higher the number, the more extensive the involvement. For example, $T_2N_1M_0$ means the individual has a supraglottic or subglottic extension of the primary tumor with normal or impaired mobility (T_2), a single node on one side (N_1), and no known metastasis (M_0) [10]. If there is no evidence of tumor (T_0), no involvement of lymph nodes

Table 1.2 Tumor-node-metastasis (TNM) classification for laryngeal cancer staging

Primary tumor (T)	Staging
T_x	Tumor that cannot be assessed by rules
T_0	No evidence of primary tumor
Supraglottis	
TIS	Carcinoma in situ
T_1	Tumor confined to region of origin with normal vocal cord mobility
T_2	Tumor involving adjacent supraglottic site(s) or glottis without vocal cord fixation
T_3	Tumor limited to larynx with fixation and/or extension to involve postcricoid area, medial wall of pyriform sinus, or pre-epiglottic space
T_4	Massive tumor extending beyond the larynx to involve oropharynx, soft tissues of neck, or destruction of thyroid cartilage
Glottis	
TIS	Carcinoma in situ
T_1	Tumor confined to vocal cord(s) with normal mobility (may involve anterior or posterior commissures)
T_2	Supraglottic and/or subglottic extension of tumor with normal or impaired cord mobility
T_3	Tumor confined to the larynx with cord fixation
T_4	Massive tumor with thyroid cartilage and/or extension beyond the confines of the larynx
Subglottis	
TIS	Carcinoma in situ
T_1	Tumor confined to the subglottic region
T_2	Tumor extension to vocal cords with normal or impaired cord mobility
T_3	Tumor confined to the larynx with cord fixation
T_4	Massive tumor with cartilage destruction, extension beyond the confines of the larynx, or both
Nodal involvement (N)	
N_x	Nodes cannot be assessed
N_0	No clinically positive nodes
N_1	Single clinically positive homolateral node <3 cm in diameter
N_2	Single clinically positive homolateral node 3–6 cm in diameter; multiple clinically positive homolateral nodes, none >6 cm in diameter; or metastasis in bilateral or contralateral lymph nodes, none >6 cm in diameter
N_{2a}	Single clinically positive homolateral node 3–6 cm in diameter
N_{2b}	Multiple clinically positive homolateral nodes, none >6 cm in diameter
N_3	Massive homolateral node(s), bilateral nodes, or contralateral node(s)
N_{3a}	Clinically positive homolateral nodes, none >6 cm in diameter

N_{3b} Bilateral clinically positive nodes (in this situation, each side of the neck should be staged separately; that is, N_{3b}: right, N_{2a}: left, N_1)

Distant metastasis (M)

M_x	Not assessed
M_0	No (known) distant metastasis
M_1	Distant metastasis present

Stage grouping

Stage I	$T_1N_0M_0$
Stage II	$T_2N_0M_0$
Stage III	$T_3N_0M_0$
	T_1 or T_2 or T_3, N_1, M_0
Stage IV	T_4, N_0 or N_1, M_0
	Any T, N_2 or N_3, M_0
	Any T, any N, M_1

Residual tumor (R)

R_0	No residual tumor
R_1	Microscopic residual tumor
R_2	Microscopic residual tumor

Source: Reprinted with permission from the American Joint Committee for Cancer Staging and End Results Reporting: Manual for Stages of Cancer (4th ed). Philadelphia: Lippincott, 1992;39.

(N_0), or no known metastasis (M_0), the corresponding symbol is omitted (e.g., the above example, $T_2N_1M_0$, would be written as T_2N_1).

TREATMENT OPTIONS

Laryngeal cancer is treatable with the individual use or combined use of radiation therapy, surgery, and chemotherapy [1, 2, 4, 8]. A number of factors are taken into consideration to select the best treatment option. The exact site, extent, and type of primary tumor have a direct effect on the physician's treatment recommendation. Relevant to the decision are the individual's age, medical history, and personal perceptions about cancer and treatment [3].

Radiation Therapy

If the tumor is small and superficial, radiation therapy alone has a good chance of eliminating the tumor [3, 4, 8]. Radiation therapy alone may be the treatment of choice for inoperable tumors or for other reasons that prevent surgical intervention [3, 4]. When used preoperatively, radiation therapy is expected to reduce the size of the tumor [3, 15]. Preoperative irradiation frequently results in hardening of the tissues, which can interfere with the surgical procedure and delay healing [4, 7]. In postoperative applications, radiation therapy destroys any cancer cells that may remain within the tissues [3, 4, 15]. Swelling of the tissues (edema) with airway obstruction is a potential side effect of postoperative radiation therapy [4].

A study published in *The New England Journal of Medicine* showed that patients who smoke during the course of radiation therapy experience lower response rates and have shorter survival periods than their nonsmoking counterparts [16]. Based on the results of this study, patients should be advised to stop smoking before beginning radiation therapy.

Hypothyroidism has been identified in 30–40% of individuals who receive external radiation therapy to the thyroid gland or pituitary gland [17, 18]. All patients with laryngeal cancer should undergo evaluation of thyroid function before and after radiation therapy.

The standard course of radiation treatment is 5 days per week extending over a 5- to 6-week period [3, 15]. The effect of radiation is to kill all fast-growing cells, among which are the targeted cancer cells. Also included are the fast-growing cells of hair, tooth roots, the digestive tract, and fingernail beds. Radiation makes no distinction between the "bad" and "good" fast-growing cells. As a consequence of the death of digestive tract cells, some patients experience nausea, vomiting, extreme fatigue, sore throat, dry mouth, sensitive tongue, loss of sense of taste or smell, and thickened mucus [3, 7]. On occasion, the gums shrink, resulting in ill-fitting dentures. The radiated skin of the neck often becomes red and dry [3, 7], interfering with tactile sensation as well as placement of the electrolarynx. Most of these side effects of radiation therapy lessen with time [3].

Surgery

Surgery may be the optimal method for tumor removal. The location of the tumor and its size determine the type of surgery required [4].

Phonosurgery

Laser excision may be used to remove a tumor that is small, superficial, and confined to the level of the vocal folds (glottis) [3, 19]. After this procedure, the individual does not lose the voice; vocal quality may or may not be affected.

Partial and Hemilaryngectomy

If the tumor is contained within the larynx, the physician may perform a limited removal of tissue—a partial or hemilaryngectomy. In a partial procedure, only one vocal cord or part of a vocal cord is excised [3]. In a hemilaryngectomy, at least half the larynx is surgically removed using vertical or sagittal sectioning [4]. Half the thyroid cartilage, a true vocal fold, the vocal process of the arytenoid cartilage, or the entire arytenoid cartilage are sacrificed [4].

Nasal respiration is maintained; the patient is able to breathe in the normal manner. The postoperative voice is characterized as hoarse, breathy, and low in volume [3, 4]. Some patients experience difficulty swallowing [4].

Supraglottic Laryngectomy

Tumors involving structures above the level of the vocal folds (i.e., epiglottis, false vocal folds, hyoid bone, and upper portions of the thyroid cartilage) are surgically removed using supraglottic laryngectomy [4]. Because the true vocal folds are preserved, the patient usually has a normal voice [4]. Removal of the structures superior to the larynx interferes with the normal swallow; thus, the individual must learn compensatory movements for swallowing [4]. Supraglottic laryngectomy has the best chance for success when it is limited to the immediate supraglottic region [8].

Near-Total Laryngectomy (Shunt)

In select cases in which the tumor has not involved the posterior commissure, at least one arytenoid and ventricle may be spared during the surgical removal of the larynx [4]. An internal, lung-powered shunt connecting the trachea and pharynx is created using a strip of laryngeal tissue, pharyngeal tissue, or both [4, 20]. The shunt, lined with mucosa and innervated by the recurrent laryngeal nerve, resists aspiration or stenosis [20]. Depending on the location of the cancer and the subsequent surgical procedure, nasal or stomal respiration may result [20]. Postoperatively, modified voicing is produced when lung air is forced through the shunt into the pharynx [4, 8, 20]. Therapeutic intervention is helpful to address optimal coverage of the stoma, articulation, rate, and phonation [20].

Total Laryngectomy

When laryngeal cancer is advanced, the surgical procedure of choice is total laryngectomy [4]. A surgical incision is made into the neck and the entire laryngeal mechanism is removed—from the hyoid bone to the upper two to three rings of the trachea [21–23]. Structures removed include the hyoid bone; epiglottis; thyroid, cricoid, and arytenoid cartilages; upper two to three rings of the trachea; and surrounding musculature, including the strap muscles [21–23].

During the surgery, the trachea loses its connection with the pharynx and oral cavity and is brought forward to create an opening superior to the sternal notch at the front of the neck [21–24]. The opening in the neck is called a *stoma* and is ½–¾ in. in diameter [2]. For a period after the surgery, a tracheostomy tube preserves the new airway [3, 22, 23]. The laryngectomee—now permanently a neck breather—breathes, coughs, and sneezes through the stoma [2, 15, 22, 23, 25] (compare the pre- and postoperative anatomy in Figure 1.1). Due to the loss of the vocal mechanism, the laryngectomee must learn an alternate way of communicating [4] (a discussion of oral communication options is found in Chapter 3).

Total Laryngectomy with Radical Neck Dissection

If the cancer has regionalized to the lymph nodes in the neck, more extensive surgery is required [4]. After the total laryngectomy is performed, the cervical

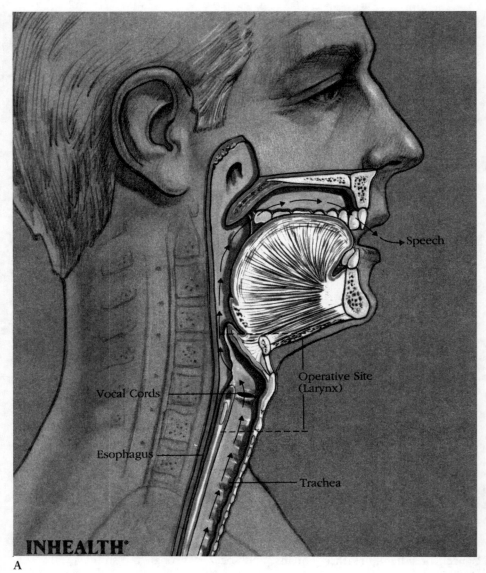

A

Figure 1.1 A. Before laryngectomy, the individual breathes in through the nose and mouth. Air returns from the lungs via the trachea to the larynx where voicing occurs. B. After laryngectomy, the individual breathes, coughs, and sneezes through the stoma, an opening in the neck. (Reprinted with permission of InHealth Technologies. Postlaryngectomy Training Aid Set. Carpinteria, CA: InHealth Technologies, 1995.)

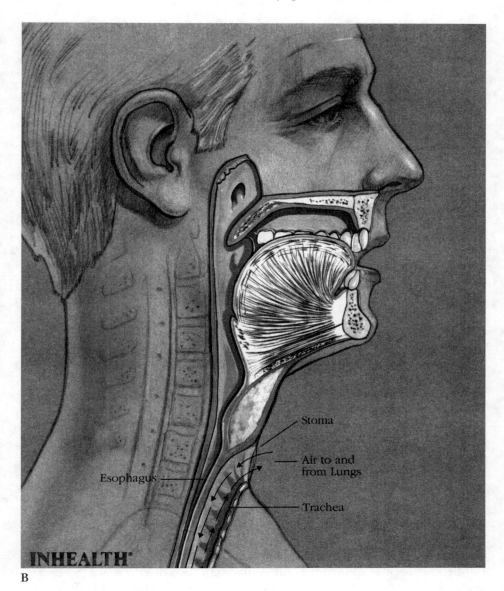

Stoma

Air to and
from Lungs

Esophagus

Trachea

INHEALTH®

B

lymph nodes are removed from one or both sides of the neck [21]. In a radical
neck dissection, the sternocleidomastoid muscle, internal jugular vein, and
spinal accessory nerve (cranial nerve XI) are sacrificed in addition to the cervical lymph nodes [26]. In a modified radical neck dissection, all lymph nodes
are removed; however, one or more of the nonlymphatic structures are preserved [26]. Other structures that may be surgically removed are the omohy-

oid muscle, external carotid artery, lobe of the thyroid gland, and sub-mandibular gland [21].

If cranial nerves V (trigeminal), X (vagus), and XII (hypoglossal) are affected, oral sensory function (i.e., touch, taste) and lingual motor movements for articulation may be impaired. The laryngectomee may also experience dysphagia, paralysis of the soft palate, jaw deviation, and facial pain. Removal of the sternocleidomastoid muscle interferes with head rotation. If cranial nerve XI (spinal accessory) is severed, the laryngectomee experiences a painful, dropped shoulder with restricted movement [4, 27].

Surgical Removal of Adjacent Structures in Addition to Total Laryngectomy

Cancerous invasion of head and neck structures other than the larynx require additional surgical intervention. Partial removal of the pharynx, esophagus, or tongue can significantly alter the patient's anatomy, create scar tissue, and interfere with swallowing. After extended surgery, the laryngectomee may have limited potential for achieving intelligible alaryngeal speech [4, 7].

Surgical Removal of the Larynx in the Absence of Cancer

In a few rare cases, surgical removal of the larynx occurs in the absence of cancer. Possible etiologies include traumatic injury to the neck, severe stenosis of the airway, aspiration due to a failed partial or hemilaryngectomy, or any other condition that compromises the individual's ability to safeguard the respiratory tract [4].

Chemotherapy

Chemotherapy is used to reduce a large tumor before radiation therapy or surgery [3, 4]. Chemotherapy may also be used for cancer that has metastasized [3, 4]. During chemotherapy, a chemical is injected into the bloodstream or ingested orally [3]. The chemical enters the bloodstream and attacks fast-growing cells. Again, the healthy fast-growing cells are affected as well as the cancer cells.

Typically, the individual receives 1 week of chemotherapy, 2 weeks of rest, and another week of chemotherapy culminating in surgery [4], or the physician may elect to perform surgery first and follow with a schedule of chemotherapy [4]. Because chemotherapy treats the entire body, the side effects are more widespread. The laryngectomee may experience lowered resistance to infection, lethargy, nausea, loss of appetite, weight loss, and skin problems [3, 4].

PROGNOSIS

The importance of early detection of cancer cannot be emphasized too strongly. When detected and treated in the early stages of development, laryngeal cancer is one of the most curable cancers, with a reported 95% successful treatment rate [2, 24]. Delayed diagnosis means poorer prognosis for survival [4].

Individuals treated for laryngeal cancer are at the greatest risk for recurrence in the first 2–3 years postoperatively. The recurrence of cancer after 5 years is rare and usually indicates a new primary malignancy. Periodic postoperative visits with the otolaryngologist are crucial to maximize good health and successfully manage any complications.

The 5-year survival rate following treatment for laryngeal cancer is 68% for white Americans and 52% for black Americans [1, 4]. Cultural attitudes, lifestyle, and behavioral patterns are suggested as logical reasons for this disparity. Environmental conditions (e.g., living and working in industrial and high-smog areas) coupled with certain culturally rooted dietary patterns [1, 5], a higher rate of alcohol and tobacco use (including smokeless tobacco) [1, 5], lack of health care insurance [5], and poor education about the warning signs of cancer are all considered risk factors [1]. Since 1988, the American Cancer Society has been active in funding community service programs that provide cancer education for the medically underserved population in the United States [4].

INFORMING THE PATIENT OF THE DIAGNOSIS AND TREATMENT OPTIONS

It is the physician's responsibility to inform the patient of the diagnosis of cancer and the recommended treatment—that is, radiation therapy, surgery, and chemotherapy [12]. The patient learns from the physician that the larynx will be removed and an alternate method of communication is needed. Ideally, the physician makes a referral to the speech-language pathologist (SLP) for preoperative counseling [2, 4, 12]. Salmon [28] estimates less than one-half of all laryngectomees receive preoperative counseling from an SLP.

THE IMPORTANCE OF PREOPERATIVE COUNSELING BY THE SPEECH-LANGUAGE PATHOLOGIST

Preoperative contact between the SLP and the individual is important for a number of reasons. First, it provides an opportunity to provide basic information and answer questions about the laryngectomy procedure and alaryngeal speech rehabilitation [2, 4, 12, 21, 29, 30]. The SLP should begin by asking the individual and his or her family what they know about the impending surgery. This leads to a general and simplified explanation of selected topics—for example, altered method of breathing, the loss of the larynx and voicing, the "normal" presence of nasogastric and intravenous tubes postoperatively, and tracheostoma care [12, 29, 30]. Imagery and anatomic illustrations (such as those shown in Figure 1.1) should be used to facilitate understanding [28, 29]. Communication options—the artificial larynx, esophageal speech, and tracheoesophageal speech [2, 4, 24, 29, 30]—are reviewed briefly. The SLP should know whether the physician's plans include placement of the tracheoesophageal prosthesis. Immediate postsurgical communication should also be discussed; writing or a communication book are used until the physician approves initiation of other methods [12, 29, 30].

Second, a supportive atmosphere establishes a positive relationship between the SLP and the individual [2, 24, 29, 30]. If at all possible, the family is encouraged to attend the session [2, 4, 12]. The term *family* is used here in its broadest sense and includes "significant others" in the laryngectomee's life as well as persons related by blood or marriage. The family support system for the laryngectomee is a critical component in the rehabilitation process. These are the individuals who have the potential to encourage and support the laryngectomee in his or her adaptation to postoperative changes and learning of a functional communication method. The more informed the family is about alaryngeal speech rehabilitation and the more they are included in the process, the more likely they are to cooperate as members of the team. Two publications, *Self-Help for the Laryngectomee*, by Edmund Lauder, and *Looking Forward . . . . A Guidebook for the Laryngectomee*, by Robert L. Keith, are suggested as take-home reading material because they have been written expressly for laryngectomees and their families.

Third, a preoperative meeting allows the SLP to analyze the individual's habitual speech pattern for future reference [4, 24, 29]. An audio recording of connected speech provides a long-term record of the individual's preoperative speech characteristics and intelligibility. The individual is asked to provide his or her name, address, and the date, followed by a reading of a standard passage. If the individual cannot read, he or she can engage in conversation about a familiar topic—for example, occupation, family members, or a special interest. Conditions for intelligibility of alaryngeal speech production are based, in part, on the same factors as those for preoperative speech intelligibility: articulatory precision, dialectal differences between the speaker and the listener, competing noise, complexity of subject content, level of message redundancy (e.g., phonetic, linguistic, and environmental), and rate of speech [31]. Are there errors of substitution, omission, distortion, or addition? If possible, any articulatory imprecision due to habituation (e.g., loose dentures) or to a lack of physiologic control of the articulators (e.g., dysarthria associated with parkinsonism or a poststroke condition) should be determined. An examination of the oral structures may be conducted at this time or deferred until the postoperative evaluation (see Chapter 2, "The Oral Examination"). Intelligibility may be influenced by the presence of a regional dialect or foreign accent [12]. Speech rhythm, or the temporal features of speech, differs from one language to another and influences meaning as well as intelligibility. Speech rhythm encompasses *accent* (syllabic stress within words), *emphasis* (stressed word or words within a phrase or sentence), *phrasing* (placement of silent intervals between phrases), *intonation* (rising and falling pitch within the utterance), and *rate* (number of syllables or words produced within a specified time period) [29, 31]. As appropriate, the tape of the laryngectomee's preoperative speech pattern may be used as a model for alaryngeal speech production [29].

Fourth, determination of cognitive function, audiologic status, and reading and writing levels assists in preparation of a postoperative rehabilitation plan [4, 12]. Educational and cognitive levels, occupational status, and recreational interests influence the selection of an oral communication method [7] (see Chapter 3) as well as the vocabulary to be used in therapy. If the individual has a history of neurologic impairment (e.g., head trauma, cerebrovascular disease, or chronic alcoholism), adjustments in the level of vocabulary used for instruction and practice stimuli may be needed. Significant hearing loss can interfere with the individual's ability to follow directions as well as self-monitoring skills during therapy [4, 32]. The selection of educational materials to give to the laryngectomee (e.g., written instructions and word lists) depends on his or her reading level. Legible handwriting means the individual has an immediate method of communicating after surgery; otherwise a personalized communication book needs to be constructed [12, 30].

The SLP should bring closure to the consultation by summarizing the key points and reassuring the individual and family that the alaryngeal speech rehabilitation process will begin as soon as possible after the surgery at the surgeon's recommendation [12, 28, 30]. The SLP's name and office telephone number should be given to the laryngectomee or his or her family in case they have further questions or concerns.

REFERENCES

1. American Cancer Society. Cancer Facts and Figures—1997. Atlanta: American Cancer Society, 1997;1, 4, 16, 22.
2. Case JL. Clinical Management of Voice Disorders (2nd ed). Austin, TX: PRO-ED, 1991;226, 247.
3. National Institutes of Health. What You Need to Know About Cancer of the Larynx. Bethesda, MD: National Cancer Institute, 1993;4.
4. Casper JK, Colton RH. Clinical Manual for Laryngectomy and Head and Neck Cancer Rehabilitation. San Diego: Singular, 1993;1.
5. Battle DE. Communication Disorders in Multicultural Populations. Boston: Andover, 1993;213.
6. Rohe DE. Loss, Grief and Depression After Laryngectomy. In RL Keith, FL Darley (eds), Laryngectomee Rehabilitation (3rd ed). Austin, TX: PRO-ED, 1994;487.
7. Lewin JS. Special Problems of the Alaryngeal Speaker. In RL Keith, FL Darley (eds), Laryngectomee Rehabilitation (3rd ed). Austin, TX: PRO-ED, 1994;283.
8. DeSanto LW, Pearson BW. Factors in the Choice of Treatment of Patients with Laryngeal Cancer. In RL Keith, FL Darley (eds), Laryngectomee Rehabilitation (3rd ed). Austin, TX: PRO-ED, 1994;63.
9. King P, Fowlks E, Pierson G. Rehabilitation and adaptation of laryngectomy patients. Am J Phys Med 1968;47:192.
10. Union International Centre le Cancer (UICC). Manual of Clinical Oncology. Berlin: Springer, 1987;22.
11. Wynder EL, Covey LS, Marbuchi K, et al. Environmental factors in cancer of the larynx, a second look. Cancer 1976;38:1591.
12. Doyle PC. Foundations of Voice and Speech Rehabilitation Following Laryngeal Cancer. San Diego: Singular, 1994;58, 98.

13. American Cancer Society. Rehabilitating Laryngectomees. Atlanta: American Cancer Society, 1990.
14. American Joint Committee for Cancer Staging and End Results Reporting: Manual for Stages of Cancer (4th ed). Philadelphia: Lippincott, 1992;39.
15. American Cancer Society. First Steps: Helping Words for the Laryngectomee. Atlanta: American Cancer Society, 1995;4.
16. Browman GP, Wong G, Hodson I. Influence of cigarette smoking on the efficacy of radiation therapy in head and neck cancer. N Engl J Med 1993;328:159.
17. Turner SL, Tiver KW, Boyages SC. Thyroid dysfunction following radiotherapy for head and neck cancer. Int J Radiat Oncol Biol Phys 1995;31:279.
18. Constine LS. What else don't we know about the late effects of radiation in patients treated for head and neck cancer? Int J Radiat Oncol Biol Phys 1995;31:417.
19. Colton RH, Casper JK. Understanding Voice Problems: A Physiological Perspective for Diagnosis and Treatment (2nd ed). Baltimore: Williams & Wilkins, 1996;178, 247.
20. Thomas JE, Keith RL, Pearson BW, DeSanto LW. Speech Rehabilitation After Near-Total Laryngectomy. In RL Keith, FL Darley (eds), Laryngectomee Rehabilitation (3rd ed). Austin, TX: PRO-ED, 1994;93.
21. CIBA. The Larynx. Summit, NJ: CIBA Pharmaceutical Company, 1964;96.
22. DeWeese DD, Saunders WH. Textbook of Otolaryngology (5th ed). St. Louis: Mosby, 1997.
23. Cheesman AD. Surgical Management of the Patient. In Y Edels (ed), Laryngectomee: Diagnosis to Rehabilitation. Rockville, MD: Aspen, 1983;36.
24. Boone DR, McFarlane SC. The Voice and Voice Therapy (5th ed). Englewood Cliffs, NJ: Prentice-Hall, 1994;216.
25. American Cancer Society. Rescue Breathing for Laryngectomees and Other Neck Breathers. Atlanta: American Cancer Society, 1995;5.
26. Robbins KT, Medina JE, Wolfe GT, et al. Standardizing neck dissection terminology. Arch Otolaryngol Head Neck Surg 1991:117;601.
27. Gilmore SI. The Physical, Social, Occupational, and Psychological Concomitants of Laryngectomy. In RL Keith, FL Darley (eds), Laryngectomee Rehabilitation (3rd ed). Austin, TX: PRO-ED, 1994;425.
28 Salmon SJ. Pre- and Postoperative Conferences with Laryngectomees and Their Spouses. In RL Keith, FL Darley (eds), Laryngectomee Rehabilitation (3rd ed). Austin, TX: PRO-ED, 1994;133.
29. Murrills G. Pre- and Early Postoperative Care of the Laryngectomee and Spouse. In Y Edels (ed), Laryngectomee: Diagnosis to Rehabilitation. Rockville, MD: Aspen, 1983;58.
30. Reed CG. Surgical-prosthetic techniques for alaryngeal speech. Commun Disord 1983;8:109.
31. Calvert DR. Descriptive Phonetics (2nd ed). New York: Thieme, 1986;163.
32. Gates GA, Ryan W, Cantu E, Hearne E. Current status of laryngectomee rehabilitation: II. Causes of failure. Am J Otolaryngol 1982;3:8.

2

The New Laryngectomee

Surgery for laryngeal cancer results in significant changes in the laryngectomee's anatomy and physiology. Equally important is the influence surgery has on the laryngectomee's communicative, psychological, sociological, and economic well-being. *Adjustment* becomes the daily byword. Appreciation of the overall impact that laryngeal cancer has on the laryngectomee as well as his or her family enhances the effectiveness of the speech-language pathologist (SLP) in the early stages of the alaryngeal speech rehabilitation process.

IN THE HOSPITAL: ISSUES RELATED TO ANATOMIC AND PHYSIOLOGIC CHANGES

The laryngectomee is moved to the recovery room after surgery and then, depending on hospital policy and the patient's medical status, is transferred to the surgical floor of the hospital. Swelling of the throat as a result of the surgery prevents normal swallowing; the laryngectomee has a nasogastric tube in place for receiving nourishment [1]. An intravenous tube may also be present [1]. The average hospital stay is 10 days. During that time, the swelling reduces, and the laryngectomee is usually able to resume eating orally [1]. Complications such as fistula, hemorrhage, pulmonary infection, stenosis, rupture of the carotid artery, and heart or pulmonary problems may prolong hospitalization.

A tracheostomy tube is placed in the stoma during the healing process. The nursing staff teaches the laryngectomee how to remove and clean the device. Some laryngectomees continue to wear the tracheostomy tube after going home, and some use a stoma button; however, most laryngectomees function without the tube or button [2].

After surgery, the lungs produce increased mucus. The nursing staff shows the laryngectomee how to suction the mucus from the stoma. Eventually, the laryngectomee is able to cough the mucus from the lungs without assistance.

Laryngeal surgery alters the human anatomy. The laryngectomee experiences a number of physiologic changes as a result of the surgery, and it is important to discuss their significance with the patient. A summary of anatomic and physiologic changes in the laryngectomee is presented in Table 2.1.

Table 2.1 Anatomic and physiologic changes in the laryngectomee

---

Altered breathing. The laryngectomee breathes and coughs through an opening in the neck called a stoma. A stoma cover acts as a filter, and it retains moisture and warms the air entering the trachea.

Reduced airway protection. The laryngectomee must wear stoma protection to keep foreign substances out of the airway.

Water and the stoma. Precautions must be taken to keep water out of the stoma, the trachea, and the lungs.

Lifting and bearing down limitations. Intra-abdominal air pressure can be achieved by tightening the abdominal muscles and covering the stoma with the finger while attempting to exhale.

Nose blowing. Compensatory methods (e.g., tongue pumping; suctioning with a bulb syringe) can be used to remove mucus from the nose.

Reduced smell and taste. Fanning air into the nostrils may improve the sense of smell and stimulate salivation.

Altered eating patterns. A well-balanced diet is needed to maintain appropriate body weight, regain strength, and rebuild normal tissues. Eating smaller but more frequent meals throughout the day may be helpful.

Limited neck and shoulder movements. Physical therapy may assist in the improvement of neck and shoulder mobility.

Altered Breathing

After removal of the larynx and surrounding musculature, the top of the trachea is brought forward between the clavicles and superior to the sternum, or breastbone. An opening is made to the outside of the body, and the top of the trachea is sutured in place. The laryngectomee will breathe through this permanent opening, the stoma, rather than through the nose or mouth. This anatomic alteration interrupts the normal pattern for processing air as it is taken into the body (see Figure 1.1).

According to Zemlin [3], several things happen to the air that enters the body through the nose and mouth during normal respiration. First, the air is warmed to body temperature as it passes along the walls of the respiratory tract on its way to the lungs. Second, moisture is added to the air via mucous glands located along the respiratory passages. Third, impurities in the air are filtered out by tiny hair-like cilia that sweep debris back up the respiratory passage away from the lungs and toward the oral and nasal cavities. The end result is warmed, moistened, filtered air entering the lungs [3, 4].

During respiration in the laryngectomee, air enters the body at the level of the stoma. The passageway to the lungs is virtually cut in half, and there is insufficient distance for the air to be sufficiently warmed, moistened, or filtered. The laryngectomee is particularly susceptible to problems caused by breathing cold, hot, or dry air—respiratory dryness and irritation accompanied by nonproductive coughing [5].

The laryngectomee learns to compensate for the loss of preconditioned air by using humidification. Among the techniques available are the following:

- Wearing a heat and moisture exchanger such as the Stoma-Vent or HumidiFilter Heat/Moisture Exchanger (InHealth Technologies [Carpinteria, CA]) (see Appendix A)
- Sleeping in a room with a humidifier or vaporizer
- Keeping the stoma cover moistened
- Creating a sauna effect by closing the bathroom door and running hot water in the basin or bathtub for several minutes as needed
- Drinking plenty of water to replenish the body's fluid and avoiding substances that have a drying effect (e.g., caffeine, antihistamines, decongestants) and diuretics (e.g., milk and milk products)

Protection of the Airway

Laryngectomy changes more than the method of breathing. The primary biological function of the larynx is to maintain the airway, prevent foreign matter from entering the airway, and valve the airway to build up intra-abdominal pressure [3]. With the larynx removed, these functions are interrupted.

With the larynx in place, foreign substances are quickly blown out of the airway by coughing or throat clearing. This is accomplished by *valving* (closing the vocal folds), building up subglottic air pressure, and then forcefully exhaling (coughing) or releasing short bursts of air while vocalizing (throat clearing) [3]. In the laryngectomee, coughing occurs through the stoma rather than through the mouth. Coughing is poorly controlled because the individual cannot valve the airway [5]. The laryngectomee learns to place a tissue over the stoma to deflect the air and mucus while at the same time covering the mouth for the appearance of conformity. Throat clearing is not possible in the laryngectomee because of the inability to pass short bursts of air from the lungs into the pharynx.

Because the laryngectomee is no longer able to protect the airway from foreign objects and substances, the stoma must be covered. Laryngectomees can choose among a variety of cloth and foam stoma covers, turtleneck shirts, dickeys, scarves, and specialized jewelry (see Appendix A). All of these devices are intended to prevent the entry of objects into the stoma—for example, hair, lint, buttons, insects, paper, and dust.

Patients can, unfortunately, learn the importance of wearing a stoma cover the hard way. Bob, a laryngectomee in our alaryngeal speech group, was particularly resistant to our advice and refused to wear a stoma cover of any kind. He walked into his neighbor's garage while wood was being cut with an electric saw. As a result of inhaling the wood dust, he developed pneumonia. Within the following year, while redecorating a room, Bob accidentally splashed paint into his uncovered stoma. A trip to the emergency room was required for removal of the paint. A bit wiser from experience, he now wears a stoma cover regularly.

Care of the Stoma In and Around Water

Keeping water out of the stoma requires thinking ahead and compensating for the loss of laryngeal valving abilities. On a daily basis, the laryngectomee is in the greatest danger of inhaling water during a shower. Most laryngectomees report that a washcloth folded in fourths and held against the stoma while rinsing their head effectively keeps the stoma clear of water. A commercial stoma shield is also available (see Appendix A). A soak in the tub is acceptable as long as the laryngectomee remembers to keep the stoma above the water line. Most laryngectomees choose not to swim due to risk of aspirating water; however, there are swimming devices (e.g., the LARKEL snorkel [Seidel Medizin Gauting-Buchendorf, West Germany]) for more adventurous clients [6] (see Appendix A).

Paul, before joining our alaryngeal speech group, decided to resume his daily swim after being released from the hospital after his laryngectomy. Either he had not been warned about the water-in-the-stoma hazard or he forgot, but Paul put on his swim trunks, walked to the poolside, and dived in. He recalls sinking to the bottom of the pool and looking up through the water at the lifeguard peering in at him. Paul was rescued and, amazingly, suffered no ill effects. He did not return to swimming but switched to golf—a "drier pastime" as he put it.

Another of the laryngectomees in our group, Peter, an avid fly fisherman, headed for the Russian River north of San Francisco for vacation. While fly casting alone, he slipped on algae-covered rocks into the chilly waters. The highway runs parallel to that part of the river, and luckily, a passing motorist saw him fall in and made a timely rescue. Peter returned from his trip with pictures of his string of beautiful mountain trout and a story to tell his grandchildren.

Lifting and Bearing Down Activities

For the individual with a larynx, lifting and bearing down involve tightening of the vocal folds to trap the subglottic air and allow intra-abdominal pressure to build [7]. Surgical removal of the larynx leaves the laryngectomee unable to "hold" his or her breath. The consequence of not being able to lift heavy objects may be no more than a nuisance (or a terrific excuse!) unless the laryngectomee is employed in a position that requires lifting.

The laryngectomee faces a more immediate problem related to the act of bearing down. Movement of the bowels (defecation) requires build up of intra-abdominal pressure. The laryngectomee learns a variety of ways to compensate (e.g., increase the amount of fruit and fiber in the diet, use stool softeners, and gently press-roll the lower abdomen with both hands). Tensing the abdominal muscles combined with covering the stoma with a finger while attempting to exhale may be successful [4]. If these strategies fail, the laryngectomee should be advised to consult with his or her physician.

Blowing the Nose

Blowing the nose is generally considered a lost skill because lung air cannot be forced up through the nasal cavity. A compensatory method, relaxing the soft palate and using the tongue to pump oral air into the nasal cavity, is one way of "blowing the nose" [6]. An infant ear syringe placed in the nostril is helpful for suctioning mucus from the nose, according to several of our laryngectomees. Roberts [5] suggests cleaning the nose using tissues or cotton-tipped swabs followed by application of a petroleum-based lubricant to prevent dryness and irritation.

Reduced or Absent Senses of Taste and Smell

The interaction of smell and taste is important for regulating appetite and food intake [1, 5]. Olfactory receptors in the nasal cavities detect food odors drawn in through the nostrils during normal breathing. The signals are relayed to the brain, triggering the perception of hunger, and, in turn, stimulating salivation. To activate the tongue's taste buds, food substances must be dissolved. Saliva assists in this process [8].

From 80% to 90% of laryngectomees experience loss of smell [9, 10]. Laryngeal surgery does not destroy the sense of smell; rather, it interferes with the *process* of smelling [5, 6, 11]. Rerouting air into the stoma bypasses the olfactory receptors that lie in the nasal cavity. Without air movement in the nose, the individual cannot smell. Some laryngectomees have discovered that fanning air into their noses as they lean over a plate of food may stimulate smell as well as salivation. Damsté [6] describes the use of a compensatory pumping action of the tongue similar to that taught during esophageal speech training. The soft palate is relaxed, and instead of pumping air into the esophagus, the laryngectomee diverts air into the nasal cavity, which may enhance the sense of smell.

Approximately half of all laryngectomees report reduced taste [9, 10]. Radiation therapy can reduce saliva production, resulting in dryness of the mouth and throat. The combination of interrupted smell and taste plus limited salivation have a direct effect on the patient's eating patterns.

Altered Eating Patterns

According to Diedrich and Youngstrom [12], approximately one-third of all laryngectomees report that it takes them longer to eat. Increased gastrointestinal symptoms, such as bloating, pain, and flatulence, occur in approximately 70% of laryngectomees [9, 12]. Dysphagia is a problem for one-third of laryngectomees [9, 12]. One-half of all laryngectomees have difficulty drinking from a water fountain or sipping soup from a spoon [12].

The laryngectomee may need assistance from a nutritionist to develop a well-balanced diet for the maintenance of appropriate body weight, regaining strength, and rebuilding of normal tissues. Dysphagia therapy includes consideration of medication to increase or compensate for saliva production. A soft diet using sauces, gravies, soups, pudding, and high-protein milkshakes may be recommended [1]. Roberts [5] suggests increasing fluid intake with meals; using artificial saliva or applying vegetable oil to the tongue; and avoiding caffeine, diuretics, and antihistamines or decongestants. The laryngectomee usually has success eating smaller but more frequent meals throughout the day [1].

Limited Neck and Shoulder Movements

During radical neck dissection, the spinal accessory nerve is sacrificed, interrupting innervation to the trapezius and the sternocleidomastoid muscles [13]. Damage to the trapezius muscle results in a dropped shoulder, loss of strength, and reduced arm movement [1, 9]. Impaired rotation of the head is a symptom of sternocleidomastoid muscle function loss [1, 9]. Physical therapy, by physician referral, may benefit the laryngectomee who has these symptoms [14].

IN THE HOSPITAL: COUNSELING THE LARYNGECTOMEE AND THE FAMILY

Counseling is an essential component in helping the patient and his or her family members express and understand their emotional needs after laryngectomy. Fear, anger, depression, and guilt frequently surround the loss. Questions need to be answered by a knowledgeable and supportive listener. The SLP should be prepared to help the laryngectomee deal with feelings of self-loss, being handicapped, dependence on others, heightened sense of aging, and increased awareness of mortality. The laryngectomee and his or her family may have concerns about how to interact with relatives, friends, and strangers. If the laryngectomee is unable to maintain his or her former employment, the family must deal with the potential economic crisis. For the laryngectomee who has the option of returning to work, communication as well as social obstacles deserve discussion.

Concerns about self-image and interrelationships are not uncommon for patients of either gender [9, 10, 15]. Because society places considerable emphasis on the attractiveness of the female body, the female laryngectomee may have particular anxieties about her appearance. In addition to the physical disfigurement caused by surgery, the *quality* of the artificial voice—whether its source is the artificial larynx, esophageal speech, or tracheoesophageal (TE) speech—is considered low-pitched, husky, and masculine [9, 16]. In Gardner's study of female laryngectomees [17], 35% of the women blamed their surgical scars and stoma for reduced attractiveness, 23% felt laryngectomy made them less feminine, and 16% reported difficulty expressing affection. Almost 50% of these women's husbands expressed revulsion and irritation in connection with the loss of their wives' voices.

On a positive note, couples who enjoy a healthy marital relationship before the laryngectomy tend to maintain such a relationship after surgery [9, 18]. Stack [19] surveyed 29 female laryngectomees, and 82% of the women reported the laryngectomy had not negatively influenced their marital relationship.

An expanded discussion of counseling laryngectomees and their families about anatomic and physiologic changes, diet, personal hygiene, and problem solving appears in Chapter 8, "Group Therapy." Within the group setting, laryngectomees and their families are encouraged to address fears of aging, death, and recurrence of cancer, as well as loss of communication, independence, power, and self.

IN THE HOSPITAL: ESTABLISHING A COMMUNICATION SYSTEM

The physician examines the laryngectomee and determines eligibility for speech therapy. Timely and satisfactory healing is a significant factor in giving approval for alaryngeal speech rehabilitation.

The goal of the SLP is to establish a communication system as early as possible, preferably while the laryngectomee is hospitalized. In the initial stages of the rehabilitation process, devices such as a communication board, "magic slate" (with plastic stylus—chalk dust may be hazardous to the stoma), pencil and paper, finger and hand signals, or a Cooper-Rand (Luminaud [Mentor, OH]) mouth-type artificial larynx are recommended [20] (see Appendix A).

With the physician's permission and referral, a veteran laryngectomee may be invited to visit the new laryngectomee. The International Association of Laryngectomees (IAL) is affiliated with the American Cancer Society and has a list of individuals who have received special training for making such hospital visits [21, 22]. The visiting laryngectomee's presence conveys a powerful message to the new laryngectomee: "I am surviving nicely, thank you." If a visit from another laryngectomee is not possible, the new laryngectomee and his or her family should be informed about the IAL and various laryngectomee support groups in their area. The American Cancer Society is a rich source of information for the SLP and the laryngectomee and his or her family (see Appendix A).

INTAKE INTERVIEW AND CONSULTATION

For many reasons, the SLP may not have the opportunity to interact with the laryngectomee and his or her family preoperatively or postoperatively (while still in the hospital setting). The time between the diagnosis and surgery may be limited, a referral for pre- or postoperative counseling may not be made, or the individual may choose not to follow the physician's advice. The first meeting with the SLP may not occur until after the laryngectomee has been discharged from the hospital and has received clearance from the physician to begin alaryngeal speech training. Under these circumstances, the intake interview and consultation take place in the SLP's clinic.

Molyneaux and Lane [23] identified the goals of effective interviewing: information gathering, information giving, expression and exploration of feelings, problem solving, and planning for future action. An SPL's preliminary meetings with the laryngectomee and his or her family have the potential to serve all of these functions.

Information Gathering

One of the goals of the interview is to obtain factual information about the laryngectomee's background in terms of occupation, education, operative, physical and social factors, and communication patterns (Figure 2.1). This information is valuable for providing direction for alaryngeal speech training [24].

Occupation and Education

Knowledge of the laryngectomee's occupation and educational level offers insight into the person's cognitive status and influences the selection of vocabulary used in therapy. If the laryngectomee plans to return to work, therapy goals can be established that address communication needs within the work setting.

Operative Factors

The extent of surgery offers clues to the recovery of communication abilities. For example, because one vocal cord is usually spared in a partial or hemilaryngectomy, the individual is expected to achieve a breathy, hoarse, and somewhat low-pitched voice. Radical neck dissection associated with total laryngectomy frequently results in reduced neck and shoulder movements, which may interfere with placement of the artificial larynx or finger valving of the stoma during TE speech. More extensive surgery that includes the pharynx, esophagus, and/or tongue suggests potential difficulty mastering esophageal speech methods [14, 25].

Swelling of neck tissues after radiation therapy may dictate, at least temporarily, the use of an intra-oral artificial larynx. Hardening of the tissues in the neck contribute to decreased sensation after radiation therapy [1, 14, 25]. The laryngectomee may not feel the placement of the artificial larynx against the neck. In addition, radiation frequently shrinks alveolar tissue in the mouth, resulting in loose dentures that can cause articulatory imprecision. There are many side effects associated with radiation therapy and chemotherapy; the laryngectomee who is undergoing either procedure sometimes elects to delay active speech therapy until after completion of treatments.

The laryngectomee should be encouraged to contact the physician with any reported postoperative complications—for example, bleeding from the stoma, difficulty sleeping, swallowing problems, or sudden weight loss.

Physical Factors

Coexisting physical conditions (e.g., gastroesophageal reflux disease) pose potential difficulties in achieving esophageal speech [26]. Respiratory inefficiency interferes with the laryngectomee's ability to clear secretions effectively, often

Alaryngeal Speech Clinic

Date_____

Name_____   Physician_____
Spouse_____   Address_____
Address_____   _____
              _____   Phone_____
Phone_____   Referred by_____
Birth date_____ Age____ Sex____   Clinician_____
Occupation(s)_____
Education_____

Operative Factors
   Date of surgery_____
   Presurgical complaints (e.g., hoarseness, coughing up blood)_____
   _____
   Extent of surgery (e.g., total laryngectomy, radical neck dissection)_____
   _____
   Radiation, chemotherapy, other treatment procedures (pre- or postoperative)_____
   _____
   Postoperative complications (including hygiene, sleeping, diet, swallowing)_____
   _____
   _____

Physical Factors
   General physical condition_____
   Coexisting conditions (e.g., diabetes, high blood pressure, heart disease, gastroesopha-
     geal reflux)_____
   Upper respiratory condition (e.g., allergies, asthma, emphysema, chronic obstructive
     pulmonary disease)_____
   _____
   Medication(s) (identify condition prescribed for)_____
   _____
   Hearing (+ date of last hearing test)_____
   Smoking/alcohol habits (pre- and postoperative)_____
   _____

Social Factors
   Client's attitude (e.g., optimistic, depressed, need for psychological counseling)_____
   _____
   Sociability of client (preoperatively: a "talker" or a "listener"? Have social activities
     changed postoperatively?)_____
   Vocational aspects_____
   Spouse/family attitudes (e.g., reactions to laryngectomy, expectations, potential for
     support)_____

Figure 2.1   Intake interview for the laryngectomee.

Communication

Preoperative speech pattern (e.g., regional dialect, foreign language and/or accent, dysfluency, articulation disorder)_____

Current communication status (e.g., gestures, writing, artificial larynx)_____
_____

Reading and writing skills_____
_____

Other factors affecting speech (e.g., stroke, parkinsonism, multiple sclerosis, amyotrophic lateral sclerosis)_____
_____

Figure 2.1   (continued)

resulting in mucus buildup. The laryngectomee with asthma, emphysema, or chronic obstructive pulmonary disease is probably not a good candidate for a TE prosthesis (TEP) because (1) TE speech production relies on adequate pulmonary support and flow and (2) thick mucus may block the passage of air through the prosthesis [27]. Undesirable side effects of certain medications impede the success of alaryngeal speech rehabilitation. Antihistamines, for example, are known to cause dryness of the mucous membranes as well as decreased alertness. A significant hearing loss compromises the laryngectomee's ability to self-monitor for stoma noise [28, 29]. Many laryngectomees report smoking their last cigarette before their surgery. A relatively small number of laryngectomees resume smoking postoperatively, jeopardizing their chances for survival. Rohe [13] suggests that a history of chronic alcohol abuse places the laryngectomee at greater risk for physical and mental health problems. These laryngectomees "remain at high risk for return to use of alcohol as a means of coping with their losses."

Social Factors

Family attitudes about alaryngeal speech rehabilitation are indicators of the support the laryngectomee will receive in the home environment while learning an alternate method of communication. Expectations for level of participation in group activities are based on the sociability of the individual preoperatively (i.e., a "listener" versus a "talker"). The direction and success of therapy will be influenced by the laryngectomee's willingness to take risks and his or her ability to adapt to new situations.

Communication Patterns

When the SLP has the opportunity to counsel the laryngectomee preoperatively, an audio recording of the patient's laryngeal speech is available for reference.

Otherwise, the SLP must depend on the laryngectomee or his or her family to report the preoperative speech pattern. The patient should be asked about articulatory precision, dialectal differences, articulation errors, fluency, and the presence of dysarthria. Was intelligibility affected by any of these factors? Any neurologic components that may affect the speech (e.g., stroke, parkinsonism, multiple sclerosis, or amyotrophic lateral sclerosis) should be noted.

The means and success of the laryngectomee's current communication (e.g., by finger and hand gestures, writing, or use of the artificial larynx) should be determined. At what level are the laryngectomee's reading and writing skills? Adjustments in therapy materials must be made for the laryngectomee who has a visual impairment or is illiterate.

Information Giving

Another objective of these initial meetings is to provide accurate, helpful, and appropriate information to the laryngectomee and his or her family [24]. The American Cancer Society has an excellent selection of materials available (see Appendix A). The laryngectomee should be encouraged to obtain a copy of Lauder's book, *Self-Help for the Laryngectomee* [2]. In our clinic, we have assembled a teaching-demonstration kit that contains a number of items relevant to the new laryngectomee: neck and oral types of electrolarynges (with charged batteries), several styles of TEPs and valves, a sampling of cloth and foam stoma covers, information about Medic Alert (bracelet and wallet identification), a recent *International Association of Laryngectomees News*, and the telephone number of the local New Voice Club. We use a sketch pad set of anatomic drawings (InHealth Technologies) illustrating pre- and postlaryngectomy anatomy, esophageal speech, electrolarynx use, and the TEP (see Appendix A). These drawings can be personalized for the laryngectomee to take home.

Expression and Exploration of Feelings

The SLP should strive to create an accepting environment in which the laryngectomee and his or her family are invited to express and explore their emotions. Freedom to reveal negative as well as positive emotions without fear of judgment heightens awareness and acceptance of underlying feelings [30]. Becoming a laryngectomee involves emotional pain, and there is nothing we can do or say that will lessen the pain. The feelings of the laryngectomee and his or her family need to be accepted for what they are: a very normal reaction to a catastrophic situation. The emotions are an integral part of dealing with "the loss of the way things were before the diagnosis of cancer." The grieving process has begun; the laryngectomee and his or her family are embarking on a complex journey involving a variety of emotions and attempts to cope with the loss. Denial and resistance give way to feelings of anger, inadequacy, guilt, vulnerability, and confusion as the laryngectomee and his or her family move toward a state of acceptance [30].

Problem Solving

As laryngectomees and their families explore the feelings associated with the significant changes in their lives, problems will be identified and acknowledged. Yet another function of the SLP-laryngectomee relationship is the identification of solutions to these problems. A client-centered approach allows the SLP, the laryngectomee, and the family to work together to identify possible options and discuss the consequences of each with respect to the current circumstances. Throughout the therapeutic relationship, the laryngectomee and his or her family are invited to explore issues that are meaningful to their lives (see Chapter 8, "Group Therapy" for further discussion).

Planning for Future Action

The ultimate responsibility for changing behavior or devising a plan of action rests with laryngectomees and their families. Performed skillfully, this arrangement promotes client growth and *empowers*, rather than *rescues*, the laryngectomee.

Accountability and the Intake Interview

To ensure consistent service delivery to all laryngectomees and their families, Salmon [24] has developed a checklist for pre- and postoperative laryngectomee consultations. In Figure 2.2, the items on the checklist are related to information gathering, information giving, expression and exploration of feelings, problem solving, and planning for future action. Salmon suggests placing a copy in each laryngectomee's clinic file as a matter of record keeping.

THE ORAL EXAMINATION

The purpose of the oral examination is to determine structural and functional adequacy for speech production [31], regardless of whether the laryngectomee is going to use an artificial larynx, TE speech, or esophageal speech. Intelligibility ranks high in importance in the development of alaryngeal speech. Articulation is the single most important factor in determining speech intelligibility [31].

An example of the oral examination form is found in Figure 2.3. The oral examination must be systematic and swift [31]. The following equipment is needed: a flashlight, a tongue depressor, disposable gloves, and a mirror. The laryngectomee should be seated comfortably in a chair, and the SLP should be positioned so that his or her eyes are level with the laryngectomee's mouth. This positioning avoids having the laryngectomee tilt his or her head back, an angle that is unnatural and that may interfere with accuracy of observation. As with all procedures that involve the potential for mucous membrane or skin contact with blood, body fluids, or tissues containing blood, the SLP must observe universal precautions developed by the Centers for Disease Control [32] (Figure 2.4). The Occupational Safety and Health Administration has modified these

Patient's name:_____

	Date completed	By whom

I. Preoperative consultation

   A. Review medical chart. Is primary TEP planned? _____ _____

   B. Confer with both patient and spouse. Begin by asking facts they can relate about the upcoming surgery. _____ _____

   C. Underscore that patient will breathe differently and the voice box will be removed. _____ _____

   D. Discuss alternatives for postoperative communication and test legibility of patient's writing. _____ _____

   E. Estimate length of surgery and prepare spouse for intensive care unit and patient's appearance. _____ _____

   F. Outline postop services provided by speech-language pathologist and set date for first postop appointment. _____ _____

   G. Inform about the availability of a counselor, social worker, chaplain, VA pension representative, etc. _____ _____

   H. Write consultation report and place in medical chart. _____ _____

   I. If necessary, investigate referral sources for alaryngeal speech therapy. _____ _____

II. Postoperative consultation

   A. First visit

      1. Give patient packet of selected literature from American Cancer Society, Easter Seals, VA, etc. _____ _____

      2. Show patient and spouse various types of stoma covers. _____ _____

      3. Furnish addresses, prices, and patterns for commercially available types of stoma covers. _____ _____

      4. Discuss Medic Alert information: "Neck breather" to be engraved on back of bracelet and printed on billfold card. _____ _____

      5. Refer to appropriate counselor.

      6. Request permission to write IAL and New Voice Club to place patient's name on newsletter mailing lists. _____ _____

   B. Second visit

      1. Discuss literature provided at first visit. _____ _____

      2. Show film or videotape that demonstrates esophageal speech and TEP speech. _____ _____

Figure 2.2 Checklist for pre- and postoperative laryngectomee consultations. (TEP = tracheoesophageal prosthesis; VA = Veterans Administration; IAL = International Association of Laryngectomees.) (Reprinted with permission from SJ Salmon. Checklist for pre- and postoperative laryngectomee consultations. Presented at the Thirty-Sixth International Association of Laryngectomees Voice Institute. Hot Springs, AR, 1996.)

	Date completed	By whom

3. Request permission to arrange visit(s) from alaryngeal speaker(s) (and spouse when appropriate) trained by American Cancer Society for hospital visits. _____ _____

4. Notify head nurse of scheduled time for visit(s). _____ _____

5. Record visit(s) in medical chart. _____ _____

C. Third visit

1. Show film or videotape that demonstrates artificial larynx devices. _____ _____

2. Have variety of devices displayed during the film or video and orient the patient and significant other to them. _____ _____

D. Other visits

1. Discuss visit(s) from trained hospital visitors. _____ _____

2. Help select an appropriate artificial larynx device and begin instruction about use. _____ _____

3. When possible, issue or loan an artificial larynx device after instruction, but before hospital discharge. _____ _____

4. Loan patient booklets (e.g., *Self-Help for the Laryngectomee*, by Edmund Lauder and *Looking Forward .... A Guidebook for the Laryngectomee*, by Robert L. Keith). _____ _____

5. Provide patient with written appointment schedule for outpatient appointments. _____ _____

6. Record each visit in medical chart and the type of artificial larynx device recommended and/or loaned. _____ _____

Figure 2.2   (continued)

precautions to meet the needs of SLPs and audiologists. A summary of infectious diseases of potential concern to the practicing SLP appears in Table 2.2. Guidelines for infection control are listed in Table 2.3.

Lips

Labial structure, function, and motility should be assessed. The symmetry of the lips at rest and during stretch and purse activities should be noted. Is the laryngectomee able to capture and hold air in the cheeks? Adequate lip movement and tight lip seal are required for the production of bilabial obstruents /p/ and /b/ as well as for the injection method for sonorants (i.e., /w/, /l/, /r/, /j/, /m/, and /n/) and vowels.

Oral Examination

Scoring: WNL = Within normal limits   ARS = Asymmetry on right side
           D = Deviation noted   ALS = Asymmetry on left side
           C = Concern   NA = Not applicable
           NO = Not observed

I. Lips
____ Structure   Note symmetry at rest, weakness, drooling.
____ Condition   Note chapping, bleeding.
____ Frenum   Tug on upper lip; adequate for bilabial productions?
____ Stretch   Observe symmetry during smile or production of /i/ as in "me."
____ Purse   Observe symmetry during pucker or production of /u/ as in "boo."
____ Alternating   Note symmetry during rapid repetitions of /u-i/.
____ Seal   Capture air in cheeks; move from side to side with lips closed.
____ Other   Observation:_____

II. Dentition
Natural teeth
____ Structure   Are all teeth present? If not, note missing teeth:_____
____ Health   Note presence of staining, cavities, bleeding or puffy gums.
Dental appliances
____ Partials   Note upper or lower partials:_____   Fit_____
____ Full dentures Note upper or lower full dentures:_____   Fit_____
____ Other   Observation:_____

III. Hard palate
____ Structure   Note scarring, bluish coloration, repaired cleft palate.
____ Other   Observation:_____

IV. Soft palate
____ Structure   Note symmetry at rest, scarring, atrophy.
____ Mobility   On production of /ɑ/ as in "odd"; Note symmetry during elevation.
____ Control   Do liquids escape into the nose during swallow?
____ Sucking   Is laryngectomee able to suck through straw, sip from spoon?
____ Other   Observation:_____

V. Tongue
____ Structure   Note symmetry at rest, scarring, atrophy, weakness.
____ Elevation   With mandible open, is tongue tip able to touch upper lip?
____ Depression   Does tongue tip extend beyond lower lip?
____ Protrusion   Does tongue tip extend past anterior teeth for production of /θ/ as in "thumb"?
____ Retraction   Is tongue drawn into the posterior oral cavity?
____ Lateralization With mandible still, move tongue from left to right.
____ Anterior strength   Push tongue against tongue depressor held at center of lips.
____ Lateral strength   Push tongue against tongue depressor held to each cheek.

Figure 2.3 The purpose of the oral examination is to determine whether structure and function of the oral mechanism are adequate for speech production.

VI. Diadochokinesis

____ (pʌtʌkʌ)　　　8 sets/10 secs.

VII. Swallow pattern

____ Liquid　　　Do liquids escape at the lips, through the nose, or into the trachea?

____ Solid　　　Are solids swallowed easily? Are there problem consistencies?

____ Other　　　Observation:_____

VIII. Mandible

____ Structure　　　Note symmetry at rest, scarring.

____ Open-close　　　Note symmetry during opening, closing. Check temporomandibular joint for clicking.

IX. Neck

____ Structure　　　Note symmetry at rest, scarring, swelling, tenderness, radical neck dissection.

____ Lateralization　　　Note range of movement to the left and right.

____ Stoma size　　　Note size in approximate diameter:_____

____ Breathing　　　Is breathing audible, labored?

____ Other　　　Observation: _____

X. Additional observations

____ Articulation　　　Note imprecision, substitutions, omissions, regional dialect, or foreign accent:_____

____ Oral habits　　　Note nail biting, lip biting, cheek biting:_____
_____

Figure 2.3　(continued)

Dentition

The absence of any natural teeth and the presence of any staining, cavities, bleeding, or puffy gums should be noted. If partials or dentures are worn, their location and fit should be recorded. Missing teeth or loose dentures can interfere with articulatory precision.

Hard and Soft Palates

The shape and width of the hard palate and the presence of any scarring should be noted. The SLP should inspect the velum for symmetry at rest and note any scarring. It should be determined whether the laryngectomee has experienced any difficulty with liquids coming through his or her nose during swallowing. Is the laryngectomee able to suck through a straw or sip from a spoon? The client should be instructed to produce /ɑ/ with the mouth open as the SLP observes for symmetric lifting of the soft palate. Velopharyngeal inadequacy may interfere

Figure 2.4
The speech-language-pathologist conducts an oral examination observing universal precautions developed by the Centers for Disease Control.

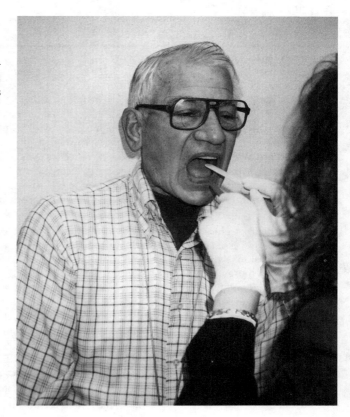

with the acquisition of esophageal speech by allowing air from the oral cavity destined for the esophageal sphincter to escape into the nasal cavity.

Tongue

With the laryngectomee's mouth open, the tongue should be observed at rest for size and symmetry of structure, and any scarring, atrophy, or weakness (see Figure 2.4). Agility of tongue movements during depression, elevation, protrusion, retraction, and lateralization activities is a critical predictor of the laryngectomee's articulatory skills. Imprecise tongue movements may indicate a need for oral agility and strengthening exercises.

Diadochokinesia

The laryngectomee should be asked to repeat /pʌtʌkʌ/ as rapidly as possible for approximately 30 seconds. Even without voicing, the number of "sets" performed can be observed. Adequacy is judged at 8 sets in 10 seconds.

Table 2.2 A summary of infectious diseases of potential concern to the practicing speech-language pathologist (SLP)

Acquired immunodeficiency syndrome (AIDS)
- The human immunodeficiency virus (HIV) is the virus that causes AIDS, a fatal disease for which there is neither a cure nor a vaccine.
- Statistics show an estimated 17 million people worldwide have the virus; by the year 2000, 30–40 million people are predicted to be infected by the virus.
- Transmission is considered to be through contact with bodily fluids, primarily blood. There is minimal evidence of transmission through saliva, although oral lesions could produce blood in the saliva. In a reported incident, a health care worker contracted HIV through exposure of ungloved, chapped hands to infected blood [33].
- SLPs are at extremely low risk for contracting HIV through work-related activities, even though they are exposed to saliva, cerumen, mucous membranes, and tears.

Hepatitis B
- Hepatitis B is a highly contagious virus that may damage the liver and can be fatal.
- There are an estimated 200,000 newly infected persons in the United States annually.
- Transmission is via blood or mucus; the hepatitis B virus is capable of surviving for 7 days or more on contaminated instruments or surfaces.
- SLPs are at greater risk of being exposed to hepatitis B than to HIV. Three types of vaccine are available.

Tuberculosis (TB)
- TB is a bacterial infection that attacks the lungs. TB may lead to disability or death.
- The incidence of TB in the United States is on the rise.
- Transmission is possible through contact with saliva and by breathing contaminated air.
- SLPs are at particular risk for contracting TB during interactions with AIDS patients and foreign immigrants from countries in which TB is common. Tests are available to detect whether one has been exposed to the bacteria.

Cytomegalovirus (CMV)
- CMV is also known as the herpes virus. CMV is a major source of infection for newborn infants and may cause birth defects or death. CMV is harmless to healthy children and adults approximately 90% of the time.
- SLPs may be exposed to CMV through contact with blood, saliva, or mucus from an infected child. CMV is a potential hazard to the unborn child of the pregnant SLP.

Herpes simplex
- Herpes simplex is a highly contagious virus evidenced by canker sores, cold sores, herpetic conjunctivitis, and herpetic lesions on the fingers and hands.
- Transmission is via saliva, blood, mucus, or exudate from the sores.
- SLPs are at high risk for exposure to herpes simplex because of the oral manifestations of the disease.

SLP = speech-language pathologist.
Source: Adapted from RJ Kemp, RJ Roeser, DW Pearson, BB Ballachanda. Infection Control for the Professions of Audiology and Speech-Language Pathology. Chesterfield, MO: Oaktree Products, 1996;17.

Table 2.3   Guidelines for infection control

Universal precautions have been developed by the Centers for Disease Control and are used by health facilities nationwide to prevent transmission of blood-borne pathogens. Universal precautions assume all body fluids, especially blood or fluids containing blood, are infectious and should be treated as such. Precautions must be taken in all interactions that involve potential for mucous membrane or skin contact with blood, body fluids, tissues containing blood, or potential spills or splashes from them.

Handwashing is the single most important defense against the spread of infection. The SLP should wash his or her hands in the following situations:
- After removing gloves
- Before and after oral examinations
- Before and after performing any personal body function
- Before and after physical contact with clients
- Between clients
- Immediately and thoroughly if potentially contaminated with blood or body fluids
- When arriving and before leaving a setting
- When hands are obviously soiled

Protocol for handwashing. For thorough, effective handwashing
- Remove rings from the fingers before washing
- Use medical-grade liquid antibacterial soap under running water
- Work up a lather using vigorous mechanical action to include hands, wrists, and forearms
- Continue handwashing for 15 seconds if not grossly contaminated
- Rinse hands thoroughly and gently blot dry with a paper towel
- Use towel to turn off faucet

Use *gloves* when there is the potential to contact blood, body fluids, mucous membranes, and broken skin during the performance of invasive procedures, such as
- An oral examination
- Dysphagia assessment and therapeutic procedures
- Introducing a laryngeal mirror into the mouth (e.g., for purposes of oral stimulation, oral exercises, or indirect laryngoscopy)
- Manipulation of the oral structures during articulation therapy
- Touching the stoma for cleaning
- Placement of a tracheoesophageal prosthesis or housing

Protocol for wearing gloves. The following procedures should be observed:
- Use tight-fitting latex or vinyl gloves
- Change gloves after contact with each client
- Bandage any open cuts or sores on hands before putting on gloves
- If a glove is accidentally torn, immediately wash hands
- Double-glove if the client is known to be infected with HIV or hepatitis B
- Remove gloves in a way that prevents ungloved fingers from contacting contaminated glove surface
- Discard gloves in trash before exiting room

Additional precautions. In addition to gloves, wear goggles or a face shield during procedures likely to generate droplets of blood or body fluids via coughing, drooling, and so forth (e.g., placement of the tracheoesophageal prosthesis). Position the laryngectomee so that you are not sitting in the direct path of mucus coughed from the stoma.

Table 2.3 (continued)

To clean and decontaminate spills or splashes of blood or body fluids
- Wear gloves, goggles, and gown
- Use disposable toweling and remove visible materials
- Decontaminate areas of flooding with liquid germicide
- Clean surfaces using 10% bleach solution and disposable toweling
- Disinfect contaminated equipment (e.g., laryngeal mirrors, microphones, prostheses and inserters, artificial larynxes) and materials (e.g., objects, pens, pencils)
- Immediately launder all contaminated clothing and effects
- When performing cardiopulmonary resuscitation, use a mouthpiece/resuscitation/ventilation device to eliminate the need for mouth-to-mouth or mouth-to-stoma action

SLP = speech-language pathologist.
Source: Adapted from RJ Kemp, RJ Roeser, DW Pearson, BB Ballachanda. Infection Control for the Professions of Audiology and Speech-Language Pathology. Chesterfield, MO: Oaktree Products, 1996;17.

Diadochokinetic rate is another indicator of oral agility, calling into play rapid alternating movements of the tongue and lips.

Swallow Pattern

The laryngectomee should be observed while he or she swallows a sip of water. Does the water escape through the lips or nose or leak into the trachea (evidenced by coughing)? The client should be offered a cracker and observed for any difficulties swallowing. The laryngectomee should be asked if there are any problematic food consistencies (e.g., beef). Swallowing difficulties are not uncommon after radiation therapy and some types of surgery to treat head and neck cancer.

Mandible

As the laryngectomee opens and closes his or her jaw, symmetry of jaw movement should be noted. Does the laryngectomee experience any pain in the temporomandibular joint?

Neck

Radiation frequently leaves neck tissues red, swollen, and painful to the touch. As the laryngectomee turns his or her head to the left and then to the right, the range of movement should be noted. Surgical removal of strap muscles and scar tissue may limit the extent of head turning. The SLP should note the approximate diameter of the stoma. Laryngectomees with exceptionally small stomas may experience audible breathing and typically are not good candidates for TEPs.

Additional Observations

Articulation difficulties, such as substitutions or omissions, can interfere with intelligibility of speech. Intelligibility may also be influenced by regional dialect or foreign accent.

AUDIOMETRIC EVALUATION

Audiometric assessment of the laryngectomee before the initiation of alaryngeal speech training is essential. Hearing loss can have a significant effect on the success of alaryngeal speech rehabilitation [28]. High-frequency hearing loss is common among laryngectomees 60 years old or older. Speech proficiency, particularly for the fricatives, is at risk when the laryngectomee's ability to receive auditory feedback is impaired. Stoma noise, a high-frequency signal, is the result of air turbulence within the trachea and detracts from alaryngeal speech. The laryngectomee with a high-frequency loss is unable to effectively self-monitor for, and thus reduce, excessive stoma noise [29]. The presence of hearing loss is an important variable in the direction and planning of alaryngeal speech therapy.

REFERENCES

1. National Institutes of Health. What You Need to Know About Cancer of the Larynx. Bethesda, MD: National Cancer Institute, 1993;18.
2. Lauder E. Your New Voice. In J Lauder (ed), Self-Help for the Laryngectomee. San Antonio, TX: Lauder, 1994;6.
3. Zemlin WR. Speech and Hearing Science: Anatomy and Physiology (3rd ed). Englewood Cliffs, NJ: Prentice-Hall, 1988;100, 227.
4. Maragos N. Anatomy and Physiology of the Laryngectomee. In RL Keith, FL Darley (eds), Laryngectomee Rehabilitation (3rd ed). Austin, TX: PRO-ED, 1994;72.
5. Roberts NK. Nursing Intervention for the Laryngectomee: Management of Change in Self-Care Practices Following Hospitalization. In RL Keith, FL Darley (eds), Laryngectomee Rehabilitation (3rd ed). Austin, TX: PRO-ED, 1994;124.
6. Damsté PH. Smelling and Swimming after Laryngectomy. In RL Keith, FL Darley (eds), Laryngectomee Rehabilitation (3rd ed). Austin, TX: PRO-ED, 1994;555.
7. Prater RJ, Swift RW. Manual of Voice Therapy. Boston: Little, Brown, 1984;257.
8. Kapit W, Macey RI, Meisami E. The Physiology Coloring Book. San Francisco: Harper Collins, 1987;99.
9. Gilmore SI. The Physical, Social, Occupational, and Psychological Concomitants of Laryngectomy. In RL Keith, FL Darley (eds), Laryngectomee Rehabilitation (3rd ed). Austin, TX: PRO-ED, 1994;412.
10. Wallen V, Webb B. A survey of background characteristics of 2,000 laryngectomees: a preliminary report. Mil Med 1975:140;532.
11. Tatchell RH, Lerman JW, Wyatt J. Olfactory ability as a function of nasal air flow volume in laryngectomees. Am J Otolaryngol 1985;6:426.
12. Diedrich WM, Youngstrom KA. Alaryngeal Speech. Springfield, IL: Thomas, 1966;70.
13. Rohe DE. Loss, Grief, and Depression after Laryngectomy. In RL Keith, FL Darley (eds), Laryngectomee Rehabilitation (3rd ed). Austin, TX: PRO-ED, 1994;488.

14. Casper JK, Colton RH. Clinical Manual for Laryngectomy and Head and Neck Cancer Rehabilitation. San Diego: Singular, 1993;53.
15. Snidecor JC. Speech Rehabilitation of the Laryngectomized (2nd ed). Springfield, IL: Thomas, 1968;173.
16. Aronson AE. Clinical Voice Disorders (2nd ed). New York: Thieme, 1985;382.
17. Gardner WH. Adjustment problems of laryngectomized women. Arch Otolaryngol 1966:83;31.
18. Natvig K. Laryngectomees in Norway. Study #5: problems in everyday life. J Otolaryngol 1984:13;15.
19. Stack F. The Feminine Viewpoint on Being a Laryngectomee. In RL Keith, FL Darley (eds), Laryngectomee Rehabilitation (2nd ed). San Diego: College-Hill, 1986;263.
20. Doyle PC. Foundations of Voice and Speech Rehabilitation Following Laryngeal Cancer. San Diego: Singular, 1994;116.
21. American Cancer Society. First Steps: Helping Words for the Laryngectomee. Atlanta: American Cancer Society, 1995;14.
22. Salmon SJ. Laryngectomee Visitations. In RL Keith, FL Darley (eds), Laryngectomee Rehabilitation (2nd ed). San Diego: College-Hill, 1986;149.
23. Molyneaux D, Lane VW. Successful Interactive Skills for Speech-Language Pathologists and Audiologists. Rockville, MD: Aspen, 1990;14.
24. Salmon SJ. Pre- and Postoperative Conferences with Laryngectomees and Their Spouses. In RL Keith, FL Darley (eds), Laryngectomee Rehabilitation (2nd ed). San Diego: College-Hill, 1986;144.
25. Lewin JS. Special Problems of the Alaryngeal Speaker. In RL Keith, FL Darley (eds), Laryngectomee Rehabilitation (3rd ed). Austin, TX: PRO-ED, 1994;283.
26. Wolfe RB, Olson JE, Goldenberg DD. Rehabilitation of the laryngectomee: the role of the distal esophageal sphincter. Laryngoscope 1971:81;1971.
27. Bosone ZT. Tracheoesophageal Fistulization/Puncture for Voice Restoration: Presurgical Considerations and Troubleshooting Procedures. In RL Keith, FL Darley (eds), Laryngectomee Rehabilitation (3rd ed). Austin, TX: PRO-ED, 1994;362.
28. Martin DE, Hoops HR, Shanks JC. The relationship between esophageal speech proficiency and selected measures of auditory function. J Speech Hear Res 1974:74;80.
29. Martin DE. Pre- and Postoperative Anatomical and Physiological Observations in Laryngectomy. In RL Keith, FL Darley (eds), Laryngectomee Rehabilitation (2nd ed). San Diego: College-Hill, 1986;85.
30. Luterman DM. Counseling Persons with Communication Disorders and Their Families (3rd ed). Austin, TX: PRO-ED, 1996;66.
31. Emerick LL, Haynes WO. Diagnosis and Evaluation in Speech Pathology (3rd ed). Englewood Cliffs, NJ: Prentice-Hall, 1986;68.
32. Kemp RJ, Roeser RJ, Pearson DW, Ballachanda BB. Infection Control for the Professions of Audiology and Speech-Language Pathology. Chesterfield, MO: Oaktree Products Inc., 1996;17.
33. Centers for Disease Control. Healthcare workers and AIDS. MMWR June 23, 1987.

3

Oral Communication Options

DECIDING THE OPTIMAL TECHNIQUE

The ultimate goal of alaryngeal speech rehabilitation is to help the laryngec-tomee develop functional, intelligible speech [1]. The laryngectomee has three primary methods of oral communication from which to choose: (1) artificial larynx speech, (2) esophageal speech, and (3) tracheoesophageal (TE) speech. Selecting a communication technique ultimately rests with the laryngectomee; however, the physician and the speech clinician are important and influential partners in the decision-making process [2–5]. The speech-language pathologist (SLP) is responsible for providing information about the communication options and allowing the laryngectomee freedom to make an informed choice based on needs and abilities [2, 5–7].

ARTIFICIAL LARYNGEAL SPEECH

The artificial larynx is a viable alternative to esophageal and TE speech [6]. Selection of an artificial larynx is a highly individualized process and, at best, represents a compromise among a number of determining factors: physical needs, proficiency, availability of the devices, personal preference, and initial cost and maintenance [2].

Two types of artificial larynges are available: (1) pneumatic and (2) bat-tery operated.

Pneumatic Artificial Larynx

The pneumatic speech aid directs lung air from a rubber or steel cup placed over the stoma into a tube directed into the mouth [4, 8, 9]. The Tokyo artifi-cial larynx (Clyde Welch [Omaha, NE]), an example of such a device, requires competent lung power and abdominal support. The inexpensive unit comes in a do-it-yourself kit and includes a variety of rubber, plastic, and metal stoma cups, plastic tubing, and small squares of rubber. Pitch is controlled by placing

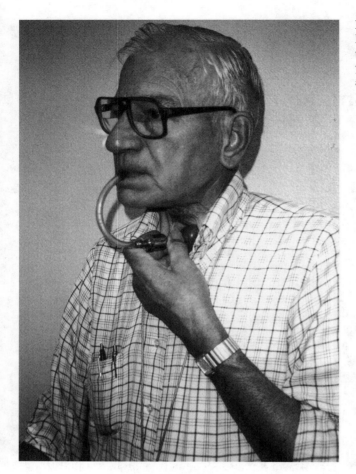

Figure 3.1
Intraoral placement for the Tokyo artificial larynx (Clyde Welch [Omaha, NE]).

varied thicknesses and widths of the rubber strip in the vibrator housing before use [8–10]. Varying breath pressure affects both pitch and loudness [8–10].

Advantages of the Pneumatic Artificial Larynx

The primary advantages of the pneumatic artificial larynx are that it is relatively low in cost and requires no batteries [10, 11]. The laryngectomee's lung air vibrates the rubber diaphragm, creating a sound that resembles a hoarse rather than a mechanical voice. Because placement for the pneumatic artificial larynx is intraoral (Figure 3.1), the device may be used successfully in the presence of neck tissue that is edematous, thick, scarred, or fibrotic.

Disadvantages of the Pneumatic Artificial Larynx

Manual dexterity is a requirement for efficient use of the pneumatic artificial larynx. The laryngectomee must be able to form a good seal over the stoma while simultaneously directing the air tube into the oral cavity [11]. Precise articulation is necessary due to the presence of the plastic tube in the mouth. Extensive surgery of the tongue or palate may interfere with articulatory precision. During speech, the stoma cup must be periodically lifted from the stoma for air intake and then repositioned [10]. Sound production may be hindered by the accumulation of saliva in the oral tube or mucus from the lungs in the stoma cup [8]. Adequate lung pressure as well as abdominal support are needed to maintain airflow through the housing to vibrate the rubber strip and produce sound. An individual in frail health or with respiratory insufficiency, such as chronic obstructive pulmonary disease, would not be a good candidate for use of a pneumatic device [8]. A problem common to all artificial larynges is the use of one hand for operation of the unit, denying the laryngectomee simultaneous use of both hands.

Battery-Operated Artificial Larynx

The battery-operated artificial larynx is used more often than the pneumatic device. Battery-operated artificial larynges are divided into two subtypes: neck and intraoral [8]. The power source for the neck-type device is a battery that vibrates a metal or plastic head on the artificial larynx. This vibrating head is placed against the laryngectomee's neck (or cheek). As the tone resonates in the hypopharynx and oral cavity, the laryngectomee uses the articulators to shape the sound into meaningful speech. The laryngectomee has a wide variety of neck-type battery-operated devices from which to select—for example, the Servox Inton Electronic Speech Aid (Siemens Hearing Instruments [Prospect Heights, IL]) (Figure 3.2), the TruTone Electronic Speech Aid (Griffin Laboratories [Temecula, CA]) (Figure 3.3), the Nu-Vois Artificial Larynx (Mountain Precision Manufacturers [Boise, ID]) (Figure 3.4), the OptiVox Artificial Larynx (Bivona Medical Technologies [Gary, IN]), the SPKR Artificial Larynx (UNI Manufacturing Company [Ontario, OR]) and the ROMET Speech Aid (ROMET [Missoula, MT]) (see Appendix A). All of these artificial larynges have adjustments for pitch and loudness.

Postsurgically, the laryngectomee may develop a fistula or experience pain or tenderness in the neck region. Furthermore, the neck tissue may become swollen, hardened, and thickened, resulting in reduced transmission of sound using the neck-type artificial larynx. Under these circumstances, an intraoral electronic device may be selected [4, 11]. All the neck-type battery-operated artificial larynges can be adapted for oral use by the fitting of a plastic tube to the metal or plastic head (intraoral adapter). The Cooper-Rand Electronic Speech Aid (Luminaud [Mentor, OH]) (Figure 3.5) is designed specifically for intraoral use [10]. An electronically generated sound enters the mouth via a plastic tube attached to a small hand-held tone generator [8, 9, 11]. Pitch and loudness controls are located on the pulse generator [8].

A relatively new technologic contribution to alaryngeal speech rehabilitation is an intraoral device called the Ultra Voice (Health Concepts [Malvern,

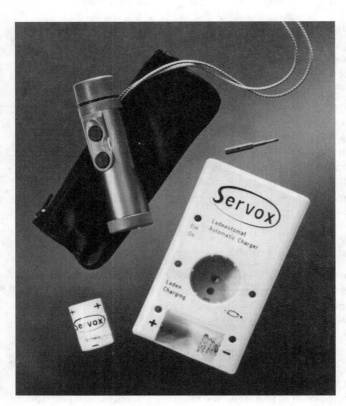

Figure 3.2
The Servox Inton Electronic Speech Aid (Siemens Hearing Instruments [Prospect Heights, IL]) comes with battery, dual charger, and leather storage pouch. (Reprinted with permission of InHealth Technologies. 1996 Professional Catalog: Blom-Singer Voice Restoration Systems. Carpinteria, CA: InHealth Technologies, 1996;10.)

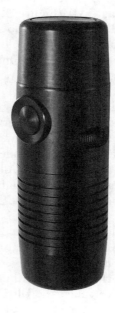

Figure 3.3
The TruTone Electronic Speech Aid (Griffin Laboratories [Temecula, CA]) is equipped with a single pressure-sensitive button for natural voice intonation. The unit is lightweight, made of durable impact-resistant materials, and operates on rechargeable or 9-V batteries. The speech aid comes with an oral adapter. (Reprinted with permission of Griffin Laboratories.)

Figure 3.4
Constructed of high-impact materials, the Nu-Vois Artificial Larynx (Mountain Precision Manufacturers [Boise, ID]) weighs less than 5 oz, including the battery. The unit is equipped with pitch and volume control and is designed to operate on rechargeable 9-V batteries. An intraoral adapter is included with the kit.

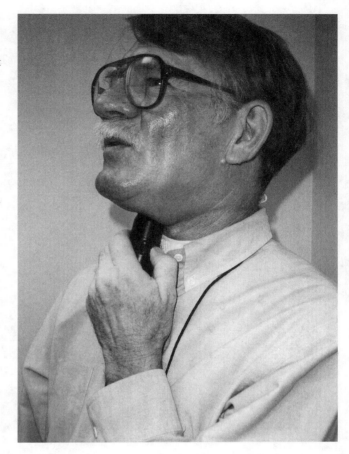

PA]). The oral unit is custom built as a denture or a palatal retainer. Three basic components are built into the oral unit: a loudspeaker, an electronic circuit for pitch and volume control, and rechargeable batteries. The oral unit is protected from saliva, food, and liquids by a silicone membrane. Manipulating the button on the handheld remote control turns the oral unit on or off, adjusts tone for inflection, and increases or decreases loudness (i.e., whisper mode). A demonstration video of the Ultra Voice is available from Health Concepts (see Appendix A).

Advantages of the Battery-Operated Artificial Larynx
Controversy exists in the literature as to whether the use of an artificial larynx facilitates or inhibits the learning of esophageal speech [7, 12]. In our alaryngeal speech class, none of the laryngectomees has deferred learning esophageal speech because he or she *preferred* to use the artificial larynx. The artificial larynx is comparatively easy to master when contrasted with esophageal speech [5,

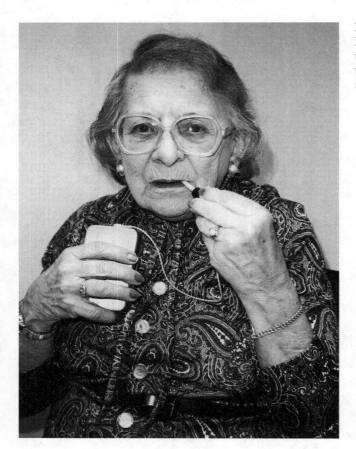

Figure 3.5
Intraoral placement for the Cooper-Rand Electronic Speech Aid (Luminaud [Mentor, OH]).

7, 11]. Training with the artificial larynx can begin within days of surgery [6, 11]. In the first few sessions, the laryngectomee learns the basics of coordinating the on-off switch with articulation and placement of the unit intraorally or on the neck or cheek. Although practice is required to achieve proficiency, the laryngectomee regains access to functional oral communication almost immediately [4, 7]. The anxiety associated with being unable to communicate is relieved. With the artificial larynx in hand, the laryngectomee who wants to pursue additional esophageal or TE speech training does so without the frustration of "waiting to communicate" [4, 8, 11].

Most of the electronic speech aids have volume control, allowing the laryngectomee to be heard in noisy environments and by hearing-impaired listeners [2, 5–7, 12]. Many of the artificial larynges also have pitch control for individual preferences. The sound from the electronic speech aids transfers satisfactorily over the telephone [7, 12].

The artificial larynx is an acceptable communication alternative when the laryngectomee experiences physical or psychological conditions that interfere with learning esophageal or TE speech. Severe hearing impairment, advanced age, extensive oral-pharyngeal-esophageal surgery, and limited access to rehabilitative services are a few of the conditions that may necessitate use of the artificial larynx [12].

Disadvantages of the Battery-Operated Artificial Larynx

Most users of the electronic artificial larynx object to the mechanical or buzzing sound produced and the unwanted attention it attracts to the speaker in public [5, 7, 11]. The unit must be held in one hand during use, interfering with two-handed activities, such as driving, taking photographs, writing while holding the telephone, and cooking [7]. The laryngectomee must demonstrate sufficient hand and finger dexterity to operate the on-off switch and the pitch and volume controls on the unit.

Traditionally, artificial larynges have been bulky and somewhat awkward to carry [7]. Most artificial larynges are sturdily built to withstand frequent daily use. Current production models are lightweight (some weigh less than 5 oz), compact (as short as 4 in. long and 1 in. in diameter), and made with high-impact materials to resist breakage. Most artificial larynges come with a safety strap to place around the neck. Failure to use the strap can result in dropping the artificial larynx, often causing permanent damage. Repairs may be costly and inconvenient, and unless the laryngectomee has a borrowed or backup unit, communication may be difficult during the repair period [7].

Spontaneity is also hindered; the laryngectomee must choose between keeping the artificial larynx in hand in anticipation of speaking or continuously putting the unit away and retrieving it on demand [7]. The battery in the artificial larynx may fade at inopportune times, so the laryngectomee must carry a charged spare battery.

The neck (or cheek) tissue must be pliable enough to allow transmission of the electronically induced vibrations into the hypopharynx and oral cavity [2]. Surgical intervention may have left the surface of the neck too irregular to make a good seal with the head of the artificial larynx. If the neck tissues are hard and fibrous, consideration must be given to either cheek placement or the use of an oral-type speech aid.

A specific disadvantage of the oral-type speech aid is that the plastic tube may interfere with tongue movements, resulting in articulatory imprecision [2]. In addition, some laryngectomees experience dysarthric tongue movements as a result of surgery [2]. The introduction of a plastic tube into the oral cavity only intensifies the articulatory difficulties. Saliva may block the plastic tube and, in some cases, damage the mechanism of the artificial larynx [2].

The initial investment in an artificial larynx may be substantial; however, there are units available in all price ranges. Some telephone companies (e.g., Pacific Bell of California) offer an artificial larynx as an assistive device option to their customers. The local American Cancer Society may have a limited supply of rebuilt, donated artificial larynges for short-term loan or at reduced cost. Depending on the speech unit, the laryngectomee may need to purchase a charger and several rechargeable batteries or keep a supply of disposable replacement batteries on hand.

ESOPHAGEAL SPEECH

During a total laryngectomy, the larynx is removed and the top of the trachea attached to the sternal area [13]. The pharynx is shaped into a tubular form and attached directly to the esophagus. The point at which the hypopharynx joins the esophagus is referred to as the pharyngoesophageal (PE) segment [13, 14]. This segment, located at the level of C4–C7, is composed of striated muscle: the cricopharyngeus muscle, the lower strands of the inferior pharyngeal constrictor, and the superior esophageal sphincter [13, 15, 16]. The PE segment is the neoglottis—the "new" vibrator—for voicing during esophageal speech [14, 15, 17]. The esophagus becomes the reservoir of air for voice production [13, 14, 17].

At rest, the air within the nasal, oral, and pharyngeal cavities has positive air pressure in contrast to the negative air pressure that exists in the esophagus [14]. Before esophageal speech attempts, the air pressure in the esophagus is –4 mm Hg to –7 mm Hg below atmospheric pressure [14, 18, 19]. Thus, the air pressure is positive above and negative below the PE segment.

There are two primary processes for moving air through the PE segment and into the esophagus for esophageal speech production: (1) injection and (2) inhalation [14, 15, 18, 20]. *Injection* occurs when positive air pressure is increased in the oral cavity via movements of the lips and tongue, forcing air through the closed PE segment into the esophagus [18]. When the air is in the upper portion of the esophagus, tightening of the surrounding thoracic muscles and abdominal muscles moves the air back up over the PE segment, vibrating the PE segment and creating sound. The sound is given resonance in the oropharyngeal and nasal cavities, and articulation of specific syllables and words occurs [14].

There are two subtypes of the injection process based on the manner of articulation: (1) the injection method for obstruents and (2) the injection method for sonorants and vowels. Plosives, fricatives, and affricates are all obstruents, because during their production, the breath stream is partially or totally obstructed. In contrast, sonorants (i.e., nasals, glides, and lateral /l/) and vowels are made with a relatively unobstructed flow of air.

Injection Method for Obstruents

The *injection method for obstruents* uses the production of plosives, fricatives, and affricates to increase the positive air pressure within the oral cavity [14, 21]. The intraoral air pressure builds behind the point of articulatory contact until it is sufficient to overcome the resistance of the closed PE segment [5, 14]. The air is forced past the PE segment into the esophagus [13, 15]. Return of the air from the esophagus to the oral cavity vibrates the PE segment for voicing. Doyle [5] discusses the contribution of tongue and lip muscle strength to air pressure buildup and compression of the oropharyngeal cavity during articulation. Deidrich and Youngstrom [15] observed that the fricative sound for /s/ occurred simultaneously with the injection of air into the esophagus. Other writers refer to this method as consonant press or injection, "Dutch method" of air injection, and plosive injection [14, 18, 20].

The injection method for obstruents is an effective means of charging the esophagus with air for words that begin with an obstruent (e.g., peach, stop, or chat). According to Weiss et al. [22], the percentage of occurrence of obstruents in English is approximately 36%. In conversational speech, the phrases or sentences are likely to be interspersed with obstruents; thus, the laryngectomee may increase duration of speaking time by learning to inject air on these obstruents [13, 14, 23].

Injection Method for Sonorants and Vowels

The laryngectomee cannot rely solely on the injection method for obstruents because all words do not begin with a plosive, fricative, or affricate. In fact, sonorants and vowels represent 62% of English productions [22]. To be a proficient esophageal speaker using the injection method, the laryngectomee must also learn the *injection method for sonorants and vowels*. A lip or tongue seal is used to trap the air and the tongue moves the air into the pharynx. Other authors have referred to this type of injection method as tongue pumping, glossopharyngeal press, and glossopharyngeal closure [13–15, 18, 20]. The pumping action of the tongue along the length of the hard and soft palates decreases the size of the oral cavity. The compressed air forces the PE segment open (by overcoming muscular resistance), or the PE segment relaxes and the air slips into the esophagus [14]. Velopharyngeal closure is required to prevent air escape into the nasal cavity [13, 14, 18].

Inhalation Method

The *inhalation method* occurs when negative pressure is increased below the level of the PE segment so that air in the oral cavity is sucked rather than forced into the upper esophagus [14]. The lips and tongue are not actively involved in the inhalation method, although the velopharyngeal port may be closed or open [13, 15, 18, 20]. The laryngectomee takes in a quick breath via the stoma. The rapid intake of air through the stoma further lowers the air pressure in the thoracic cavity where the esophagus is located [14]. Negative air pressure falls to approximately −15 mm Hg, creating a vacuum effect [13, 20]. A significant difference in air pressure is created between the oral cavity (above the PE segment) and the esophagus (below the PE segment). To equalize the air pressure, air flows from the oral and nasal cavities into the pharynx, past the PE segment, and into the esophagus. The PE segment must be relaxed voluntarily during the inward air flow [13, 18]. The PE segment then closes, trapping the air in the esophagus. Once air is in the esophagus, the procedure for producing sound parallels that of the injection process. Abdominal muscles and the muscles surrounding the PE segment are contracted, moving the air up over the PE segment. Air return is also facilitated by the air pressure in the esophagus, the recoiling and elastic properties of the esophagus, diaphragmatic tension, and abdominal muscle contractions [13, 18]. The vibrated air returns to the oral and nasal cavities for articulation and resonation.

Advantages of Esophageal Speech

There are several important advantages to using esophageal speech. First, esophageal speech requires no initial investment in equipment, maintenance, or repair costs. Second, because there are no external devices, the laryngectomee's hands are free to perform other functions [5, 11]. Third, Bennett and Weinberg [24] found that esophageal speech was preferred to the mechanical sound produced by the artificial larynx. Fourth, many proficient esophageal speakers develop the ability to manipulate their pitch, intensity, and rate during speech, resulting in improved communication technique [11].

Although the primary methods of esophageal speech, injection and inhalation, are discussed separately, many esophageal speakers use both methods of air intake [14, 15, 18, 20]. Either method may be introduced to the laryngectomee first [20]. Some laryngectomees develop a preference for one method. The esophageal speaker may learn the inhalation method as the primary method yet benefit from the injection method for obstruents when producing plosives, fricatives, and affricates within context [5]. Neither method is superior to the other [15], and the SLP's responsibility is to encourage experimentation among the methods [14, 20].

Disadvantages of Esophageal Speech

The laryngectomee's decision to learn esophageal speech does not guarantee success. The literature is replete with discouraging statistics regarding the development of acceptable esophageal speech. The estimate of laryngectomees who fail to acquire functional esophageal speech ranges from 40% [25–27] to 74% [28]. Salmon [8] and King et al. [29] estimate the figure at close to 60%.

Casper and Colton [11] describe individuals who may be inappropriate candidates for esophageal speech therapy "as patients with extensive pharyngeal, esophageal, lingual, and/or mandibular resection; patients whose medical status is otherwise compromised; patients with significant hearing loss; patients who have chosen to have a tracheoesophageal fistulization; and patients who have no desire to learn esophageal speech." Gilmore [30] offers six categories of factors that prevent patients from learning esophageal speech with the caveat that these factors generally coexist and interact: physical, social, occupational, psychological, training, and idiopathic. Physical factors include hearing loss, motor speech disorders, surgical complications, and concurrent medical conditions. The laryngectomee may experience a reduction in income, recognition, and social status, and a loss of normal interactions with family, friends, and society. Breathing changes, coughing, mucus, cosmetic alterations, and noises/mannerisms associated with air intake are reminders of the disability. Occupational factors may include changes in employment—for example, forced retirement, unemployment, demotion, or transfer. Psychological factors—for example, emotions, attitudes, and behaviors—are associated with the laryngectomee's efforts to deal with loss and grief related to having had cancer. The competence and effectiveness of the members of the alaryngeal rehabilitation team have a direct effect on the laryngectomee's acquisition of esophageal speech. Finally, Gilmore states there are idiopathic, or unexplainable, factors that prevent an individual from acquiring esophageal speech.

There may be substantial time and financial commitments to learning esophageal speech [5, 11]. Although the laryngectomee may experience early success in achieving esophageal voicing, considerable time is needed to refine articulatory precision, increase duration of utterances, and develop appropriate rate and phrasing.

Compared with the laryngeal speaker, the esophageal speaker is at a disadvantage in terms of pitch, loudness, rate of speech, and intelligibility. The fundamental frequency for esophageal speech, regardless of gender, is approximately 65 Hz, or one-half that of the normal adult male laryngeal speaker [5, 31, 32]. For the female laryngectomee, having a fundamental frequency of 65 Hz means that her voice is two octaves lower than the voice of her female laryngeal-speaking counterpart [5, 11]. Furthermore, esophageal speech is 6–10 dB less in intensity than laryngeal speech [2, 11, 32], making intelligible speech difficult under conditions of competing noise [33]. The speaking rate of the laryngectomee tends to be slower than the laryngeal speaker [11, 34]; Snidecor and Curry [35] reported an average of 113 words per minute in their superior esophageal speakers. Shanks [33] suggests a rate of 100–110 words per minute, or two-thirds the average rate for laryngeal speakers (150–165 words per minute), as a reasonable goal. Intelligibility ratings by untrained listeners for esophageal speech range from 54.9% [36] to 78.5% [37] at the word level and from 54% [38] to 75.1% [39] at the sentence level. Casper and Colton [11] reported an overall 71.3% intelligibility rating for 10 studies involving listener comprehension of esophageal speech. Listeners tend to misinterpret voiced-unvoiced consonant productions; however, voiced consonants are understood more readily than unvoiced consonants [40]. A more complete discussion of intelligibility factors and esophageal speech appears in Chapter 6.

TRACHEOESOPHAGEAL SPEECH

To provide lung air for TE speech, the physician performs tracheoesophageal fistulization (TEF) during the laryngectomy or as a later, secondary procedure [5, 11, 41, 42]. A variety of surgical procedures are used to create the fistula (opening) between the trachea and the esophagus. In one method, an illuminated endoscope is inserted via the mouth into the esophagus. An opening in the front of the endoscope (the side near the TE wall) acts as a light guide for the surgeon. Using a needle, the surgeon creates a fistula near the top of the trachea into the anterior wall of the esophagus below the PE segment. The positioning of the endoscope prevents accidental puncture of the posterior esophageal wall.

After TEF, the physician has two options for fitting the TE prosthesis (TEP). The first alternative is to secure a No. 14 French catheter in the fistula for 7–10 days if fistulization occurs at the time of laryngectomy or for 3–4 days if it occurs as a secondary procedure [42]. At the end of the waiting period, the TEP is inserted in the opening between the posterior tracheal wall and the anterior esophageal wall [42]. The second option is to fit the laryngectomee with the TEP at the time of fistulization.

Design of the Tracheoesophageal Prosthesis

The TEP is a hollow silicone tube [43] with a shaft available in various lengths to span the diameter of the trachea [5] (Figure 3.6). A strap for securing the device to the neck is located at the tracheal end of the prosthesis (Figure 3.7). A retention collar snaps into place on the esophageal side of the fistula to prevent leakage [43]. All prostheses have a one-way valve designed to allow air to pass from the lungs into the esophagus and to resist aspiration of fluids from the esophagus into the trachea [5, 11, 41, 43]. The esophageal end of the prosthesis is available with a duckbill tip and slit valve or a low-pressure tip with inner flapper valve. The physician determines the type of prosthesis most appropriate for the individual.

InHealth Technologies (Carpinteria, CA) manufactures three styles of Blom-Singer voice restoration prostheses: Low Pressure, Duckbill, and Indwelling Low Pressure (Figure 3.8). Bivona Medical Technologies (Figure 3.9) manufactures a variety of devices for TE restoration of the voice, including the Bivona Ultra Low Resistance voice prosthesis, the Bivona Duckbill voice prosthesis, and the Bivona-Colorado voice prosthesis. Bivona is also a distributor of the PROVOX Low Resistance voice prosthesis featuring a one-piece molded valve. The prosthesis is reported to be resistant to *Candida* (yeastlike fungi) growth and can be maintained with the prosthesis in place.

How the Tracheoesophageal Prosthesis Works

Air pressure is exerted to produce sound. Air is expelled from the lungs into the trachea and diverted via the prosthesis into the esophagus if the stoma is occluded by a thumb, finger (Figure 3.10), or tracheostoma valve [5, 11, 42]. Once in the esophagus, the air moves superiorly causing the PE segment to vibrate [11]. The vibrated air moves into the pharyngeal, oral, and nasal cavities and is given resonance. The articulators form the sound into meaningful speech.

The tracheostoma valve is designed to eliminate the need to cover the stoma with a finger during speech production [5, 11, 41–43]. The tracheostoma valve is worn in addition to the voice prosthesis. One version of the valve is the

Figure 3.6
Components of the tracheoesophageal voice prostheses available from InHealth Technologies (Carpinteria, CA). A. Low Pressure Voice Prosthesis. B. Traditional Duckbill Voice Prosthesis. (Reprinted with permission of InHealth Technologies. 1996 Professional Catalog: Blom-Singer Voice Restoration Systems. Carpinteria, CA: InHealth Technologies, 1996;3.)

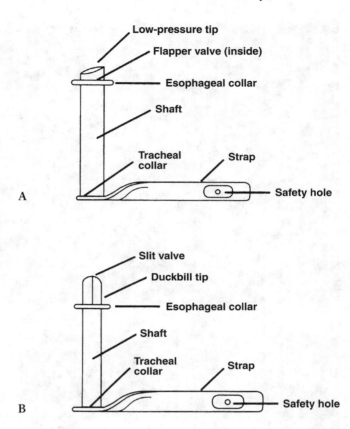

Figure 3.7
The Blom-Singer Duckbill Voice Prosthesis (InHealth Technologies [Carpinteria, CA]). Note the strap of the prosthesis taped securely against the neck.

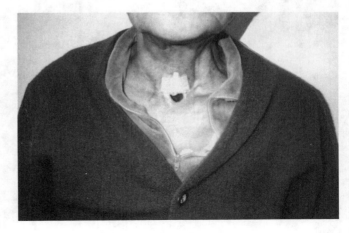

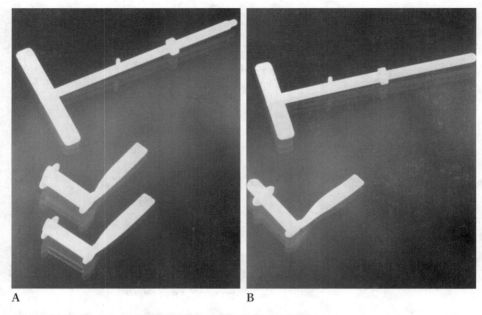

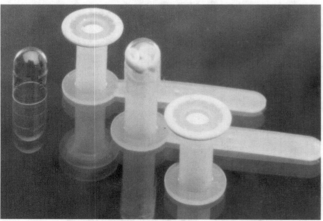

Figure 3.8 Three styles of Blom-Singer voice restoration prostheses are available from InHealth Technologies (Carpinteria, CA). A. Low Pressure Voice Prosthesis with insertion stick. B. Duckbill Voice Prosthesis with insertion stick. C. Indwelling Low Pressure Voice Prosthesis is placed by the physician or speech clinician and maintained without removal.

Figure 3.8 (*continued*).
D. The Blom-Singer Adjustable Tracheostoma Valve (InHealth Technologies
[Carpinteria, CA]) allows hands-free
operation of the stoma for speech while
using one of the three types of voice
prostheses. (Reprinted with permission of InHealth Technologies. 1996
Professional Catalog: Blom-Singer Voice
Restoration Systems. Carpinteria, CA:
InHealth Technologies, 1996;2, 3, 4.)

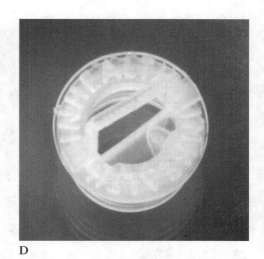

D

Blom-Singer Adjustable Tracheostoma Valve (InHealth Technologies) (see Figure 3.8). Clear housing is attached to the skin surrounding the stoma with silicone adhesive. The silicone valve assembly snaps into the center of the housing. A cross bar permits adjustment of the valve to accommodate various levels of air pressure produced during physical exertion. A slight increase in exhalation blocks the exit of the air to the outside via the stoma. Instead, air is redirected through the prosthesis and into the esophagus. The Blom-Singer Adjustable Tracheostoma Valve, when used with the Blom-Singer HumidiFilter System, is reported to improve heat and moisture exchange and reduce dryness, mucous secretions, and coughing [42, 44] (see Appendix A).

Bivona Medical Technologies manufactures the Tracheostoma Valve II with a unique spring-action valve (see Figure 3.9). Differential sensitivity to the individual laryngectomee's respiratory needs is achieved using interchangeable valves. The Barton-Mayo Tracheostoma button (Bivona Medical Technologies) is designed to be worn with the voice prosthesis and allows hands-free TE speech without the use of potentially irritating skin adhesive [43].

Care, Cleaning, and Maintenance of the Tracheoesophageal Prosthesis

Care and maintenance of the voice prosthesis is determined by the type of device inserted. The traditional duckbill or low-pressure voice prosthesis is removed, cleaned with soap and water, and reinserted by the laryngectomee or family member on a daily basis [42, 43]. Also available is an indwelling low-pressure voice prosthesis that is worn for extended periods of time and is replaced by the physician or speech clinician [42, 43]. The silicone material discourages accumu-

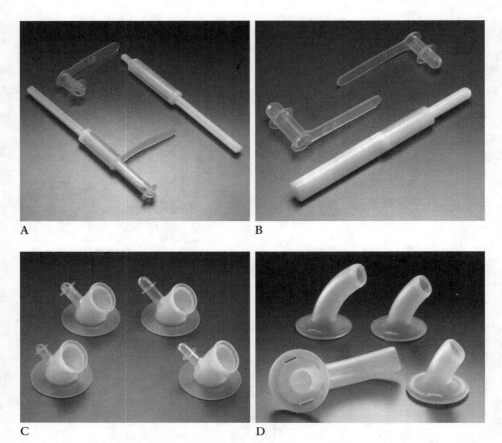

A   B

C   D

Figure 3.9 A variety of devices for tracheoesophageal restoration of the voice is offered by Bivona Medical Technologies (Gary, IN). A. Bivona Ultra Low Resistance voice prosthesis with insertion device. B. Bivona Duckbill Voice Prosthesis with insertion device. C. The Bivona-Colorado voice prosthesis is a self-retaining prosthesis and button in one system and offers a choice of duckbill or ultra low resistance stem style. D. Bivona tracheostoma vent manufactured of biocompatible silicone. E. Tracheostoma valve available with Ultra Light, Light, Medium, and Firm valve assemblies. F. Tracheostoma Valve II with interchangeable springs to adjust sensitivity to airway pressures. (Reprinted with permission of Bivona Medical Technologies. 1996 Voice Restoration Products and Supplies Catalog. Gary, IN: Bivona Medical Technologies, 1996;3, 6, 7, 9, 10.)

lation and solidification of mucus [43]. With the prosthesis in place, the interior or shaft can be flushed using a water-filled pipet.

Leakage of fluid from the esophagus into the trachea via the prosthesis is the primary indicator that the prosthesis needs replacement [41]. A buildup of *Candida* on the esophageal end of the prosthesis is frequently the culprit [5, 41–43]. An

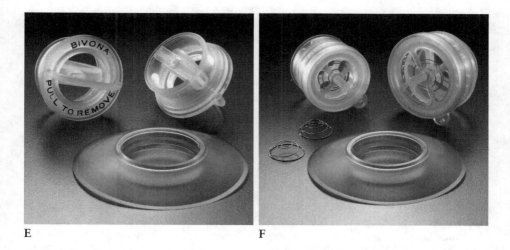

E   F

Figure 3.10
This laryngectomee is
using two fingers to
occlude the stoma for
speaking with a tracheo-
esophageal prosthesis.

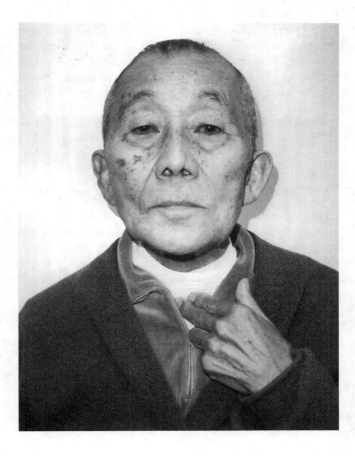

increase in the growth of *Candida* has been observed in laryngectomees who have undergone radiation therapy or chemotherapy [41]. Use of nystatin (Nystatin Oral Suspension) has been credited with reducing yeast colonization on the TE valve, significantly increasing the life of the prosthesis [45, 46].

Emergency care requires the laryngectomee to carry a catheter, stent, or spare prosthesis at all times. If the prosthesis becomes dislodged or is removed and not replaced, the fistula can close sufficiently within a few hours to prevent reinsertion of the prosthesis [5, 11]. Surgical reopening of the fistula may be required.

Advantages of Tracheoesophageal Speech

Many physicians and speech clinicians attest to the relative ease and rapidity of learning to use TE speech [11, 47–49]. Reported success rates for restoration of the voice, as measured by intelligibility and fluency, have ranged from 88% [49] to as high as 93% [32]. TE speech has been found effective for laryngectomees who have difficulty developing esophageal speech [47–49]. TEF restores the laryngectomee's access to more than 2,000 cc of lung air for speech production [41]. Overall measurements indicate that, compared with the esophageal speaker, the TE speaker demonstrates increased duration of speech production, improved intensity levels, and the potential for pitch variation [32, 41, 50]. The speech rate of the TE speaker appears to be greater than that of the esophageal speaker but less than that of the laryngeal speaker [50].

Use of the tracheostoma valve eliminates the need for finger closure of the tracheostoma during speech [5, 11, 41–43] and frees the individual to engage in everyday two-handed activities such as driving, cooking, photography, typing, and gardening.

Disadvantages of Tracheoesophageal Speech

Care and maintenance of the fistula, prosthesis, and stoma valve can be time consuming, particularly for the laryngectomee who removes the prosthesis on a daily basis [41, 47]. The cost of the prosthesis and accessory items for routine care and daily maintenance can be considerable. Good cognition, manual dexterity, and good eyesight are necessary components in the care and use of the prosthesis [11, 41, 47]. Respiratory function must be adequate to support speech production [41, 47].

One hand is frequently used for valving the stoma. Many laryngectomees experience problems maintaining the seal on the valve housing and must occlude the stoma manually [41, 47]. According to Gilmore [47], many medical complications may interfere with success of TE speech: "*Candida*, aspiration, vertebral osteomyelitis, pneumonia, stomal irritation, esophageal perforation, tracheal mucositis, mediastinitis, paraesophageal abscess, allergic reactions to the tape or the prosthesis, esophageal stenosis, and gastroesophageal reflux."

In the presence of a hypertonic or hypotonic PE segment, TE speech may not be achieved. Esophageal insufflation testing, in which air is introduced into the esophagus in an attempt to vibrate the PE segment [5, 11, 41], identifies individuals at risk for failure to develop TE speech [5, 51]. Additional procedures are available to correct a hypertonic PE segment and facilitate TE speech (e.g., pharyngeal myotomy, pharyngeal plexus block or neurectomy, and esophageal dilation) [5, 51].

CONCLUSION

The primary purpose of alaryngeal speech rehabilitation is to assist the laryngectomee in the development of functional, intelligible speech. A summary of the oral communication methods for the alaryngeal speaker appears in Table 3.1. The physician and the speech clinician have completed the education of the laryngectomee for this level of the rehabilitation process. The laryngectomee is now in the position to make an informed decision regarding the communication technique that best meets his or her needs and abilities.

After exposure to the various communication methods, the laryngectomee frequently elects to learn more than one of the techniques [3, 5, 6, 8]. All six of the laryngectomees currently enrolled in our alaryngeal speech group use the artificial larynx and either esophageal or TE speech. Two of the laryngectomees in our alaryngeal speech class have opted to use the artificial larynx, esophageal speech, *and* TE speech because each method satisfies different communication needs. The TEP is compatible with other forms of alaryngeal speech; the presence of the prosthesis does not interfere with the learning or use of the artificial larynx or esophageal speech methods [41, 42].

The next step in the rehabilitation process is to begin instruction for the selected alaryngeal speech method(s). A systematic approach to therapy facilitates the acquisition of intelligible speech by providing the clinician an objective method for analyzing and modifying the laryngectomee's behaviors. In Chapter 4, the concept of a hierarchical approach to teaching alaryngeal speech is explained.

Table 3.1 A summary of oral communication methods for the alaryngeal speaker

Oral communication method and how it works	Advantages	Disadvantages
Artificial larynx		
Pneumatic type		
Lung air is directed from the stoma to the oral cavity via tube	Low-cost, do-it-yourself kit	Manual dexterity needed
	No batteries	Must maintain good stomal seal
Vibration of rubber diaphragm creates hoarse voice	Hoarse versus mechanical voice	Articulation precision needed
Articulators shape the sound into speech	Bypasses fibrotic or painful neck tissue	Saliva may clog oral tube
Pitch and loudness controlled via varied breath pressure	Relatively easy to learn	Good respiratory health needed
		Uses one hand to operate
Battery-operated neck type		
Vibrating head driven by battery is held against neck or cheek	Relatively easy to learn	Articulation precision needed
	Volume adequate for hearing-impaired listeners and noisy environments	Fibrotic or painful neck tissue may prevent use
Tone resonates in oral cavity		Has mechanical sound
Articulators shape the sound into speech	Adjustable pitch control	Uses one hand to operate
	Intelligible on telephone	Manual dexterity needed
Adjustments for pitch and loudness control	Newer units lightweight	Some units are bulky and awkward
	Resistant to breakage	Initial cost can be high
	Sometimes loaners are available from American Cancer Society or telephone company	Repairs can be costly and inconvenient
		Supply of batteries needed
Battery-operated oral type	Relatively easy to learn	Saliva may clog oral tube
Vibrated air is directed into the oral cavity via a plastic tube	Bypasses fibrotic or painful neck tissue	Has mechanical sound
	Available for use immediately following surgery	Tube may interfere with articulation and intelligibility
Articulators shape the sound into speech	Adjustable pitch and volume control	Manual dexterity needed
Adjustments for pitch and loudness control	In some cases, can be converted to neck type	Uses one hand to operate
		Initial cost can be high
		Repairs can be costly and inconvenient
		Supply of batteries needed
Battery-operated oral type: Ultra Voice (Health Concepts [Malvern, PA])		
Remote control–operated oral unit is placed in custom-built denture/retainer	Relatively easy to learn	Uses one hand to operate remote control
	Bypasses fibrotic or painful neck tissue	Articulation precision needed
Articulators shape the sound into speech	Adjustable pitch and volume control	Initial cost is very high

Table 3.1 (continued)

Oral communication method and how it works	Advantages	Disadvantages
Adjustments for pitch and volume control	Sound superior to neck-type electrolarynges Whisper mode available	Repairs can be costly and inconvenient
Esophageal speech *Injection method for obstruents* Production of plosives, fricatives, and affricates increase positive air pressure in the oral cavity Air is forced into the PE segment to the esophagus Returning air vibrates the PE segment, producing sound Articulators shape the sound into speech	*For all methods of esophageal speech* No initial investment in equipment, maintenance or repair costs Both hands are free No equipment to keep track of Esophageal quality preferred over mechanical sound of the artificial larynx More natural form of communication	*For all methods of esophageal speech* Substantial time commitment to learn 60% failure rate Inappropriate for individuals who have had extensive surgery or have significant hearing loss Investment in speech therapy may be substantial Less intelligible than laryngeal speech
Injection method for sonorants and vowels Lip or tongue seal traps air Tongue moves air into the PE segment to the esophagus Returning air vibrates the PE segment, producing sound Articulators shape the sound into speech		Articulation precision needed Female esophageal speech two octaves lower than female laryngeal speech 6–10 dB less in intensity than laryngeal speech Slower speaking rate than laryngeal speech
Inhalation method Rapid intake of air via stoma increases negative air pressure in esophagus Air flows from oral and nasal cavities into PE segment to the esophagus Returning air vibrates the PE segment, producing sound Articulators shape the sound into speech		
TE speech *TEP* A hollow silicone tube is inserted in the fistula created between the posterior wall	Lung air is accessed rather than injection/inhalation of air as in esophageal	Uses one hand to valve stoma Fistula can close quickly;

Table 3.1 (continued)

Oral communication method and how it works	Advantages	Disadvantages
of the trachea and the anterior wall of the esophagus. Air from the lungs is shunted into the esophagus. Air vibrates the PE segment, producing sound Articulators shape the sound into speech	speech TE speech quality preferred over mechanical sound of the artificial larynx TE speech duration greater than that for esophageal speech; phrasing and rate are closer to laryngeal speech Improved intensity levels More natural form of communication Relatively easy to learn; 88–93% success rate Indwelling low-pressure TEP available for extended wear	may require surgical procedure to reopen Good cognition, visual acuity, and respiratory health needed Manual dexterity for valving (in some cases for removal, cleaning, and placement) Risk of aspiration if TEP becomes dislodged Surgical expense; subsequent supplies and maintenance required Articulation precision needed *Candida* growth can decrease life of prosthesis Hypertonic or hypotonic PE segment may interfere with TE speech production
Tracheostoma valve Additional device worn with the TEP Eliminates need for finger or thumb occlusion for speech Valve is activated by slight increase in force of exhalation	Allows hands-free operation of the stoma for TE speech Adjustable valve for varying levels of physical activity Barton-Mayo (Bivona Medical Technologies [Gary, IN]) Tracheostoma button is adhesive free	Manual dexterity needed to apply valve Adhesive material is difficult to apply; does not always secure properly Risk of skin irritation from adhesive material

PE = pharyngoesophageal; TE = tracheoesophageal; TEP = tracheoesophageal prosthesis.

REFERENCES

1. Berry WR. Approaches to Treatment. In SJ Salmon, LP Goldstein (eds), The Artificial Larynx Handbook. New York: Grune & Stratton, 1978;116.
2. Berry WR. Indications for the Use of Artificial Larynx Devices. In SJ Salmon, LP Goldstein (eds), The Artificial Larynx Handbook. New York: Grune & Stratton, 1978;17.
3. Berry WR. Attitudes of Speech Pathologists and Otolaryngologists About Artificial Larynges. In SJ Salmon, LP Goldstein (eds), The Artificial Larynx Handbook. New York: Grune & Stratton, 1978;40.

4. Lerman JW. The Artificial Larynx. In SJ Salmon, KH Mount (eds), Alaryngeal Speech Rehabilitation for Clinicians by Clinicians. Austin, TX: PRO-ED, 1991;29.
5. Doyle PC. Foundations of Voice and Speech Rehabilitation Following Laryngeal Cancer. San Diego: Singular, 1994;121, 144, 189.
6. Duguay MJ. Why Not Both? In SJ Salmon, LP Goldstein (eds), The Artificial Larynx Handbook. New York: Grune & Stratton, 1978;3.
7. Goldstein LP. The Artificial Larynx: Pro and Con. In SJ Salmon, LP Goldstein (eds), The Artificial Larynx Handbook. New York: Grune & Stratton, 1978;11.
8. Salmon SJ. Artificial Larynx Speech: A Viable Means of Alaryngeal Communication. In Y Edels (ed), Laryngectomy: Diagnosis to Rehabilitation. Rockville, MD: Aspen, 1983;143.
9. Salmon SJ. Artificial Larynges: Types and Modifications. In RL Keith, FL Darley (eds), Laryngectomee Rehabilitation (3rd ed). Austin, TX: PRO-ED, 1994;155.
10. Blom ED. The Artificial Larynx: Past and Present. In SJ Salmon, LP Goldstein (eds), The Artificial Larynx Handbook. New York: Grune & Stratton, 1978;57.
11. Casper JK, Colton RH. Clinical Manual for Laryngectomy and Head and Neck Cancer Rehabilitation. San Diego: Singular, 1993;56, 107.
12. Rothman HB. Acoustic Analysis of Artificial Laryngeal Speech. In A Sekey (ed), Electroacoustic Analysis of Alaryngeal Speech. Springfield, IL: Thomas, 1982;95.
13. Diedrich WM. Anatomy and Physiology of Esophageal Speech. In SJ Salmon, KH Mount (eds), Alaryngeal Speech Rehabilitation for Clinicians by Clinicians. Austin, TX: PRO-ED, 1991;2.
14. Edels Y. Pseudo-Voice—Its Theory and Practice. In Y Edels (ed), Laryngectomy: Diagnosis to Rehabilitation. Rockville, MD: Aspen, 1983;112.
15. Diedrich WM, Youngstrom KA. Alaryngeal Speech. Springfield, IL: Thomas, 1977;37, 59.
16. Zemlin WR. Speech and Hearing Science: Anatomy and Physiology (2nd ed). Englewood Cliffs, NJ: Prentice-Hall, 1988;274.
17. Martin DE. Pre- and Postoperative Anatomical and Physiological Observations in Laryngectomy. In RL Keith, FL Darley (eds), Laryngectomee Rehabilitation (3rd ed). Austin, TX: PRO-ED, 1994;79.
18. Duguay MJ. Esophageal Speech Training: The Initial Phase. In SJ Salmon, KH Mount (eds), Alaryngeal Speech Rehabilitation For Clinicians by Clinicians. Austin, TX: PRO-ED, 1991;48.
19. Dey FL, Kirchner JA. The upper esophageal sphincter after laryngectomy. Laryngoscope 1961;71:99.
20. Salmon SJ. Methods of Air Intake for Esophageal Speech and Their Associated Problems. In RL Keith, FL Darley (eds), Laryngectomee Rehabilitation (3rd ed). Austin, TX: PRO-ED, 1994;222.
21. Shanks JC. Evoking esophageal voice. Semin Speech Lang 1986;7:1.
22. Weiss CE, Gordon ME, Lillywhite HS. Clinical Management of Articulatory and Phonologic Disorders (2nd ed). Baltimore: Williams & Wilkins, 1987;49.
23. Gardner WH. Laryngectomee Speech and Rehabilitation. Springfield, IL: Thomas, 1971;38, 94.
24. Bennett S, Weinberg B. Acceptability ratings of normal, esophageal, and artificial larynx speech. J Speech Hear Res 1973;16:608.
25. Putney EJ. Rehabilitation of the post-laryngectomized patient. Ann Otol Rhinol Laryngol 1958;67:544.
26. Martin H. Rehabilitation of the laryngectomee. Cancer 1963;16:823.
27. Gardner WN, Harris HE. Aids and devices for laryngectomees. Arch Otolaryngol 1961;73:145.
28. Gates GA, Ryan W, Cooper JC, et al. Current status of laryngectomee rehabilitation: I. results of therapy. Am J Otolaryngol 1982;3:1.

29. King PS, Fowlks EW, Pierson GA. Rehabilitation and adaptation of laryngectomy patients. Am J Phys Med 1968;47:192.
30. Gilmore SI. Failure in Acquiring Esophageal Speech. In SJ Salmon, KH Mount (eds), Alaryngeal Speech Rehabilitation For Clinicians by Clinicians. Austin, TX: PRO-ED, 1991;194.
31. Martin DE. Evaluating Esophageal Speech Development and Proficiency. In RL Keith, FL Darley (eds), Laryngectomee Rehabilitation (3rd ed). Austin, TX: PRO-ED, 1994;334.
32. Robbins J, Fisher HB, Blom ED, Singer MI. A comparative acoustic study of normal, esophageal, and tracheoesophageal speech production. J Speech Hear Disord 1984;49:202.
33. Shanks JC. Developing Esophageal Communication. In RL Keith, FL Darley (eds), Laryngectomee Rehabilitation (3rd ed). Austin, TX: PRO-ED, 1994;211.
34. Hoops HR, Noll JD. Relationship of selected acoustic variables to judgments of esophageal speech. J Commun Disord 1969;2:1.
35. Snidecor JC, Curry ET. Temporal and pitch aspects of superior esophageal speech. Ann Otol Rhinol Laryngol 1959;68:623.
36. Shames GH, Font J, Matthews J. Factors related to speech proficiency of the laryngectomized. J Speech Hear Disord 1963;28:273.
37. Kalb MB, Carpenter MA. Individual speaker influence on relative intelligibility of esophageal and artificial larynx speech. J Speech Hear Disord 1981;46:77.
38. Clayton S. Relationships Among Word and Sentence Intelligibility: Global Ratings of Esophageal Speech Skill. Master's thesis. Michigan State University, East Lansing, 1976.
39. Hoops HR, Curtis JF. Intelligibility of the esophageal speaker. Arch Otolaryngol 1971;93:300.
40. Hyman M. An experimental study of artificial larynx and esophageal speech. J Speech Hear Disord 1955;20:291.
41. Bosone ZT. Tracheoesophageal Fistulization/Puncture for Voice Restoration: Presurgical Considerations and Troubleshooting Procedures. In RL Keith, FL Darley (eds), Laryngectomee Rehabilitation (3rd ed). Austin, TX: PRO-ED, 1994;359.
42. Blom ED. Tracheoesophageal speech. Semin Speech Lang 1995;16(3):191.
43. Roberts NK. Nursing Intervention for the Laryngectomee: Management of Change in Self-Care Practices Following Hospitalization. In RL Keith, FL Darley (eds), Laryngectomee Rehabilitation (3rd ed). Austin, TX: PRO-ED, 1994;121.
44. Crum R. Attachment of the adjustable tracheostoma valve and housing from the view of a laryngectomee. Orl-Head Neck Nurs 1996;14(1):15.
45. Blom ED (ed). Correct use of Nystatin. Clin Insights 1995;1:1.
46. Blom ED, Singer MI. Disinfection of silicone voice prostheses. Arch Otolaryngol Head Neck Surg 1986;112:1303.
47. Gilmore SI. The Physical, Social, Occupational, and Psychological Concomitants of Laryngectomy. In RL Keith, FL Darley (eds), Laryngectomee Rehabilitation (3rd ed). Austin, TX: PRO-ED, 1994;400.
48. Singer MI, Blom ED. An endoscopic technique for restoration of voice after laryngectomy. Ann Otol Rhinol Laryngol 1980;89:529.
49. Singer MI, Blom ED, Hamaker RC. Further experience with voice restoration after total laryngectomy. Ann Otol Rhinol Laryngol 1981;90:498.
50. Trudeau M. The Acoustical Variability of Tracheoesophageal Speech. In RL Keith, FL Darley (eds), Laryngectomee Rehabilitation (3rd ed). Austin, TX: PRO-ED, 1994; 383.
51. Blom ED, Singer MI, Hamaker RC. An improved esophageal insufflation test. Arch Otolaryngol Head Neck Surg 1985;111:211.

4

Teaching Alaryngeal Speech: A Hierarchical Approach

The acquisition of alaryngeal speech is an educational process for the laryngectomee. The laryngectomee, who spoke preoperatively with little or no awareness of how speech was produced, must now learn and consciously apply an alternative method of communication. The success of alaryngeal speech depends on many factors internal to the laryngectomee—for example, medical, physical, cognitive, and psychological conditions. Speech training, a determinant external to the laryngectomee, is the primary responsibility of the speech-language pathologist (SLP) in the alaryngeal speech rehabilitation process. The SLP's role is to help the laryngectomee learn a functional method of communication. The competency and the efficiency with which the clinician administers the treatment protocol is a major factor in facilitating the acquisition of intelligible alaryngeal speech.

Noted researcher-clinicians in speech pathology, such as Brookshire [1], LaPointe [2, 3], Mowrer [4], and Rosenbek [5], have adapted behavior modification techniques from the writings of learning theorists for use with a variety of speech and language disorders. The design of a programmed behavior modification approach allows the clinician to analyze the laryngectomee's productions and to apply operant procedures systematically to modify behavior. Stimuli are selected carefully to control the response. Target responses are identified and criteria established to move the laryngectomee through successive approximations—small, intermediate steps—progressing toward the target, or terminal, behavior. Goals and procedures are explained and described with each activity. If needed for clarity, the desired behavior is modeled. Evaluation of the laryngectomee's responses includes visual (mirror), auditory (verbal and audiotape), and tactile (touch) feedback. In the initial phase of treatment, the laryngectomee relies on the SLP to provide feedback. Every correct response is acknowledged by reference to the specific behavior(s). Direct suggestions are made for improving the behavior after every incorrect response. In the intermediate and advanced phases of treatment, emphasis is placed on the laryngectomee's development of self-evaluation and self-correction skills. Taking control of one's speech productions is intrinsically reinforcing.

UNDERSTANDING THE THERAPY HIERARCHY

Efficient alaryngeal speech requires frequent and regular practice of specific target behaviors. After the identification of therapy goals, a step-by-step arrangement of therapy activities is followed. In a hierarchical approach, speech activities are organized into a series of stimuli that increase in length and difficulty as the laryngectomee masters each level. By maintaining a minimum performance level of 70–80% accuracy during every activity, the laryngectomee experiences successful productions or behaviors seven or eight out of 10 times. If the laryngectomee is performing below 70–80% accuracy, the task is considered too difficult, and adjustments are made to facilitate target performance. The criterion to move up to the next step on the hierarchy is 90% accuracy over three consecutive sets of stimuli (10 trials each). If behavioral change does not occur, the treatment approach is ineffective and must be altered to suit the needs of the individual.

For each therapy activity, a score sheet is used to record client responses. Activity score sheets are provided to assist the clinician in leading the laryngectomee through a series of exercises designed to develop proficient alaryngeal speech (see Chapters 5–7 for score sheets individualized by alaryngeal speech method). Regardless of the speech method, setting up the therapy activity requires knowledge of the laryngectomee's performance level. Once the goals are identified, therapy begins with the initial phase at the lowest level of production. For purposes of explaining the use of the activity score sheet, Figure 4.1 shows an activity score sheet for teaching artificial larynx speech.

Practice activities are divided into three *phases*: initial, intermediate, and advanced. In the initial phase of teaching alaryngeal speech, one goal per activity is identified for practice. In the example (see Figure 4.1), only one goal— placement of the artificial larynx—is identified. In the intermediate phase, the laryngectomee attends to two goals within the same activity—for example, placement *and* articulatory precision. In the advanced phase, the laryngectomee monitors for all the goals within the same activity, a skill important to communicating in the natural environment. The laryngectomee moves through the three phases (initial, intermediate, and advanced) at each level of production (e.g., Level I: two- to four-syllable words and phrases) before proceeding to the next level of production (e.g., Level II: five- to seven-syllable words and phrases).

Therapy *goals* are based on known characteristics of intelligible speech for a particular alaryngeal speech method. In the next three chapters, goals are identified and instructions given for teaching use of the artificial larynx, esophageal speech, and tracheoesophageal (TE) speech. Included are techniques for solving problems frequently associated with the teaching of these behaviors. In the example (see Figure 4.1), the identified goal is *placement of the artificial larynx.*

Name___Example_____ Date_____

Phase:
- ■ Initial (one goal)
- ❏ Intermediate (two goals)
- ❏ Advanced (multiple goals)

Goal(s):
- ■ Placement
- ❏ "On" Control
- ❏ Articulation
- ❏ Rate and phrasing
- ❏ Nonverbal behaviors

Level of production: Unrestricted phonetic context:
- ■ I. Two- to four-syllable phrases
- ❏ II. Five- to seven-syllable phrases
- ❏ III. Eight-syllable phrases or more
- ❏ IV. Oral reading of paragraphs
- ❏ VI. Structured conversation
- ❏ VII. Spontaneous conversation

Monitoring:
- ■ Clinician
- ❏ Laryngectomee/clinician
- ❏ Laryngectomee

	Stimuli Appendix: **D** Level: **1** Set: **1**	Trial No. **1**	Comments
1	Act your age.	+	Verbal reminder
2	Do a good job.	+	Verbal reminder
3	Quick and easy	–	Excess buzzing
4	Hurry up.	+	Verbal reminder
5	No parking	+	Self-corrected
6	Skip lunch.	–	Excess buzzing
7	Come as you are.	+	Verbal reminder
8	Let's get started.	+	Self-monitored
9	Forget it.	–	Excess buzzing
10	What did you say?	+	Verbal reminder
	Total correct	7	
	Percent correct	70%	Repeat task with Set 2 of Appendix D, I.

+ = correct; – = incorrect.

Figure 4.1 Activity score sheet for teaching artificial larynx speech.

The *level of production* represents the length of utterance and the phonetic context. The composition and length of stimuli are chosen based on the method of alaryngeal speech being practiced. Because the production of artificial larynx speech does not depend on specific consonants and vowels, the phonetic context of the stimuli is unrestricted, meaning any consonant and vowel combination may be used. Phonetic context is unrestricted during TE speech and during the use of combined esophageal speech methods as well. The stimuli for the practice of these alaryngeal speech methods is found in Appendix D. The stimuli for individual methods of air intake in esophageal speech *do* employ restricted phonetic context. The injection method for obstruents uses the contacts made during the production of unvoiced and voiced consonants to move air into the esophagus; stimuli using the restricted phonetic context for this method are found in Appendix F. Stimuli for the injection method for sonorants and vowels and for the inhalation method are restricted to the use of sonorants and vowels and exclude the use of obstruents (see Appendix G). The rationale for using restricted phonetic contexts in the teaching of esophageal speech methods is further discussed in Chapter 6.

In the example for teaching artificial larynx speech (see Figure 4.1), the level of production is identified as two- to four-syllable phrases using unrestricted phonetic context. A level of production is chosen in which the laryngectomee produces the target behavior, *placement*, with 70–80% accuracy. At this level of accuracy, the correct response is strengthened, and the laryngectomee is motivated to continue practicing. The criterion to move to the intermediate phase is 90% accuracy for three consecutive sets of stimuli at the two- to four-syllable phrases and sentences level of production.

The development of *self-monitoring skills* is an important component of alaryngeal speech rehabilitation. Laryngectomees who are able to self-monitor and self-correct have the potential to manage and perfect their speech beyond the scheduled therapy sessions.

In the initial phase, clinician feedback, with suggestions for improvement, is provided (see Figure 4.1). The laryngectomee is encouraged to participate in analyzing the production. In the intermediate phase, the laryngectomee is invited to self-monitor before receiving clinician feedback. The laryngectomee is expected to self-monitor accurately for each production in the advanced phase. During the intermediate and advanced phases, self-monitoring skills for speech goals are applied to interactions with people other than the clinician (e.g., family members, fellow laryngectomees, and the general public) and to other environments (e.g., small groups, on the street, at the mall, on the telephone, and in the car).

After determining the goal(s) and the appropriate level of production, a set of 10 *stimuli* is selected and entered in the 10 blanks provided (see Figure 4.1). The laryngectomee is asked to produce the utterance. Scoring is binary; the response is either correct (+) or incorrect (–). A more sophisticated level of scoring can be used—that is, designating whether a correct response was immediate, delayed, assisted, or self-corrected (for further details, see the multidimensional scoring system developed by Porch [6]). A space is provided for the SLP's comments regarding the laryngectomee's productions.

The use of prefabricated word and phrase lists allows the laryngectomee to concentrate on the *goal*—placement of the artificial larynx—without the distraction of having to generate an original utterance. Built into the stimulus materials is vocabulary common to everyday usage. The laryngectomee gains skill and confidence through performance of structured activities with the clinician in a protected environment.

Regular reassessment of the laryngectomee's speech progress occurs and is recorded in the client's chart. The laryngectomee and his or her family are involved in discussions about speech improvement. Some laryngectomees progress through the activity hierarchy rapidly and with a high rate of success. Others need additional time to acquire alaryngeal speech and benefit from the highly structured stimulus-response-reinforcement arrangement of therapy. The important point is that the laryngectomee works through the phases at each level of production at a pace that is challenging, yet comfortable. The laryngectomees in our group are encouraged to practice routinely and not make comparisons between their progress and the progress of other laryngectomees in the group.

In the example (see Figure 4.1), the laryngectomee experienced 70% successful placement of the artificial larynx during the production of two- to four-syllable phrases. The clinician noted extraneous buzzing of the electrolarynx as the cause of errors. Correct responses were preceded by a verbal reminder five times. On completion of the task, the clinician gave direction for the next activity: continue at the same level of production with the next set of stimuli. Accountability through good record keeping is a critical variable in the teaching of alaryngeal speech. For the programmed behavior modification program to work effectively, systematic and careful records must be kept. Further discussion of accountability via evaluation, lesson planning, and report writing is found in Chapter 9.

LENGTH AND FREQUENCY OF TREATMENT SESSIONS

The laryngectomee's physical and mental endurance have an influence on the length as well as the frequency of the therapy sessions. Availability of the clinician, accessibility of the therapy site, financial considerations, and the extent of therapy also determine the scheduled duration and frequency of sessions.

The length of the therapy session depends on the laryngectomee's attention span and level of endurance. The laryngectomee must be able to focus on an activity for short periods of time before becoming distracted. Physical endurance may be limited for a variety of reasons, including recovery from the surgery, radiation, or chemotherapy; an accompanying health condition, such as emphysema; or advanced age. For the client who fatigues easily or has a limited attention span, individual activities are kept short, and the entire length of the session may not extend past 15–20 minutes. If the laryngectomee is learning more than one method of communication—for example, using the artificial larynx *and* esophageal speech—alternating speech methods from one activity to the next offers respite. Two laryngectomees may be paired in a turn-taking situation; one laryngectomee rests while the other laryngectomee responds. As the laryngectomee's tolerance for therapy increases, the length of individual sessions increases and the frequency of the sessions decreases.

Accessibility of the therapy site is an important variable for the laryngectomee. While still hospitalized, the laryngectomee is likely to experience short, frequent visits from the staff SLP (and other members of the rehabilitation team). After the laryngectomee has returned home, therapy session attendance becomes influenced by the distance between the therapy site and the individual's home, transportation issues (e.g., parking, bus schedules, taxi expense, elevator and wheelchair access, dependence on a relative or friend), weather conditions (e.g., rain, cold, snow), and competition with other rehabilitation appointments (e.g., doctor, radiology, physical therapy).

In very few cases does the laryngectomee have unlimited financial resources to pay for alaryngeal speech rehabilitation. Medical expenses, loss of wages during recovery, and forced retirement can change the laryngectomee's financial status after surgery. In a survey of more than 3,000 laryngectomees, Horn [7] reported 66% suffered loss of income related to their laryngectomized condition; 19% were forced to borrow money to pay medical expenses; and 17% relied on the spouse's income for financial support. Medical insurance is unlikely to cover alaryngeal speech therapy services fully. Various therapy options are available to the laryngectomee. The American Cancer Society (see Appendix A) is an excellent resource for locating the nearest International Association of Laryngectomees (IAL) Club, a local university or speech and hearing clinic may provide low-cost therapy services to the community, or the SLP may consider offering small-group therapy in which laryngectomees share payment of the hourly fee.

The length of the session is also affected by the number of activities planned. As more therapy activities are included, the length of the session increases. For example, a 60-minute therapy session could incorporate a relaxation exercise, oral-facial exercises, four activities to address specific speech goals, and the assignment of home practice materials. Limiting the length of each activity to 8–10 minutes maximizes therapeutic efficiency by allowing the laryngectomee to practice a variety of goals within a specified time.

Individual therapy is highly recommended for early intervention. Two laryngectomees paired for therapy often serve as models and provide emotional support for each other. Stimulus conditions and the analysis of the laryngectomee's responses are designed to parallel those found outside the clinic environment. As the laryngectomee acquires alaryngeal speech skills, generalization of the learned behavior to more spontaneous and natural environments is encouraged via group therapy and home practice.

ARRANGEMENT OF THE THERAPY SESSION

No two therapy sessions are exactly alike. The individual needs and abilities of the laryngectomee dictate the length, frequency, and content of the sessions. This being said, there is a general sequence of events in the therapy session.

Opening the Session

The session should begin with a brief discussion of events pertaining to alaryngeal speech rehabilitation that have occurred in the laryngectomee's life since the last session. This is a good time for the laryngectomee to report results of home practice activities, ask questions, or relay information from the physician. Having been given the opportunity to express needs or concerns, the laryngectomee is then ready to settle into therapy activities. In addition to, or in the absence of, an opening conversation, a relaxation exercise is used.

Relaxation Exercise

Relaxed oral-pharyngeal-esophageal musculature is essential to the production of alaryngeal speech. For esophageal speech production in particular, air is more likely to enter the esophagus and return if the pharyngoesophageal segment is relaxed [8]. In addition, relaxation exercises address secondary behaviors, such as facial grimaces, tightened shoulder muscles, and a rigid posture. An example of a 3-minute relaxation sequence is provided in Appendix B. The SLP should read aloud or tape the passage for use at the beginning of clinic and home practice sessions.

Oral-Facial Exercises

Surgical intervention may have interfered with orofacial musculature or innervation (e.g., hemiglossectomy or facial paresis). Removal of the hyoid bone requires reattachment of tongue musculature to the pharyngeal suture line; other muscle fibers of the tongue are sacrificed [9]. As a consequence, some laryngectomees may have difficulty producing certain consonant sounds due to weakness of the oral musculature. Lip, tongue, and jaw exercises designed to strengthen the oral musculature necessary for speech are provided in Appendix C. Mirror practice provides helpful visual feedback. The SLP should practice with the laryngectomee to demonstrate and reinforce correct oral movements. In some cases, a tongue depressor can be used to guide the articulators into the target position.

Goal-Directed Activities

The main segment of therapy involves practice of specific goals at the appropriate phase and level of production. The minimum performance level within each activity should be within 70–80% accuracy. If the laryngectomee is learning more than one method of communication, tasks can be alternated—for example, after working on esophageal speech the client can switch to use of the artificial larynx. When changing tasks, the SLP announces the new goal and explains the activity to the laryngectomee. Pictures or examples are used for clarity, if necessary.

Session Closure

The sequence of therapy activities should end with a task known to be successful. A more difficult level of production should not be introduced toward the end of the session when the laryngectomee is tired. It is unfair to the laryngectomee to introduce a challenging task and not resolve it before the close of the session. During the session, key words or phrases that are successful for the laryngectomee should be jotted down. At the close of the session, this list of words or phrases is provided for home practice. As a rule, practice stimuli assigned as homework have been produced in therapy with at least 80% accuracy.

The next three chapters are devoted to the teaching of alternate methods of communication. Use of the artificial larynx is presented in Chapter 5; Chapter 6 describes the techniques for facilitating esophageal speech. Teaching methods for TE speech are found in Chapter 7.

REFERENCES

1. Brookshire RH. Speech pathology and the experimental analysis of behavior. J Speech Hear Disord 1967;32:315.
2. LaPointe LL. Base-10 programmed stimulation: task specification, scoring and plotting performance in aphasia therapy. J Speech Hear Disord 1977;42:90.
3. LaPointe LL. Aphasia Therapy: Some Principles and Strategies for Treatment. In DF Johns (ed), Clinical Management of Neurogenic Communicative Disorders (2nd ed). Boston: Little, Brown, 1985;179.
4. Mowrer DE. The Behavioral Approach to Treatment. In NA Creaghead, PW Newman, WA Secord (eds), Assessment and Remediation of Articulatory and Phonological Disorders (2nd ed). New York: Macmillan, 1989;159.
5. Rosenbek JC, Lemme ML, Ahern MB, et al. A treatment for apraxia of speech in adults. J Speech Hear Disord 1973;38:462.
6. Porch BE. The Porch Index of Communicative Ability. Palo Alto, CA: Consulting Psychologists Press, 1981.
7. Horn D. Laryngectomee survey report summary. Presented at the 11th Annual Meeting of the International Association of Laryngectomees, Memphis, TN. August 1962.
8. Gardner WH. Laryngectomee Speech and Rehabilitation. Springfield, IL: Thomas, 1971;94.
9. Salmon SJ. Methods of Air Intake and Associated Problems. In RL Keith, FL Darley (eds), Laryngectomee Rehabilitation (3rd ed). Austin, TX: PRO-ED, 1994;221.

5

Using the Artificial Larynx

In this chapter, it is assumed the laryngectomee has selected an artificial larynx based on a combination of factors—physical needs, proficiency, availability of the device, personal preference, and initial cost and maintenance (see discussion of advantages and disadvantages of the artificial larynx in Chapter 3, "Artificial Larynx Speech"). The primary goal of alaryngeal speech therapy is to provide the laryngectomee with a *functional* mode of communication. Functional use of the artificial larynx means the laryngectomee has developed a reliable method of communicating information, needs, and opinions. A higher level of proficiency may be achieved by the laryngectomee who is motivated to fine tune artificial larynx speech by attending to articulatory precision, rate and phrasing, and nonverbal behaviors.

Underlying successful artificial larynx speech are five target behaviors: (1) optimal placement of the artificial larynx, (2) coordination of the "on" control with speaking, (3) articulatory precision, (4) appropriate rate and phrasing, and (5) attention to nonverbal behaviors. Each of the goals for achieving proficient artificial larynx speech is discussed in this chapter along with suggestions for teaching each skill, providing feedback, and solving problems that may occur.

GOAL ONE: OPTIMAL PLACEMENT OF THE ARTIFICIAL LARYNX

The first goal toward successful communication is placement of the artificial larynx so that the sound is transmitted into the oral cavity for maximum resonance. The artificial larynx may be positioned against the neck or cheek, intraorally, or at the stoma. Most electrolarynges are designed for neck or cheek placement; however, many devices are available with an oral adapter for intraoral use. The Cooper-Rand Electronic Speech Aid (Luminaud [Mentor, OH]) and the UltraVoice (Health Concepts [Malvern, PA]) are designed for intraoral use

71

only. An intraoral device, the Tokyo artificial larynx (available from Clyde Welch [Omaha, NE]) has no batteries or electronic components; a metal or plastic cup is placed against the stoma to capture lung air.

Neck Placement

The speech-language pathologist (SLP) should palpate the laryngectomee's neck and underside of the jaw to locate an area that is not hardened by scar tissue or the effects of radiation. The vibrating head of the artificial larynx should be placed firmly and directly against the identified "soft spot" while the laryngectomee repeats the phrase "one, two, three, four, five" or "Sunday, Monday, Tuesday." When the vibrating head of the artificial larynx is in the optimal position, the laryngectomee's "voice" is perceived as coming from the mouth and the electronic buzz is reduced (Figure 5.1).

The ideal arrangement is to have the laryngectomee hold the artificial larynx in the nondominant hand and place the unit against the same side of the neck (Figure 5.2). If the laryngectomee uses his or her nondominant hand to hold the artificial larynx, the dominant hand is free to write, gesture, drive, shake hands, and operate the telephone.

Using one hand to pass the artificial larynx to the opposite side of the neck is awkward, although some laryngectomees prefer this arrangement. The quality of the resonated sound and the laryngectomee's comfort are the overruling factors in making a decision about the hand-to-neck position.

Hearing Aids and Neck Placement

Another consideration during the search for appropriate neck placement is the presence of hearing aids. The noise produced by the artificial larynx can result in severe distortion of the hearing aid output and interfere with the laryngectomee's self-monitoring abilities [1]. If the laryngectomee wears only one hearing aid, Lerman [2] recommends placing the vibrating head of the artificial larynx on the side of the neck opposite the hearing aid, as well as adjusting the pitch downward to enhance self-monitoring abilities. Other options available to the laryngectomee are cheek placement, use of an intraoral adapter, or switching to the Tokyo artificial larynx [1].

Inconsistency in Finding Placement

Due to scar tissue, the laryngectomee may have little sensation on the neck and must rely on visual feedback as well as practiced arm and hand movements to find the best placement of the artificial larynx quickly and reliably. The SLP should offer to mark the "spot" with a pen, a piece of tape, or a colored sticker so the laryngectomee can locate the target site while practicing in front of the mirror. The laryngectomee should practice placing the vibrating head against the neck many times so that finding the best spot becomes automatic.

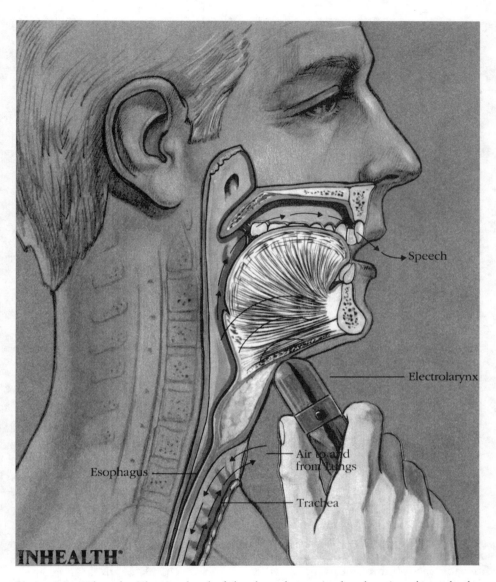

Figure 5.1 When the vibrating head of the electrolarynx is placed against the neck, the tone resonates in the hypopharynx and oral cavities. The laryngectomee uses the articulators to shape the sound into meaningful speech. (Reprinted with permission of InHealth Technologies. Postlaryngectomy Training Aid Set. Carpinteria, CA: InHealth Technologies, 1995.)

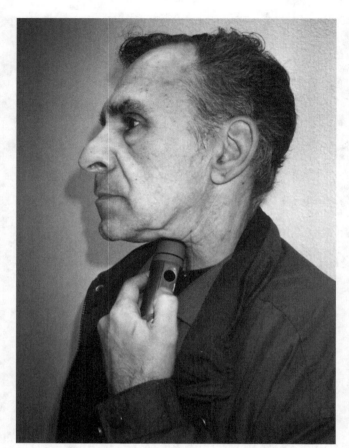

Figure 5.2
Neck placement using the Servox Inton Electronic Speech Aid (Siemens Hearing Instruments [Prospect Heights, IL]).

Improper Placement Resulting in Buzzing or Damped Sound

If placement of the vibrating head against the neck is too light, electronic buzzing occurs. If placement is too forceful, sound is damped. The laryngectomee should be re-instructed regarding optimal neck placement and practice placing the vibrating head against the palm of the hand for visual as well as tactile learning assistance. While the laryngectomee holds the artificial larynx, the SLP should guide the device into position against the neck. The laryngectomee should watch his or her reflection in the mirror during placement of the artificial larynx.

Holding the Artificial Larynx in the "Ready" Position

Sometimes the new user of the electrolarynx holds the unit against the neck or cheek in the "ready" position, even when not talking. Not only is this posture tiring for the laryngectomee, but it is visually distracting to the observer. The laryngectomee should be encouraged to practice a sequence:

1. Place the artificial larynx against the neck or the cheek or into the oral cavity.
2. Count aloud from one to five.
3. Remove the device to a resting position.
4. Find the correct placement again.

This type of practice helps the laryngectomee feel more confident about his or her ability to quickly locate the proper position for speaking.

Cheek Placement

In the presence of fibrotic tissue, scarring, tenderness, or irregularities of the neck, placement of the artificial larynx on the cheek is a viable option. Optimal placement is relatively easy to determine because there is no scar tissue on the cheek. The SLP should instruct the laryngectomee to use the nondominant hand to place the vibrating head of the artificial larynx against the cheek near the mouth (Figure 5.3) and say "one, two, three, four, five." Contact between the vibrating head of the artificial larynx and the cheek must be complete to avoid extraneous buzzing. To increase accuracy of placement, the laryngectomee should practice making vibrator-to-cheek contact over many trials.

The vibrating head of the artificial larynx is pressure sensitive. When cheek contact is too light, sound is not transmitted into the oral cavity; instead, extraneous buzzing occurs. Too much pressure against the cheek interrupts vibration. Optimal cheek placement should be demonstrated for the laryngectomee. While the laryngectomee is positioned in front of a mirror holding the artificial larynx, the SLP guides the device into position against the cheek near the mouth.

Placement Using an Intraoral Tube

Use of an intraoral tube bypasses the need to place the instrument against the neck. The laryngectomee uses the nondominant hand to place the air tube 1–2 in. into the oral cavity, positioning the tube between the side of the tongue and the molar teeth (see Figure 3.5). Using mirror feedback, the laryngectomee should practice inserting and removing the intraoral tube to learn how to find the ideal placement in the oral cavity quickly and easily.

Loss of Sound Due to Improper Placement

Placing the tube in the buccal cavity (between the teeth and the cheek) or pressing it into the tongue or the area underneath the tongue damps the sound. Tongue movements tend to be restricted and articulation impaired when the air

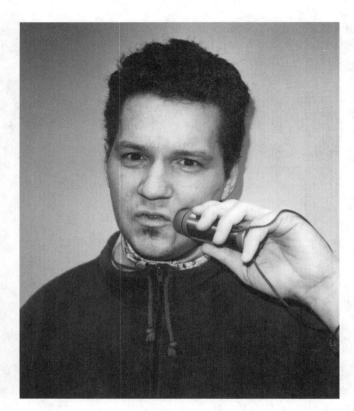

Figure 5.3
Cheek placement using the Servox Inton Electronic Speech Aid (Siemens Hearing Instruments [Prospect Heights, IL]).

tube is placed in the center of the oral cavity. The laryngectomee should be discouraged from biting down on the tube, because this interferes with mandibular movements and hinders articulatory precision.

Loss of Sound Due to Clogging of Tube with Saliva

If saliva backs up in the tube, sound is interrupted. Switching to a saliva ejector tube or adding a saliva tip to the oral end of the tube usually alleviates the problem. To decrease clogging, Salmon [1] recommends slicing the oral tip of the tube on an oblique (45-degree) angle and inserting the tube with the beveled side facing upward. The laryngectomee may also carry a supply of spare tubes and change them frequently. The intraoral tube must be cleaned and disinfected routinely as part of maintenance.

Intraoral Placement for the Ultra Voice

The "mouthpiece" of the UltraVoice is imbedded in the laryngectomee's denture or in a retainer-like prosthesis. Once the denture or prosthesis is in place, the laryngectomee must concentrate only on the operation of the hand-held control.

Stoma Placement

To operate a pneumatic device—for example, the Tokyo artificial larynx—the laryngectomee must place the stoma cup over the stoma. The cup must form a tight seal over the stoma so that air does not escape during exhalation. The oral tip is positioned in the oral cavity in the manner described in the section "Placement Using an Intraoral Tube." To take a breath during speaking, the cup is tilted slightly away from the stoma. With practice, the laryngectomee can position the stoma cup for speaking, tilt it for a quick breath, and reposition the cup to resume speaking. The Tokyo artificial larynx cannot be demonstrated by someone without a stoma; however, demonstration videotapes are available (see Appendix A).

Failure to achieve and maintain an airtight seal over the stoma during exhalation results in a hissing noise as air escapes around the edges of the stoma cup. If the leak is substantial, voicing may be lost. An assortment of stoma cups are included with the Tokyo artificial larynx. The laryngectomee should experiment to find the cup that provides best coverage of his or her stoma.

A summary of problem solving for placement of the artificial larynx appears in Table 5.1.

GOAL TWO: COORDINATION OF THE "ON" CONTROL WITH SPEAKING

Once appropriate placement is established, the laryngectomee is ready to learn how to coordinate use of the "on" control with articulation. Activation of the artificial larynx occurs simultaneously with the onset of speech movements. Step by step, the SLP should instruct the laryngectomee to do the following:

1. Find the correct placement on the neck, cheek, or in the mouth.
2. Press the "on" control on the artificial larynx and simultaneously begin articulating a phrase, for example, "one, two, three, four, five."
3. After completing the phrase, release the "on" control.
4. Return the artificial larynx to the resting position away from the neck, cheek, or mouth.

Operating an electrolarynx requires the laryngectomee to synchronize pressing or releasing the "on" control with speaking. Common errors made by the laryngectomee include the following:

- Activating the "on" control before speaking
- Beginning to speak before activating the "on" control
- Deactivating the "on" control before finishing speaking
- Continuing to activate the "on" control after finishing speaking

Table 5.1 Problem solving for placement of the artificial larynx

Problem	Solution
Neck or cheek placement	
Buzzing sound	Place the full vibrating head flat against the neck or cheek with moderate firmness.
	Place the vibrating head against supple neck tissue rather than fibrotic or scarred tissue.
Damped sound	Placement against the neck or cheek may be too forceful; reduce pressure.
Holding the artificial larynx in the "ready" position	Remove the artificial larynx to the resting position between speaking turns.
Inconsistency of placement	Mark the best "spot" with pen, tape, or a colored sticker, and observe placement in mirror during practice.
Use of hearing aids interferes with self-monitoring skills	Place the vibrating head on the side of the neck opposite the hearing aid. For bilateral hearing aids, consider using cheek placement, an intraoral adapter, or the Tokyo artificial larynx (available from Clyde Welch [Omaha, NE]).
Intraoral placement	
Damped sound	Do not place the intraoral tube in the buccal cavity area.
	Do not press the intraoral tube into the tongue.
	Do not bite the intraoral tube.
Loss of sound due to clogged oral tube	Check the tube for saliva accumulation; rinse.
	Cut the distal end of the tube (tip) at a 45-degree angle, and reinsert with beveled side up.
Holding the intraoral tube in the "ready" position	Remove the intraoral tube from the mouth to the resting position between speaking turns.
Stoma placement	
Stoma noise	Form a tight seal against the stoma to prevent air escape at the sides of the stoma cup during exhalation.

Premature or Delayed Activation of the "On" Control

If the laryngectomee presses the "on" control prematurely—that is, before beginning articulatory movements—empty buzzing of the electrolarynx is heard. If the laryngectomee begins articulating before pressing the "on" control, sound is lost and intelligibility sacrificed. Speaking and sound production must be synchronized. The SLP should use the artificial larynx to demonstrate the error to the laryngectomee. The laryngectomee should then repeat the same phrase several times to perfect his or her timing.

Premature or Delayed Deactivation of the "On" Control

Loss of voicing occurs when the "on" control is released while the laryngectomee is still articulating. If the "on" control remains pressed after the laryngectomee has finished speaking, the artificial larynx continues to produce a buzzing sound, resulting in the perception that the phrase ends in a schwa (/ə/)—for example, "What is it / that you want to know" becomes "What is it-a / that you want to know-a." The SLP should demonstrate the error and model the target behavior for the laryngectomee, or record the laryngectomee for feedback. Articulatory movements must be coordinated with the operation of the "on" control of the artificial larynx, and the laryngectomee should practice the same phrase several times.

Special note: If the laryngectomee is using the Tokyo artificial larynx, there is no "on" control. Voicing is produced as the laryngectomee exhales through the stoma cup into the tubing. During the orientation level, the laryngectomee should be encouraged to blow into the stoma cup without placing the oral tip in the mouth. With practice, the laryngectomee learns the right amount of air pressure needed to create voicing.

Special note: For the UltraVoice, manipulation of the hand-held control turns the oral unit on or off, adjusts tone for inflection, and controls loudness.

A summary of problem solving for coordinating the "on" control with speaking appears in Table 5.2.

GOAL THREE: ARTICULATORY PRECISION

Articulatory precision is key to the intelligibility of artificial larynx speech. Knowledge of the laryngectomee's pre- and postoperative speech patterns is beneficial to therapy planning. Foreign accent, regional dialect, dysarthria, or an articulation disorder can significantly affect the intelligibility of artificial larynx speech. Oral-facial exercises for the lip, tongue, and jaw (see Appendix C) and articulation drills are used to improve articulatory control and precision.

Table 5.2 Problem solving for coordination of the "on" control with speaking

Problem	Solution
Electrolarynx	
Electronic buzzing is heard before speech begins.	Press the "on" control simultaneously with the beginning of speech.
Oral speech movements begin before sound is heard; voicing is lost.	Begin speaking at the same time the "on" control is pressed.
Electronic buzzing continues after speech ends, sometimes resulting in addition of unwanted schwa (/ə/) sound.	Release the "on" control simultaneously with the conclusion of speech.
Oral speech movements continue after sound ends; voicing is lost.	Release the "on" control simultaneously with the conclusion of speech.
Pneumatic device	
Sound is heard before speech begins.	Exhale into the stoma cup simultaneously with the beginning of speech.
Oral speech movements begin before sound is heard; voicing is lost.	Begin speaking simultaneously with exhalation into the stoma cup.
Sound continues after speech ends, sometimes resulting in addition of unwanted schwa (/ə/) sound.	Cease exhalation into the stoma cup simultaneously with the conclusion of speech.
Oral speech movements continue after sound ends; voicing is lost.	Cease exhalation into the stoma cup simultaneously with the conclusion of speech.

Practicing the articulation of specific consonants adds to speech clarity. A review of the alaryngeal speech literature by Salmon [3] indicates that vowels and glides /r, w, j/ are generally perceived accurately. Consonants, particularly the obstruents (i.e., plosives, fricatives, and affricates), are not understood as well by the listener.

The lingual and labial contacts for plosives, fricatives, and affricates should be distinct and *slightly* exaggerated. Firm, energetic articulatory contacts increase the intraoral-pharyngeal air pressure needed to articulate these consonant sounds. Without the artificial larynx, the laryngectomee should practice mouthing the contacts for the obstruents. Labial contact for /p/ and lingual contacts for /t/ and /k/ should be audible. To illustrate the laryngectomee's ability to move air within the oral cavity, a piece of paper can be held in front of the laryngectomee's lips while he or she produces /p/ and watches the paper flutter, or the SLP can feel the percussion by placing the fingertips in front of the laryngectomee's lips while he or she articulates /p/ or /t/. Fricatives are normally produced with a continuous airstream from the lungs. The laryngectomee compensates by using lingual movements to compress the air within the oral and pharyngeal cavities to create turbulence.

Voiced obstruents are easier to understand than unvoiced obstruents, most likely because the artificial larynx is activated for the duration of speaking time so that all obstruents become "voiced." To produce the voiced obstruent /b, d, g, z, v, ð/ or /dʒ/ in the beginning of a phrase, the laryngectomee activates the artificial larynx simultaneously with speech production. If the voiced obstruent occurs at the end of a phrase, the "on" control is deactivated with the completion of the oral movements.

Intelligibility of the unvoiced obstruent /p, t, k, s, f, ʃ, θ/ or /tʃ/ at the beginning of a phrase is improved by making the oral movement for the sound immediately before activation of the artificial larynx. Intelligibility of an unvoiced obstruent at the end of a phrase is enhanced by deactivating the "on" control before the sharp articulatory contact for the obstruent.

A step-by-step plan for improving intelligibility of speech is an obvious outgrowth of the knowledge gleaned from listener perception studies. Specific practice is needed by the laryngectomee for the unvoiced obstruents—plosives, fricatives, and affricates. In the beginning activities, the target obstruent appears in the initial position of words. Next, practice stimuli contain the target obstruent in the final position in words. In more advanced activities, unvoiced and voiced obstruents are contrasted in minimal word pairs [1, 2, 4].

Making Voiced-Unvoiced Obstruent Distinctions

Considerable practice may be needed to coordinate activation of the artificial larynx "on" control and the production of unvoiced obstruents that occur at the beginning and at the end of phrases. If an unvoiced obstruent occurs in the beginning of the phrase—for example, /p/ in "*p*ad is the word"—pressing the "on" control prematurely causes listener confusion and the perceived phrase is "*b*ad is the word." If the phrase ends with an unvoiced obstruent—for example, /t/ in "the word is ma*t*"—failure to release the "on" control before producing the /t/ results in the listener's perception of "the word is ma*d*." Specific practice lists have been created to teach the laryngectomee coordination and timing (see Appendix E).

The carrier phrase "_____ is the word" is used for practicing phrases that *begin* with an unvoiced obstruent (see Appendix E). Carrier phrases such as "the word is _____" or "I can say _____" are used for phrases that *end* with an unvoiced obstruent (see Appendix E). The use of a carrier phrase eliminates any possible contextual cues, forcing the listener to rely solely on the production of the utterance. Contrast drills are an excellent test of the laryngectomee's ability to differentially articulate voiced and unvoiced obstruents. The control of voiced-unvoiced obstruent distinctions contributes significantly to intelligibility; time is well spent practicing to improve this skill.

Compensating for the Glottal Fricative /h/

The laryngeal speaker produces /h/ by adducting the vocal folds slightly (but not sufficiently to produce vocal fold vibration) and exhaling. Alaryngeal production of the glottal fricative /h/ is considered impossible by many laryngectomees and their SLPs because of the required continuous breath stream. Much of the time the /h/, although omitted during alaryngeal speech, is understood within the context of the utterance—for example, "Come to my 'ouse for dinner." Shanks [5] suggests substituting the /h/ with the plosive /k/ using a prolonged but less intense velar contact. The resulting sound is similar to the German word *ich*. Further reduction of the physical contact between the tongue and palate creates turbulence that closely resembles the glottal fricative /h/ [6].

Exaggeration of Articulatory Movements

The laryngectomee needs to articulate as clearly as possible without exaggerating or using unusual oral or facial movements. Articulation practice in front of the mirror allows the laryngectomee immediate visual feedback about his or her oral and facial mannerisms during speaking. This issue is discussed further in the section "Goal 5: Attention to Nonverbal Behaviors."

Imprecise Articulation and Restricted Mandibular Movement

The surgical procedure to remove the hyoid bone interrupts mandibular and lingual muscle attachments to the hyoid bone. As a result, the laryngectomee almost always presents with a dysarthric component of speech related to mandibular and lingual movements—that is, difficulty making lingual contacts and opening and closing the mouth efficiently. Oral-facial exercises assist the laryngectomee in regaining strength and precision of the oral, facial, and lingual musculature (see Appendix C). Oral-facial exercises are performed at the beginning of every session (as warm-ups) and the laryngectomee is expected to do the exercises several times daily at home.

Articulatory imprecision is a potential problem for users of intraoral adapters. The laryngectomee should avoid placing the air tube in the center of the oral cavity or in front of the tongue tip. Linguadental and lingua-alveolar productions are particularly vulnerable to blockage of tongue tip movements.

Loose Dentures

Ill-fitting dentures separate from the gums during speech and interfere with articulatory precision. If the use of a denture adhesive is unsuccessful, a referral to the dentist or prosthodontist for adjustment of the dentures is appropriate.

A summary of problem solving for articulatory precision using the artificial larynx appears in Table 5.3.

GOAL FOUR: APPROPRIATE RATE AND PHRASING

The physical quantities of duration, fundamental frequency, and intensity contribute to the prosody, or naturalness, of speech production. The duration of

Table 5.3 Problem solving for articulatory precision using the artificial larynx

Problem	Solution
Voiced-unvoiced obstruent confusion for the initial position in words	*For the battery-operated artificial larynx:* Voiced obstruents are articulated simultaneously with the activation of the "on" control. Unvoiced obstruents are articulated slightly before the activation of the "on" control. *For the pneumatic artificial larynx:* Voiced obstruents are articulated simultaneously with exhalation into the stoma cup. Unvoiced obstruents are articulated slightly before exhalation into the stoma cup.
Voiced-unvoiced obstruent confusion for the final position in words	*For the battery-operated artificial larynx:* Voiced obstruents are articulated while the "on" control is activated. Unvoiced obstruents are articulated after the "on" control is deactivated. *For the pneumatic artificial larynx:* Voiced obstruents are articulated simultaneously with exhalation into the stoma cup. Unvoiced obstruents are articulated after exhalation into the stoma cup has ceased.
Production of /h/ sound	*For all artificial larynges:* Make a prolonged but less intense velar contact for the /k/ sound, similar to the German word *ich*.
Exaggerated articulation	*For all artificial larynges:* Encourage normal lip, tongue, and jaw movements during speech production. Use mirror practice.
Imprecise articulation, restricted mandibular movement, or both	*For all artificial larynges:* Use oral-facial exercises to regain strength and precision of movement. Check fit of dentures; use denture adhesive or see a dentist/prosthodontist. *For intraoral adapters and the pneumatic artificial larynx:* Avoid placing the air tube in the center of the oral cavity or in front of the tongue tip.

speech includes measures of rate and phrasing. Articulatory movements to adjust intraoral air pressures for consonant production frequently result in reduced speech rate for the alaryngeal speaker. As previously discussed in "Goal Three: Articulatory Precision," articulatory precision is crucial to the intelligibility of artificial larynx speech. The combination of distinct articulation and a slightly slower-than-normal rate makes for improved intelligibility.

Most laryngeal speakers pause briefly between phrases. The laryngectomee learns to deactivate the artificial larynx to accommodate these natural pauses during practice of longer phrases. The SLP should suggest that the laryngectomee pause briefly wherever a comma or period would appear in written text. Early exercises to practice phrasing include marking pauses with a red pen in the text to be read. Emphasis is achieved by pausing immediately before the target word—for example, to stress the word *quart* in the sentence "I need a quart of milk," a pause is inserted before "quart": "I need a / quart of milk." A question-answer activity can be used to practice emphasis as demonstrated in the following example:

Laryngectomee:	I need a / quart of milk.
SLP:	Do you need a *gallon* of milk?
Laryngectomee:	No, I need a / *quart* of milk.
SLP:	Do you need a quart of *ice cream*?
Laryngectomee:	No, I need a quart of / *milk*.

Intermittent Activation of the "On" Control

The prosody of a phrase or sentence is disturbed when the laryngectomee presses and releases the "on" control for each syllable, producing a staccato utterance such as "be / fore / you / go." The rhythm of normal speech production should be explained: Words are not said individually but are grouped and even blended one into the other. The target phrase can be demonstrated—for example, "Before you go," as /biforjugo/. The "on" control is activated for the entire phrase.

The user of the pneumatic artificial larynx is capable of breathing short puffs of air into the intraoral tube, resulting in a broken string of words. The SLP should suggest that the laryngectomee exhale steadily into the stoma cup for the full production of each phrase.

Prolonged Activation of the "On" Control

Sometimes in longer phrases, the laryngectomee depresses the "on" control throughout the entire utterance. The monotonous, run-on outcome is often difficult to understand—for example, "countyourblessingseachdayofyourlife." An explanation and demonstration of prosody and appropriate phrasing in speech production are helpful. The longer phrase lists may be referred to for practice (see Appendix D: II and III). A red pen should be used to draw vertical lines between the words to indicate brief pauses (i.e., the "on" control deactivated). Using the example, the suggested division is "Count your blessings / each day of your life."

For the pneumatic artificial larynx user, exhalation into the stoma cup should stop between phrases. Natural pauses in written text can be marked and

Table 5.4 Problem solving for rate and phrasing during artificial larynx speech

Problem	Solution
Electrolarynx	
Staccato utterances	Mentally group words together into phrases. Activate the "on" control for the full production of each phrase.
	Mark pauses in written text and practice reading aloud, deactivating the "on" control only at the pause signs (between phrases).
Run-on utterances	Mentally group words together into phrases. Briefly deactivate the "on" control between phrases.
	Mark pauses in written text and practice reading aloud, briefly deactivating the "on" control at the pause signs (between phrases).
Pneumatic device	
Staccato utterances	Mentally group words together into phrases. Exhale into the stoma cup for the full production of each phrase.
	Mark pauses in written text and practice reading aloud, ceasing exhalation into the stoma cup only at the pause signs (between phrases).
Run-on utterances	Mentally group words together into phrases. Briefly cease exhalation into the stoma cup between phrases.
	Mark pauses in written text and practice reading aloud, briefly cease exhalation into the stoma cup at the pause signs (between phrases).

read aloud. The laryngectomee ceases exhalation into the stoma cup only at the pause marks.

A summary of problem solving for rate and phrasing during artificial larynx speech appears in Table 5.4.

GOAL FIVE: ATTENTION TO NONVERBAL BEHAVIORS

While communicating with other people, most laryngeal speakers unconsciously smile, point, cough, wink, tilt their heads, vary pitch, increase and decrease loudness, and look directly at their listener. As they learn to use the artificial larynx, some laryngectomees spontaneously resume their nonverbal accompaniment to speech production. Other laryngectomees need to practice specific nonverbal behaviors that support the perception of an engaging communicator. The laryngectomee needs to understand and use natural mannerisms complementary to speaking by using pitch and loudness variability; pausing for emphasis; using interjections such as "um," "er," or "hmm"; appropriate head nodding; facial expressions; hand gestures; and eye contact. When the laryngectomee appears relaxed and confident during speech production, the listener is more likely to attend to *what* the laryngectomee is saying rather than to *how* he or she is saying it.

Pitch Variability

In addition to rate and phrasing, pitch level (fundamental frequency) and loudness (intensity) play important roles in the perception of melodic speech. Most artificial larynges have an internal or external adjustment for pitch and loudness control. The Tokyo artificial larynx is an exception; the width and tension of the vibrating membrane determine fundamental frequency, and the amount and force of air exhaled by the lungs into the device affects pitch as well as intensity. The SLP should work with the laryngectomee to find the pitch and loudness levels that are best suited to his or her needs. The laryngectomee's gender does not always dictate the direction of pitch adjustment; some laryngectomees prefer a low pitch; others adjust the pitch to a higher frequency.

Typically, the pitch control setting remains the same throughout all communication situations. A few devices—for example, the TruTone artificial larynx (Griffin Laboratories [Temecula, CA]) (see Appendix A)—allow the laryngectomee to vary pitch during speaking by increasing or decreasing finger pressure on the control button. If the laryngectomee's artificial larynx is capable of such manipulation, he or she should practice producing declarative versus interrogative sentences as well as contrastive stress drills—for example, "*She* likes to read books," versus "She *likes* to read books," versus "She likes to read *books*" (see "Goal Four: Appropriate Rate and Phrasing").

Some laryngectomees find that pitch variability adds "color" to their speech, especially if they sing, are active in a conversation group, or engage in public speaking. One of the laryngectomees in our alaryngeal speech clinic, John, frequently spoke to large groups preoperatively. After the surgery, he was eager to regain his speaking skills. Within a few months, John mastered the use of his Servox Inton (Siemens Hearing Instruments [Prospect Heights, IL]) artificial larynx well enough that he resumed public speaking. The artificial larynx had two tone controls, one slightly higher than the other, and John learned to manipulate these controls to his benefit. When he was invited to speak to our graduate seminar in voice disorders, students remarked that, although initially aware of the artificial larynx, they quickly became engaged in the content of John's speech rather than the mechanics of how he was speaking. In an evaluation of John's presentation, students listed his facial mannerisms, eye contact with the audience, hand gestures, articulatory accuracy, pausing, and pitch changes as effective aspects of his intelligibility.

Requirements for Loudness

Different communication environments require loudness adjustments to the electrolarynx. An increase in the loudness of the artificial larynx is appropriate while dining at a noisy restaurant or engaging a hearing-impaired friend in conversation. While talking on the telephone or conversing in a quiet setting, the loudness level is set considerably lower.

In certain situations, the laryngectomee may compensate in ways other than adjusting the volume of the artificial larynx. The laryngectomee can increase listener comprehension by facing the person to boost lipreading cues, using facial expression and hand gestures, announcing the topic of conversation before speaking, rephrasing the information, or moving to a quieter environment away from ambient noise. On occasion, the volume of the artificial larynx is inappropriately loud for the situation, enough so that it draws attention to the speaker. When attending a quiet activity—for example, a church service, library, concert, theater, or lecture—the laryngectomee may choose to write a note to the intended recipient or use facial expressions or hand signals to convey intent.

The laryngectomee should be given opportunities to become competent in making pitch and loudness adjustments under the SLP's direction. The ability to operate the artificial larynx, recharge and replace the batteries, and clean and maintain the instrument provides the laryngectomee with feelings of control and independence, qualities important to successful alaryngeal speech rehabilitation.

The Good Communicator

Chapter 8, "Group Therapy," addresses social interaction issues. The foundation of our alaryngeal speech group interactions is learning to be good communicators. A good communicator is sensitive to the listener's needs, observes the rules of turn taking, stays within the time limits of the conversational situation, and checks frequently to make sure the message has been understood by the listener. Teaching and reminding the laryngectomee the habits of a considerate communicator from the early stages of artificial larynx speech adds to the laryngectomee's desirability as a communication partner.

Distracting Behaviors

Sometimes the laryngectomee involved in learning a new method of communication develops behaviors that interfere with the message and are distracting to the listener. Stoma noise, facial grimaces, head bobbing, loss of eye contact, and an overly tense posture are among the undesirable behaviors.

Stoma Noise

Prolonged exhalation is a natural part of *laryngeal* speech production. To effectively increase loudness, the laryngeal speaker relies on forced exhalation to drive air through the vocal folds. During artificial larynx speech, however, forced exhalation is no longer necessary or desirable. Strong exhalation results in stoma noise—the sound of air turbulence in the trachea. Avoidance of stoma noise is also a goal if the laryngectomee intends to learn esophageal speech. Hearing-impaired laryngectomees have difficulty hearing stoma noise and must rely on tactile feedback to monitor the air escape. The laryngectomee monitors the air exiting the stoma by placing his or her fingertips in front of, but not touching, the stoma. Judicious use of negative practice helps the laryngectomee discern between forceful and subdued exhalations. External cueing by the listener can be used to alert the laryngectomee of distracting stoma noise. A prearranged signal—for example, a raised index finger—is usually a sufficient reminder for the laryngectomee to suppress the force of exhalation.

Facial Grimaces, Head Bobbing, and Loss of Eye Contact

When mirror feedback is used during speech practice, contortions of facial and lip muscles, squinting, and erratic head movements may be more obvious to the laryngectomee. Identifying loss of eye contact is facilitated by placing a brightly colored sticker on the mirror at eye level and instructing the laryngectomee to look at the sticker while speaking. If the laryngectomee's eyes close or roll upward, the SLP should ask him or her to refocus on the sticker. Normal eye contact with the listener during spontaneous conversation occurs 80% of the time.

Excessive Muscular Tension

Several factors may contribute to muscular tension in the laryngectomee. Tenderness and stiffness related to the surgical procedure, uncertainty about the expectations of the SLP or of therapy, fear of failure, performance anxiety, and intense concentration on the task are reasons laryngectomees give to account for muscular tension. Excessive muscle tension sabotages fluent, easily produced speech. The session should begin with exercises to relax oral, facial, and shoulder muscles and promote general body relaxation (see Appendix B). Relaxation allows the laryngectomee time to move away from outside distractions and focus on therapy. Some laryngectomees also benefit from engaging in "mini" relaxations throughout the therapy session. *It is important to note that not all laryngectomees are in need of, or interested in, relaxation exercises.*

A summary of problem solving for nonverbal behaviors during artificial larynx speech appears in Table 5.5.

ACTIVITY HIERARCHY AND ARTIFICIAL LARYNX SPEECH

The learning of any new skill requires instruction and frequent practice at various levels of difficulty until competency is achieved. The rationale and general instructions for use of the therapy hierarchy appear in Chapter 4. The five goals leading to intelligible artificial larynx speech are (1) optimal placement,

Table 5.5 Problem solving for nonverbal behaviors during artificial larynx speech

Problem	Solution
Electrolarynx	
Pitch is inappropriately high or low	Make an internal or external adjustment of the unit's pitch control.
Loudness level is inappropriately high or low	Make an internal or external adjustment of the unit's volume control.
Difficulty being heard in a noisy environment or by a hearing-impaired listener	Increase the unit's volume control.
	Face the listener to boost lipreading cues.
	Use facial expression and hand gestures.
	Announce topic of conversation.
	Rephrase.
	Move to a quieter place.
Communicating in an exceptionally quiet situation	Write a note.
	Use facial expression and hand gestures.
Poor social interaction skills	Be sensitive to the listener's needs.
	Observe the rules of taking turns.
	Stay within the time limits of the conversational situation.
	Check frequently for listener comprehension.
Stoma noise	Self-monitor using tactile and auditory information.
	Decrease forceful exhalation during speech.
	Use prearranged signal as an alert of noise.
Facial grimaces, head bobbing, loss of eye contact	Practice speech while sitting in front of the mirror.
	Use prearranged signal as an alert of behavior.
Excessive muscular tension	Engage in relaxation exercises.
Pneumatic device	
Pitch is inappropriately high or low	Adjust the width and tension of the vibrating membrane—for example, a wider membrane under decreased tension lowers pitch; a narrower membrane under increased tension raises pitch.
	Evaluate the force of exhalation through the stoma cup—for example, increased air pressure results in higher pitch; decreased air pressure results in lower pitch.
Loudness level is inappropriately high or low	Evaluate the force of exhalation through the stoma cup—for example, increased air pressure results in increased loudness; decreased air pressure results in decreased loudness.
Stoma noise	Self-monitor using tactile and auditory information.
	Form a tight seal against the stoma to prevent air escape from the sides of the stoma cup during exhalation.
	Decrease forceful exhalation during speech.
	Use prearranged signal as an alert of noise.

(2) coordination of the "on" control with speaking, (3) articulatory precision, (4) appropriate rate and phrasing, and (5) attention to nonverbal behaviors. A step-by-step arrangement of therapy activities for teaching use of the artificial larynx is presented with clinical examples.

During therapy planning, an activity score sheet is prepared for each activity of the session (Figure 5.4). Practice activities for the five goals of artificial larynx speech are divided into phases: initial, intermediate, and advanced. In the initial phase, one goal per activity is identified for practice. In the intermediate phase, a combination of two goals is focused on during an activity. In the advanced phase, the laryngectomee attends to all five goals within the same activity.

The basic level of production for practicing artificial larynx speech is two- to four-syllable phrases. Short phrases are easier to produce with the artificial larynx than are single words. Considerable skill and timing are required to coordinate activation and deactivation of the "on" control with production of a single word. At the lower levels of production, the use of prepared phrases frees the laryngectomee to concentrate on appropriate placement, timing of the activation and deactivation of the "on" control, articulatory precision, rate and phrasing, and nonverbal behaviors.

When a new goal is introduced, the SLP provides the laryngectomee with feedback after each production. As the laryngectomee becomes familiar with the behavior, the SLP invites client self-monitoring before providing feedback. Ultimately, the laryngectomee is expected to reliably self-monitor. The development of self-monitoring skills is an important component of alaryngeal speech rehabilitation. Laryngectomees who are able to self-monitor and self-correct have the potential to manage and perfect their speech at all times, not just during the scheduled therapy session.

Initial Phase: An Example

In Figure 5.5, an activity score sheet for the initial phase of therapy has been completed. In the example, the client is a laryngectomee who has recently selected a neck-type artificial larynx. The initial phase is the starting point for learning to use the artificial larynx. Within the first several sessions, activities are designed to address each of the five goals for artificial larynx speech. The activity demonstrated in Figure 5.5 addresses the goal of coordinating speaking with the "on" control. The introductory level of production is Level I: two- to four-syllable phrases. A set of the two- to four-syllable phrases and sentences listed in Appendix D is selected (set 7 in this example). The stimulus items are printed on individual cards, presented as a list, or modeled (if the laryngectomee cannot read).

Because the laryngectomee is unfamiliar with the behaviors that result in correct use of the "on" control, the SLP monitors the productions and provides feedback. To ensure that the laryngectomee experiences 70–80% accuracy during the activity, the SLP must define a "correct" production. The client is instructed to activate the artificial larynx at the beginning of the phrase and deactivate the device promptly at the end of the phrase. Initially, the clinician

Name___Example_____ Date_____

Phase: ❏ Initial (one goal)
❏ Intermediate (two goals)
❏ Advanced (multiple goals)

Goal(s): ❏ Placement   ❏ Rate and phrasing
❏ "On" control   ❏ Nonverbal behaviors
❏ Articulation

Level of Unrestricted phonetic context:
production: ❏ I. Two- to four-syllable phrases   ❏ IV. Oral reading of paragraphs
❏ II. Five- to seven-syllable phrases   ❏ V. Structured conversation
❏ III. Eight-syllable phrases or more   ❏ VI. Spontaneous conversation

Monitoring: ❏ Clinician
❏ Laryngectomee/clinician
❏ Laryngectomee

	Stimuli Appendix: Level: Set:	Trial No.	Comments
1.			
2.			
3.			
4.			
5.			
6.			
7.			
8.			
9.			
10.			
	Total correct		
	Percent correct		

Figure 5.4 Activity score sheet for artificial larynx speech.

may need to provide a verbal reminder before each stimulus production. If use of the "on" control is accurate, the behavior is accepted as a correct, but assisted, response. The secondary "on" control goal becomes "The laryngectomee will coordinate use of the 'on' control with speaking 80% of the time when pre-

Name_____ Date_____

Phase: ■ Initial (one goal)
     ❏ Intermediate (two goals)
     ❏ Advanced (multiple goals)

Goal(s): ❏ Placement   ❏ Rate and phrasing
     ■ "On" control   ❏ Nonverbal behaviors
     ❏ Articulation

Level of   Unrestricted phonetic context:
production: ■ I. Two- to four-syllable phrases   ❏ IV. Oral reading of paragraphs
     ❏ II. Five- to seven-syllable phrases   ❏ V. Structured conversation
     ❏ III. Eight-syllable phrases or more ❏ VI. Spontaneous conversation

Monitoring: ■ Clinician
     ❏ Laryngectomee/clinician
     ❏ Laryngectomee

	Stimuli Appendix: **D** Level: **I** Set: **7**	Trial No. **1**	Comments
1.	Black and white	–	Premature activation
2.	Come with me.	+	Verbal reminder
3.	Everyone knows.	+	Verbal reminder
4.	Years from now	–	Premature activation
5.	Vegetable soup	+	Verbal reminder
6.	Take two aspirin.	+	Verbal reminder
7.	In front of me	+	Verbal reminder
8.	Keep it simple.	+	Self-corrected
9.	Queen mother	+	Self-corrected
10.	Smell the roses.	+	Verbal reminder
	Total correct	8	
	Percent correct	80%	Repeat task with Set 8 of Appendix D, I.

Figure 5.5 Activity score sheet for artificial larynx speech. Example: initial phase (one goal per activity). (+ = correct; – = incorrect.)

ceded by a verbal reminder." As the client learns to manipulate the "on" control appropriately, external cueing is withdrawn.

    Responses are judged as correct (+) or incorrect (–). In this activity, the client successfully coordinated the "on" control with speaking 80% of the time. In the comments section of the score sheet, the clinician has identified conditions related to the client's productions. Six of the eight correct productions were preceded by a verbal reminder from the SLP. Two of the correct productions were self-corrections by the client. At this stage of therapy, the use of verbal reminders is needed to stimulate the correct response. The laryngectomee's assisted productions are considered successive approximations leading up to the desired "unassisted correct response" designation. According to the clinician's note, this task will be repeated using set 8 of Level I: two- to four-syllable phrases (see Appendix D).

In one session, it is possible to address placement, the "on" control, articulation, rate and phrasing, and nonverbal behaviors in five *separate* activities. When a laryngectomee is working on use of the "on" control, *only* the "on" control accuracy is monitored; errors related to placement, articulation, rate and phrasing, and nonverbal behaviors are not mentioned. During articulation practice, feedback is limited to information about articulatory movements and precision. In the early stages of therapy, it is easy for the laryngectomee to become overwhelmed by too much information. Keeping the components of artificial larynx speech separate allows the laryngectomee to concentrate on one area at a time. The old saying "Divide and conquer" is relevant in this situation.

To increase teaching effectiveness, the SLP should learn to use the artificial larynx and be able to model error as well as target behavior. Demonstration is a valuable learning tool for the laryngectomee. When the target behavior is successful, the SLP should identify how success was achieved—for example, "Good timing! You pressed the 'on' control as you began speaking and released it as soon as you were finished." If the production is in error, a suggestion for improvement should be made—for example, "I heard buzzing before you started talking, like this [demonstrate premature activation of the 'on' control]. Try again. This time, start talking as you press the 'on' button."

Moving to the Intermediate Phase

During the initial phase and within the first few sessions, the laryngectomee usually moves quickly through the two- to four-syllable words and phrases level, mastering some or all of the artificial larynx goals. Differential success among the goals is common. In the example in Figure 5.5, once the client achieves 90% accuracy for each of the individual goals over three consecutive sets of stimuli at the two- to four-syllable phrase level, he is ready to enter the intermediate phase.

In the intermediate phase, the level of production remains at the two- to four-syllable phrase level. Within each activity, however, the client is expected to monitor for two goals simultaneously. In Figure 5.6, the clinician has paired two goals for the laryngectomee—placement *and* articulation—in one activity. In the intermediate phase, the SLP invites the client to self-monitor immediately after each production. The SLP then verifies or challenges the client's decision. The recorded results in Figure 5.6 show that the client was able to find appropriate placement and articulate the sounds correctly with 70% accuracy. The SLP's

Name___Example_____ Date_____

Phase: ☐ Initial (one goal)
  ■ Intermediate (two goals)
  ☐ Advanced (multiple goals)

Goal(s): ■ Placement ☐ Rate and phrasing
  ☐ "On" control ☐ Nonverbal behaviors
  ■ Articulation

Level of Unrestricted phonetic context:
production: ■ I. Two-to four-syllable phrases ☐ IV. Oral reading of paragraphs
  ☐ II. Five- to seven-syllable phrases ☐ V. Structured conversation
  ☐ III. Eight-syllable phrases or more ☐ VI. Spontaneous conversation

Monitoring: ☐ Clinician
  ■ Laryngectomee/clinician
  ☐ Laryngectomee

	Stimuli Appendix: **D** Level: **I** Set: **20**	Trial No. **1**	Comments
1.	Beat the clock.	–	Excess buzzing
2.	Call back later.	+	Verbal reminder about placement
3.	Eat your dinner.	–	Imprecise /d/
4.	That's news to me.	–	Excess buzzing
5.	Under the bed	+	Self-corrected /d/
6.	Vitamin B	+	Self-corrected
7.	While you're gone	+	Self-corrected
8.	Give to the poor.	+	Self-monitored √
9.	Heart-to-heart talk	+	Self-monitored √
10.	Live and learn.	+	Self-monitored √
	Total correct	7	
	Percent correct	70%	Repeat task with Set 21 of Appendix D, I.

Figure 5.6 Activity score sheet for artificial larynx speech. Example: intermediate phase (two goals per activity). (+ = correct; – = incorrect.)

comments indicate that the client missed two stimulus phrases due to excess buzzing of the artificial larynx, a placement problem.

Imprecise articulation was responsible for the third error. The observation that the client was able to self-monitor and self-correct six out of seven times is encouraging. The clinician's note indicates the task is to be repeated using a new set of stimuli at the same level of production. The goals and level of production remain the same until the laryngectomee is able to produce three consecutive sets of stimuli with 90% accuracy. Throughout the intermediate phase, the pairing of two of the five goals is varied at the two- to four-syllable phrase level until all combinations have been addressed in therapy activities.

Advanced Phase: A Clinical Example

The prerequisite for the client to move into the advanced phase of using the artificial larynx is 90% accuracy during a variety of paired goal activities at the two- to four-syllable phrase level. At the advanced phase level, the client attends to all five goals of artificial larynx speech within the same activity. The level of production remains at the two- to four-syllable phrase level, a relatively easy task for the laryngectomee at this stage of therapy. The difference between the advanced phase and the previous two phases is that to be "correct" in the advanced phase, the client must self-monitor for and achieve *all five goals* for each stimulus production.

Figure 5.7 illustrates the activity score sheet for the client in the advanced phase. All five goals have been marked. The client has been working at the advanced phase for several sessions and has achieved 80% accuracy for the two- to four-syllable phrase level of production. During this activity, the stimuli were chosen from Appendix D, Level I. The client enjoyed an 80% rate of accuracy. The two error productions, according to the clinician's comments, are articulation imprecision for /k/ and nonverbal behavior—that is, loss of eye contact. Early in the activity, the SLP provided verbal reminders about the "on" control. As the activity progressed, the client was able to self-monitor and self-correct more consistently. The task will be repeated at the two- to four-syllable level of production using a new set of stimuli until the client reaches 90% accuracy for all five goals over three consecutive trials. The client will then move to the next level of production, Level II: five- to seven-syllable phrases and sentences. The initial phase is reintroduced so that the laryngectomee is asked to attend to only one of the five goals of artificial larynx speech during a single activity. The systematic progression through Level II follows the same guidelines as used in the example for Level I.

CONCLUSION

The ultimate goal of postsurgical alaryngeal speech rehabilitation is to provide the laryngectomee with a functional communication method. Using a therapy hierarchy to teach artificial larynx speech, five target behaviors are practiced and refined: (1) optimal placement of the artificial larynx, (2) coordination of

Name___Example_____ Date_____

Phase: ❐ Initial (one goal)
            ❐ Intermediate (two goals)
            ■ Advanced (multiple goals)

Goal(s):   ■ Placement   ■ Rate and phrasing
            ■ "On" control   ■ Nonverbal behaviors
            ■ Articulation

Level of   Unrestricted phonetic context:
production: ■ I. Two- to four-syllable phrases   ❐ IV. Oral reading of paragraphs
            ❐ II. Five- to seven-syllable phrases   ❐ V. Structured conversation
            ❐ III. Eight-syllable phrases or more   ❐ VI. Spontaneous conversation

Monitoring: ❐ Clinician
              ❐ Laryngectomee/clinician
              ■ Laryngectomee

	Stimuli Appendix: **D** Level: **I** Set: **39**	Trial No. **2**	Comments
1.	Set the table.	+	Verbal reminder: "on" control
2.	Welcome home.	+	Verbal reminder : "on" control
3.	As good as gold	+	Self-corrected: "on" control
4.	Take my picture.	−	Articulation imprecision for /k/ in /pɪktʃɚ/
5.	Picnic basket	+	Verbal reminder: /k/ precision
6.	Obey the law.	+	
7.	My sister's son	−	Nonverbal behavior: loss of eye contact
8	Keep trying.	+	Self-corrected re: "on" control
9.	Nosy neighbor	+	Self-monitored √
10.	Rush-hour traffic	+	Self-monitored √
	Total correct	8	
	Percent correct	80%	Next: Appendix D, I: Set 40.

Figure 5.7 Activity score sheet for artificial larynx speech. Example: advanced phase (five goals per activity). (+ = correct; − = incorrect.)

the "on" control with speaking, (3) articulatory precision, (4) appropriate rate and phrasing, and (5) attention to nonverbal behaviors. Using the artificial larynx, the laryngectomee has access to a dependable method of communicating information, needs, and opinions. The proficient user of the artificial larynx conveys a clear, well-articulated message facilitated by acceptable rate, phrasing, emphasis, and loudness, and complemented by natural, nonverbal mannerisms.

The laryngectomee gains independence through effective communication skills. Being proficient in the use of the artificial larynx means the laryngectomee has the potential to express social, physical, identity, and practical needs. Happy is the laryngectomee who has the opportunity to express his or her feelings and desires, develop a sense of belonging, exercise a measure of control, protect the self, and exert influence on the environment.

REFERENCES

1. Salmon SJ. Artificial Larynx Speech: A Viable Means of Alaryngeal Communication. In Y Edels (ed), Laryngectomy: Diagnosis to Rehabilitation. Rockville, MD: Aspen, 1983;153.
2. Lerman JW. The Artificial Larynx. In SJ Salmon, KH Mount (eds), Alaryngeal Speech Rehabilitation for Clinicians by Clinicians. Austin, TX: PRO-ED, 1991;40.
3. Salmon SJ. The efficacy of speech-language pathology intervention: laryngectomy. Semin Speech Lang 1990;11(1):256.
4. Duguay M. Teaching Use of an Artificial Larynx. In WH Perkins (ed), Voice Disorders. New York: Thieme-Stratton, 1983;127.
5. Shanks JC. Developing Esophageal Communication. In RL Keith, FL Darley (eds), Laryngectomee Rehabilitation (3rd ed). Austin, TX: PRO-ED, 1994;214.
6. Hyman M. The Intermediate Stage of Teaching Alaryngeal Speech. In RL Keith, FL Darley (eds), Laryngectomee Rehabilitation (3rd ed). Austin, TX: PRO-ED, 1994;315.

6

Teaching Esophageal Speech

Of those laryngectomees who attempt to learn esophageal speech, as many as 60% fail to acquire functional esophageal speech [1, 2] (see Chapter 3, "Disadvantages of Esophageal Speech"). Improper training is listed among the reasons for failure to learn esophageal speech [3]. The competence and effectiveness of the alaryngeal speech rehabilitation team has a direct effect on the laryngectomee's acquisition of esophageal speech. For most laryngectomees, learning esophageal speech requires a substantial time commitment [4, 5]. Therapy to learn esophageal speech challenges the laryngectomee to acquire esophageal quality of voicing using the various methods of air intake, improve articulatory precision, increase duration of utterances, manipulate pitch using intonation and stress, and develop appropriate rate and phrasing [6]. Esophageal speech training should be approached in an organized and sequential manner with clearly delineated goals [7].

REVIEW OF LITERATURE SUPPORTING AN ESOPHAGEAL TRAINING HIERARCHY

Snidecor [7] outlines a nine-stage sequence for acquiring esophageal speech, suggesting the laryngectomee first learn to move the air in and out of the esophagus using "easy" vowels such as /ɑ/, /i/, and /o/. The initial stimuli are limited to plosives plus vowels (e.g., "tea") followed by functional, one-syllable words (e.g., "one" and "yes"). Two-syllable words are spoken in the fourth step. The laryngectomee progresses from producing one syllable per injection to producing two syllables per injection. Next, the laryngectomee receives audio feedback for simple three- to four-syllable phrases (e.g., "It costs too much"). At this stage, phrasing and articulatory precision are emphasized, but loudness is deferred to later stages. Snidecor constructs a hierarchy for articulation practice beginning with unvoiced consonants and advancing to contrastive drills (e.g., /bɪt/ versus /bit/). The last three stages of the hierarchy address stress using changes in pitch and loudness, reading aloud followed by active conversation, and efforts to increase rate of speaking. Cognizant of the need to compensate for disadvantages of pitch and loudness in esophageal speech, Snidecor suggests the laryngectomee stand closer to the listener in conditions of noise, hold the telephone against the lips, identify oneself as female (as appropriate) on the telephone to avoid gender confusion, and help a hearing-impaired spouse obtain a hearing aid.

Diedrich and Youngstrom [8] begin esophageal speech training by teaching the consonant method of injection: unvoiced plosives /p/, /t/, /k/, fricatives /s/ and /ʃ/, and affricate /tʃ/ are produced in consonant-vowel (CV) arrangements. Next, the inhalation method is introduced for phonation of the low-back vowel /ɑ/. The third method of air intake follows—injection using tongue pumping. Within the first few steps of therapy, the laryngectomee is introduced to the injection method for obstruents, the inhalation method, and the injection method for sonorants and vowels. Once satisfied that the laryngectomee has achieved the three methods of air intake, Diedrich and Youngstrom move into stage two, "developing efficient and intelligible speech." While practicing one-syllable words beginning with obstruents, the clinician and the laryngectomee monitor for secondary characteristics—for example, stoma noise, extraneous facial movements, and klunking (an extraneous noise that may occur during tongue pumping as air enters the hypopharynx or esophagus; a result of too much air being taken in too fast and with too much muscular tension [8]). Diedrich and Youngstrom advise against moving up the hierarchy to polysyllabic words and phrases too quickly; their emphasis is on control and stabilization at each level. The next level of stimuli includes one-syllable words beginning with sonorants, vowels, and voiced obstruents. The laryngectomee learns to blend two-syllable words and phrases using obstruents to facilitate air intake. The ability to prolong vowels is indicative of increased duration of phonation and means the laryngectomee has greater control of the air returning from the esophagus. At the three- to five-syllable level, the laryngectomee first reads passages aloud with attention to the elements of phrasing, sound blending, rate, inflection, stress, and articulation. Next, the laryngectomee produces short, spontaneous phrases and sentences in conversation. In the final stages of therapy, loudness is addressed. If loudness is attempted prematurely, inappropriate secondary behaviors frequently occur (e.g., stoma noise, increased muscle tension, and overarticulation). Digital pressure against the neck (site of the neoglottis), increased oral opening, and contraction of the abdominal muscles assist loudness. Pitch variation and inflection are practiced using emotional utterances.

Gardner [9] suggests teaching esophageal speech in phases. The stimuli of choice for initiating esophageal speech are the unvoiced plosive consonants and the fricative /s/. Instruction for the second type of injection, the tongue pump, is followed by introduction of the inhalation method. Regardless of the method of air intake, Gardner suggests frequent use of plosives to enhance speech production. Multiple productions of consonant-vowel-consonant (CVC) words using the unvoiced plosives in the initial position are encouraged. There is a consonant-by-consonant progression through two-syllable words with an unvoiced obstruent as the initiator of the second syllable (e.g., /kɪti/, /bækəp/, /dɪʃɛz/).

Injection using tongue pumping and the inhalation method is started using the vowel /ɑ/ and quickly advances to all vowels, including diphthongs.

The laryngectomee is encouraged to alternate syllable combinations (/pɑt-paɪ/) and prolong vowels to gain control of expelled air. Two-syllable words are expanded to include voiced plosives and fricatives and the affricate /dʒ/. Short phrases are introduced, and the semivowels /l/, /r/, /m/, and /ŋ/ and consonants /f/, /v/, /θ/, /ð/, /w/, and /hw/ are added. Gardner pushes for greater fluency and control of expelled air by having the laryngectomee practice polysyllabic words without plosives. Rate, melody, pitch range, inflection, and loudness are addressed in longer phrases and sentences. To achieve overall intelligibility, articulation is emphasized during vowel and consonant contrasts (e.g., /bɪt/ versus /bit/; /paɪ/ versus /baɪ/) and in final consonants (e.g., /gold/, not /gold-ə/ or /gol/). Later, in sentences, the laryngectomee practices fine distinctions in articulation (e.g., "I can say /maɪ/" versus "I can say /baɪ/").

For the laryngectomee who has acquired consistency of esophageal voicing, Hyman [10] advocates syllable drills using plosives and sibilants in CVC arrangements to enhance injection of air into the esophagus. One-syllable drills lead to multiple productions of the syllable (up to five repetitions), but Hyman cautions against pushing the laryngectomee beyond his or her capabilities.

During the syllable drills, the laryngectomee is expected to vary duration, intonation, and loudness of the syllables. Next on the hierarchy are words containing plosive and sibilant sounds in a variety of positions. A few words that begin with vowels or other consonants are introduced. The repertoire is expanded to polysyllabic words and phrases that begin with plosives and sibilants. Gradually, stimulus words and phrases that begin with vowels and other consonants are added. Finally, articulatory precision for nasals, fricatives, consonant clusters, the glottal /h/, and final consonants are addressed.

TARGETING UNVOICED AND VOICED OBSTRUENTS

For esophageal speech production of obstruents (i.e., plosives, fricatives, and affricates), intraoral and pharyngeal air is compressed by movements of the tongue (and sometimes the lips) [8]. The high intraoral air pressure involved in producing certain unvoiced obstruents (e.g., /p/, /t/, /k/, /s/, /ʃ/, and /tʃ/) and /s/ blends (e.g., /sp/, /st/, /sk/) is particularly effective for injecting air into the esophagus to provide voicing for the succeeding vowel [8, 11–14]. Diedrich and Youngstrom [8] noted that air injection from obstruents occurs in the initial (releasing) position of the syllable, not the final (arresting) position [8]. For example, air is not injected into the esophagus during the production of /k/ in the single word /stæk/. In connected speech, however, the laryngectomee may benefit from the effects of coarticulation in which one sound influences the adjacent sound. For example, in the production of /stækɪtʌp/, it is possible to inject air during the obstruents /st/, /k/, and /t/, resulting in voicing of the vowels /æ/, /ɪ/, and /ʌ/.

Air intake is apparently more difficult for voiced than unvoiced obstruents [12] because air must fill the esophageal reservoir for voicing at the same time that additional air is being compressed within the intraoral and pharyngeal cavities. The result is simultaneous explosion of the voiced consonant at the lips accompanied by esophageal phonation [8]. The laryngectomee can achieve more repetitions of CV syllables using unvoiced plosives and sibilants than he or she can using the voiced cognates (e.g., /b/ and /d/) or sonorants (e.g., /l/ and /m/) [15].

Sacco et al. [16] studied listener ratings of intelligibility of esophageal speech using perceptual confusion matrices. They found that voiced consonants were perceived correctly 76% of the time and unvoiced consonants were interpreted accurately only 60% of the time. Intelligibility ratings for unvoiced consonants decreased further when spoken during competing noise [17]. The pharyngoesophageal (PE) segment is the vibrator in esophageal speech. The PE musculature is incapable of the valving maneuvers accomplished by the vocal folds for making voiced-voiceless distinctions. Regardless of the speaker's intent, the consonant production is likely to be voiced when the PE segment has been excited by the returning air from the esophagus.

DETERMINING A VOWEL HIERARCHY

Some clinicians have recommended using certain vowels to facilitate esophageal speech acquisition. The low-back vowel /ɑ/ is often mentioned because the tongue is positioned low and in the back of the mouth in a "resting" position [8, 10]. Duguay [13] refers to use of /e/, /ɛ/, /ʌ/, /ɑ/, /ɔ/, /aɪ/, and /ɪ/ in early esophageal speech instruction. With the exception of /aɪ/ and /ɪ/, the height of the tongue is at mid or low positions in the mouth during the production of these vowels [18]. If the laryngectomee is having difficulty expelling air using the inhalation method, Duguay suggests manipulating lingual tension by experimenting with front, mid, and back vowel singletons or vowel-consonant combinations.

ORDER OF TEACHING ESOPHAGEAL SPEECH METHODS

The laryngectomee learning esophageal speech is introduced to and encouraged to try all three methods of moving air into the esophagus for vibration of the PE segment [7, 8, 9, 13, 14, 19]. As mentioned in Chapter 3 in "The Injection Method for Sonorants and Vowels," the laryngectomee cannot rely solely on the injection method for obstruents because all words do not begin with a plosive, fricative, or affricate. Words also begin with sonorants and vowels. To be a proficient user of the injection method, the laryngectomee must learn both the injection method for obstruents and the injection method for sonorants and vowels. The inhalation method enables the laryngectomee to get air into the esophagus to produce sonorants and vowels. In addition, the laryngectomee benefits from obstruents in the flow of speech. The physical contacts made in the production of obstruents injects air into the esophagus, increasing phonation time [4].

None of the methods of air intake is superior to the other [8]; either the injection method or the inhalation method may be introduced to the laryngectomee first [14]. Flexibility in the rehabilitation process is the key: If the laryngectomee is having difficulty achieving esophageal sound using one method, try another [9]. Some laryngectomees learn the inhalation method more readily than the injection methods, and some laryngectomees develop a preference for one method over the other. Snidecor [7] suggested that the superior esophageal speakers in his study used a combination of air intake methods during connected speech. Further, he observed that the dominant method of air intake varied among individual speakers.

GETTING STARTED

Esophageal speech training may begin as soon as the nasogastric tube has been removed and the physician has determined the laryngectomee does not have a fistula or any other condition with the potential to interfere with air intake [13].

The artificial larynx should have been introduced during pre-operative counseling or immediately after surgery [13]. Instruction and practice with the artificial larynx provide the laryngectomee an immediate and viable means of communication with family, hospital personnel, and the community [9]. Use of the artificial larynx tends to reduce the sense of time pressure to achieve esophageal speech as the primary method of communication [9].

The clinician should review pre- and postoperative anatomy of the oral-pharyngeal-esophageal structures with the laryngectomee (see Figure 1.1), identifying the specific structures involved in esophageal speech: the lips, tongue, hard and soft palates, pharynx, PE segment, and esophagus. At rest, the esophagus resembles a deflated balloon; during esophageal speech, the esophagus becomes an air reservoir. There are multiple methods for forcing (or sucking) air into the deflated esophagus. To successfully return air trapped in the esophagus to the oral cavity, certain conditions must exist: air pressure within the esophagus, tonus and elasticity of the esophageal walls, relaxation of the PE segment, and tension and contraction of both thoracic and abdominal muscles [13]. As air exits the esophagus, the PE segment is vibrated, producing a tone [8, 13]. The tone is resonated in the oral cavity and formed into speech sounds by movements of the lips and tongue.

While conducting the intake history or baseline evaluation, the clinician should note any sounds that are "voiced" as the laryngectomee mouths answers. The laryngectomee should be asked to recall any sounds or words voiced during whispering or speech attempts at home. If spontaneous productions have occurred, the speech-language pathologist (SLP) should request a demonstration or a description of how the sounds were produced. These spontaneous productions contain key sounds—usually one or more of the obstruents (i.e., plosives, fricatives, and affricates)—and may serve as facilitators in early esophageal speech training.

Is the laryngectomee able to inject air into and expel air from the esophagus voluntarily? If so, the clinician should request a demonstration. The sensation of fullness in the PE segment should be reinforced. Natural eructation is usually loud, short in duration, and uncontrolled. The ability to eruct, a behavior normally associated with eating, is a favorable prognostic sign for learning the inhalation method of esophageal speech. Belching, however, is generally regarded as a socially unacceptable behavior, so the use of the terms *belch* or *burp* should be avoided. With instruction, time, and practice, the laryngectomee learns to control and prolong the expelled air for the successful production of multiple syllables.

As instruction for the esophageal speech methods begins, a few general suggestions are in order:

1. The clinician should consider the cognitive and educational levels of the laryngectomee when providing esophageal speech instruction. For the session to be successful, the selection of vocabulary, the complexity of instructions, and the redundancy of information must be congruent with the intellectual abilities of the laryngectomee. Visual aids should be used to explain new terms. Instructions should be simple, stepwise, and direct. The SLP should be willing to repeat directions or to present information in a different way.

2. Visual, auditory, and tactile feedback should be included during every session. The SLP should use illustrations of the postlaryngectomy anatomy (e.g., the Postlaryngectomy Training Aid Set [InHealth Technologies, Carpinteria, CA]) or original sketches. Instructions and word lists for home practice should be written out. The clinician should demonstrate observations of the laryngectomee's behaviors (e.g., devoicing of the final consonant in words: "I hear /bɪt/ not /bɪd/") and provide audio- and videotape analysis of their productions. The laryngectomee's fingers should be placed in front of his or her mouth during the production of the plosive /p/ to monitor the exploded air. The SLP should ask the laryngectomee to think about the sensation of fullness in the neck (PE segment) during air intake.

3. After successful productions, the clinician should encourage the laryngectomee to describe the movements and use these descriptors in future instructions. Phrases generated by the laryngectomee, such as "rolled the air back with my tongue," "squeezed the air into my throat," or "popped the sound out," become facilitators for future productions.

4. The SLP should instruct the laryngectomee that the thoracic muscles surrounding the esophagus and the abdominal muscles are contracted during air expulsion. Relaxed air intake and speech productions—for example, "easy in, easy out"—should be encouraged. The SLP should de-emphasize loudness because deep inhalations coupled with forceful contraction of the abdominal muscles frequently result in stoma noise, a noisy blast of air from the stoma (see "Excessive Stoma Noise"). Not only is stoma noise distracting to the listener, but

the respiratory overexertion results in fatigue [7]. Using imagery, Shanks [20] advises laryngectomees to "turn down your fan" in reference to the stoma noise resulting from pushing the abdominal muscles in an effort to increase loudness.

5. In the early stages of learning the injection or inhalation methods of esophageal speech, the laryngectomee does not always have controlled timing of the air charge. Air then travels down the esophagus into the stomach instead of returning to the oral cavity. As a consequence, bloating frequently occurs after multiple attempts at air intake. The laryngectomee can avoid discomfort by engaging in short rather than prolonged practice sessions and refraining from eating immediately before esophageal speech practice.

The discussion in this chapter begins with specific teaching methods for the injection method for obstruents. Detailed instructions for teaching the injection method for sonorants and vowels are followed by a description of the inhalation method. Once all three methods have been introduced and the laryngectomee has reached a predetermined level of competence, the clinician is ready to combine esophageal speech methods to achieve a higher level of proficiency. Combining esophageal speech methods allows the laryngectomee to expand the length of utterance to longer phrases, sentences, oral reading of passages, structured conversation, and ultimately, spontaneous and extended conversation.

TEACHING ESOPHAGEAL SPEECH: INJECTION METHOD FOR OBSTRUENTS

The injection method for obstruents, by definition, uses plosives, fricatives, and affricates to facilitate the movement of air from the oropharyngeal cavity into the esophagus for the production of speech. The laryngectomee is asked to produce the syllable /pɑ/, making tight contact with the lips for the /p/ and opening the mouth for the /ɑ/. During the production of the obstruent, positive air pressure builds behind the point of articulatory contact in the oral cavity. The strength of lip and tongue movements literally compresses the air within the oropharyngeal cavities, forcing it through the closed PE segment into the esophagus. Tightening the thoracic and abdominal muscles returns the air to the oral cavity, vibrating the PE segment and creating sound.

Stimuli: Using a Restricted Phonetic Context with Increasing Length of Production

Using a hierarchical approach to teach the obstruent method of injection involves careful consideration of the composition of practice stimuli and the length of productions.

To increase the probability of success using the injection method for obstruents, a hierarchy of sounds has been established. Not all obstruents are equal in their ease of production; previous researchers and clinicians report that unvoiced obstruents are easier to produce than their voiced counterparts [12,

15]. Vowels produced with mid or low tongue position in the mouth are considered easier to produce than vowels produced with higher and more frontal tongue positions [8, 10, 13]. This information is important to consider when determining the hierarchy of therapy activities for the laryngectomee who is learning the obstruent method of injection.

Also to be considered is the length of utterance. In the early stages of esophageal speech training, the laryngectomee learns to control the air returning from the esophagus and, in time, to prolong the exiting air to accommodate voicing for adjacent syllables. For this reason, the hierarchy for the length of utterance begins with one-syllable words and advances to two syllables, then to three to four syllables, and finally to five- to six-syllable words and phrases.

All practice stimuli for the injection method for obstruents in esophageal speech are found in Appendix F. There are 10 levels of stimuli arranged according to a hierarchy of restricted phonetic context and the length of utterance.

Level I: One-Syllable Words Beginning with Unvoiced Obstruents Plus Mid and Low Vowels

The earliest consonant productions are limited to unvoiced obstruents: unvoiced plosives /p/, /t/, and /k/; unvoiced fricatives /f/, /s/, /ʃ/, /θ/; the unvoiced affricate /tʃ/; the /s/ blends /sp/, /st/, /sk/; and the glottal /h/ as a modified /k/. To facilitate accuracy of production, these obstruents are combined with vowels produced with mid or low tongue position in the mouth. The restricted phonetic context for vowels are the low-back vowel /ɑ/, the mid-back vowels /o/ and /ɔ/, the mid-central vowels /ʌ/ and /ə/, the low-front vowel /æ/, and the mid-front vowels /e/ and /ɛ/. A series of one-syllable words that begin with the unvoiced obstruent plus a mid- or low-back vowel appears in Appendix F, Level I. There are three sets of stimuli for each unvoiced obstruent. The laryngectomee should be directed to practice specific obstruents (e.g., /p/ words). After the sets featuring individual obstruents, there are sets of stimuli using mixed unvoiced obstruents plus mid- or low-back vowels.

Level II: One-Syllable Words Beginning with Unvoiced Obstruents Plus Other Vowels

At Level II, the unvoiced obstruents are combined with the remaining vowels. Produced with higher and more frontal tongue positions, these vowels are the high-back vowels /u/ and /ʊ/; the mid-central semivowel /ɝ/; the high-front vowels /i/ and /ɪ/; and the diphthongs /aɪ/, /aʊ/, and /ɔɪ/. A series of one-syllable words that begin with the unvoiced obstruent plus other vowels is found in Appendix F, Level II. There are lists for practice of specific obstruents (e.g., /t/ words) followed by sets of stimuli using mixed unvoiced obstruents plus other vowels.

Level III: One-Syllable Words Beginning with Voiced Obstruents Plus Mid and Low Vowels

At Level III, voiced obstruents are introduced: the voiced plosives /b/, /d/, and /g/; the voiced fricatives /v/, /z/, and /ð/; and the voiced affricate /dʒ/. Because voiced obstruents are considered more difficult to produce than unvoiced obstruents, mid- and low-back vowels are used to facilitate production. Practice lists for the individual obstruents precede the mixed voiced obstruent lists.

Level IV: One-Syllable Words Beginning
with Voiced Obstruents Plus Other Vowels

At Level IV of one-syllable productions, voiced obstruents are combined with vowels made with high or frontal tongue positions. Lists of mixed voiced obstruents plus other vowels follow lists of the individual voiced obstruent plus other vowels.

Level V: One-Syllable Words Beginning with
Unvoiced and Voiced Obstruent Blends

Advancement to Level V means the laryngectomee can produce one-syllable words initiated with unvoiced or voiced obstruents in combination with all vowels. The final practice activity at the one-syllable level of production uses mixed unvoiced and voiced obstruent blends combined with unrestricted vowels.

As previously discussed in "Review of Literature Supporting Esophageal Training Hierarchy," Diedrich and Youngstrom [8] noted that the esophageal speaker benefits from the placement of an obstruent in the releasing position of syllables. They also found that the coarticulatory effects of connected speech enabled the laryngectomee to inject air on obstruents distributed throughout the utterance. Consonants occur in the releasing and arresting positions of syllables—for example, in the word /sæt/, /s/ serves as the releaser of the syllable and /t/ is the arrester of the syllable [21]. When two or more syllables are phrased together in an utterance, their production becomes, in essence, one continuous word, with the arresting syllable of one word sometimes serving as the releaser of the following word. For example, in the utterance /stekaʊt/, /k/ arrests the first syllable and releases the second syllable. In this situation, /k/ is thought of as a double consonant because it serves two functions: It arrests the first syllable and releases the second syllable. In /stekaʊt/, air injected on the /k/ provides voicing for the diphthong /aʊ/.

Level VI: Two-Syllable Words and Phrases:
Unvoiced Obstruents

To facilitate accuracy of production at Level VI of the two-syllable level, the releasing consonant for both syllables is an unvoiced obstruent. Three practice sets for each unvoiced consonant are followed by 27 sets of mixed unvoiced consonant stimuli.

Level VII: Two-Syllable Words and Phrases:
Unvoiced and Voiced Obstruents

To increase the level of difficulty, two-syllable words with an unvoiced obstruent releasing the first syllable and a voiced obstruent releasing the second syllable are presented. Again, the laryngectomee can practice sets featuring individual unvoiced obstruents and then practice mixed sets of unvoiced plus voiced obstruent arrangements.

Level VIII: Two-Syllable Words and Phrases: Voiced Obstruents

The final activity at the two-syllable level uses voiced obstruents in the releasing position of both syllables. Specific practice for individual voiced obstruents (e.g., /b/) precedes sets of mixed voiced obstruent arrangements.

Level IX: Three- to Four-Syllable Phrases and Sentences with
Unvoiced and Voiced Obstruents in the Releasing Positions

The laryngectomee who has completed therapy activities through the two-syllable level of production has a strong foundation for practicing the injection method for obstruents. Once the laryngectomee has mastered production of unvoiced and voiced obstruents in combination with all the vowels at the two-syllable level, it is no longer expedient to separate the unvoiced-voiced components. The clinician should model the three- to four-syllable phrases and sentences for the laryngectomee in a way that emphasizes the coarticulatory effects of connected speech. The phrase "quick and easy" must be said as one continuous utterance, /kwɪkændizi/, so that the /k/ in "quick" releases the second syllable word "and," and the /d/ in "and" releases the third syllable in "easy."

Level X: Five- to Six-Syllable Phrases and Sentences with
Unvoiced and Voiced Obstruents in the Releasing Positions

As in the previous polysyllabic word lists, the obstruents in Level X are located strategically in the releasing positions of syllables to enable the laryngectomee to inject air and increase the perceived duration of the utterance. For example, the laryngectomee who uses the injection method for obstruents exclusively has a much better chance of producing the utterance /sɪkaʊtgʊdkʌmpənɪ/ than the utterance /winuwiwɜ˞ɜ˞li/. Careful examination of the first sentence reveals the opportunity to inject air for /s/ and /k/ in "seek," /g/ in "good," and /k/ and /p/ in "company." There are no obstruents in the second utterance—"we knew we were early"—leaving the laryngectomee without a method of injecting air. For this reason, the laryngectomee is encouraged to learn the injection method for sonorants and vowels or the inhalation method.

TEACHING ESOPHAGEAL SPEECH: INJECTION METHOD FOR SONORANTS AND VOWELS

The success of the injection method for obstruents depends on the occurrence of obstruents throughout the utterance. Air intake is simultaneous with the obstruent production. The injection method for sonorants and vowels does not rely on specific consonants to move intraoral air into the esophagus. Rather, lingual movements compress the intraoral air, injecting the air into the esophagus *before* speech production. Within the alaryngeal speech literature, the injection method for sonorants and vowels has several names: glossopharyngeal press, tongue pump, and glossal press [8, 14, 19].

During the injection method for vowels and sonorants, a seal is formed with the lips or tongue and the air in the oral cavity is pressed into the posterior portion of the pharynx, through the PE segment, and into the esophagus (Figure 6.1). In some individuals, air trapped by the tongue is forced posteriorly as the tongue is flattened against the hard and soft palates. Other esophageal speakers use an anterior-to-posterior rocking motion of the tongue to sweep air back. In either case, tongue action compresses air within the oral cavity and, combined with contraction of the pharyngeal walls, increases the air pressure in the hypopharynx. Adequate velopharyngeal closure is required to prevent nasal air escape.

Air return to the oral cavity is based on several factors. Increased air pressure within the esophagus (which is due to the elasticity of the normally deflated esophageal walls, positive air pressure in the thoracic cavity, diaphragmatic tension, air pressure in the stomach, and abdominal muscle contractions) overcomes the resistance of the PE segment, returning the air to the oral cavity and vibrating the PE segment [19].

Sequence and timing of labial and lingual movements are two important components for mastery of the injection method for sonorants and vowels. There are several ways to move air posteriorly and into the PE segment. The SLP should find the combination that is most successful for the individual laryngectomee. Step-by-step instructions are provided for four possible combinations.

Combination One: Lip Seal, Tongue Pump

1. Capture the ball of air in the middle of the mouth, and hold it against the hard palate with the tongue (or place the tongue in the position to make a /t/ and hold the tip and sides of the tongue firmly against the roof of the mouth).

2. Close the lips tightly.

3. Press the tongue against the hard palate and pump the ball of air out the back of the tongue into the throat.

4. As you feel the ball of air "go down" into your neck, quickly but gently push the air back up.

5. Open your mouth and say /ɑ/.

Combination Two: Lip Seal, Tongue Sweep

1. Capture the ball of air in the middle of the mouth and hold it against the hard palate with the tongue (or place the tongue in the position to make a /t/ and hold the tip and sides of the tongue firmly against the roof of the mouth).

2. Close the lips tightly.

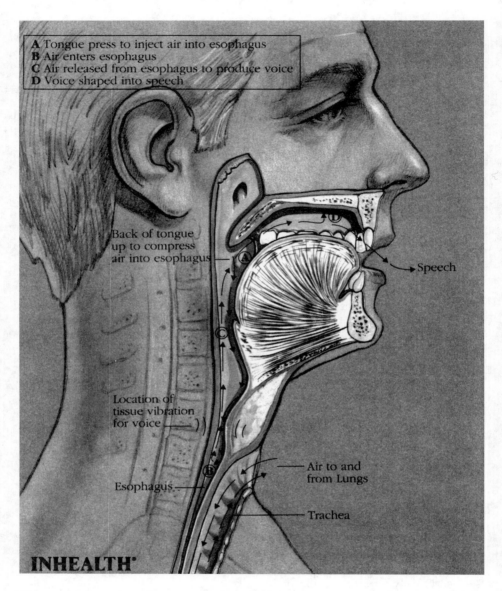

Figure 6.1 During the injection method for sonorants and vowels, tongue action combined with contraction of the pharyngeal cavity forces air into the esophagus. Return of the air vibrates the pharyngoesophageal segment to produce voice. The articulators shape the tone into speech. (Reprinted with permission of InHealth Technologies. Postlaryngectomy Training Aid Set. Carpinteria, CA: InHealth Technologies, 1995.)

3. With an anterior-to-posterior rocking motion, "roll" or sweep the ball of air back into the throat as far as you can *without* swallowing.

4. As you feel the ball of air "go down" into your neck, quickly but gently push the air back up.

5. Open your mouth and say /ɑ/.

Combination Three: No Lip Seal, Tongue Pump

1. Capture the ball of air in the middle of the mouth and hold it against the hard palate with the tongue (or place the tongue in the position to make a /t/ and hold the tip and sides of the tongue firmly against the roof of the mouth).

2. Press the tongue against the hard palate and pump the ball of air out the back of the tongue into the throat.

3. As you feel the ball of air "go down" into your neck, quickly but gently push the air back up.

4. Open your mouth and say /ɑ/.

Combination Four: No Lip Seal, Tongue Sweep

1. Capture the ball of air in the middle of the mouth and hold it against the hard palate with the tongue (or place the tongue in the position to make a /t/ and hold the tip and sides of the tongue firmly against the roof of the mouth).

2. With an anterior-to-posterior rocking motion, "roll" or sweep the ball of air back into the throat as far as you can *without* swallowing.

3. As you feel the ball of air "go down" into your neck, quickly but gently push the air back up.

4. Open your mouth and say /ɑ/.

Numerous practice tries will probably occur before the laryngectomee successfully produces /ɑ/. The SLP should be prepared to reinforce each step in terms of correct placement and sequence.

Stimuli: Using a Restricted Phonetic Context with Increasing Length of Production

The presence of an obstruent in a stimulus word assists air intake using a consonant type of injection. To avoid confusion about which method of air intake the laryngectomee is using, no obstruents appear in the stimuli lists for the injection method for sonorants and vowels. A hierarchical sequence of vowels and sonorants is used throughout the practice materials for learning the injection method for sonorants and vowels. Only mid and low vowels are used in the first level of the activity hierarchy because a lowered tongue position facilitates the return of air into the oral cavity [12, 15]. As in the injection method for obstruents, the beginning level of production is one-syllable words. The length of stimuli advances to two syllables, then to three and four syllables, and finally to five- and six-syllable words and phrases.

All practice stimuli for the injection method for sonorants and vowels in esophageal speech are found in Appendix G. There are seven levels of stimuli arranged according to a hierarchy of restricted phonetic context and the length of utterance.

Level I: One-Syllable Words Beginning with Mid and Low Vowels

The beginning level stimuli are composed of one-syllable words beginning with a restricted phonetic context of vowels: the low-back vowel /ɑ/; the mid-back vowels /o/ and /ɔ/; the mid-central vowels /ʌ/ and /ə/; the low-front vowel /æ/; and the mid-front vowels /e/ and /ɛ/. Practice sets of 10 stimuli each appear in Appendix G, Level 1.

Level II: One-Syllable Words Beginning with Other Vowels

Practice sets of one-syllable words beginning with the remaining vowels are introduced, including the high back vowels /u/ and /ʊ/; the mid-central semivowel /ɝ/; the high-front vowels /i/ and /ɪ/; and the diphthongs /aɪ/, /aʊ/, and /ɔɪ/.

Level III: One-Syllable Words Beginning with Sonorants Plus Mid and Low Vowels

At Level III of the stimulus hierarchy, the sonorants /w/, /l/, /r/, /j/, /m/, and /n/ are used in the releasing position of one-syllable words coupled with mid and low vowels. Practice lists for the individual sonorants precede the mixed sonorant lists.

Level IV: One-Syllable Words Beginning with Sonorants Plus Other Vowels

At Level IV, the sonorant consonants are combined with vowels made with high or frontal tongue positions. Following the sets featuring individual sonorants, there are sets of stimuli using mixed sonorant obstruents plus other vowels.

Level V: Two-Syllable Words Beginning with Sonorants and Vowels

Once the laryngectomee has mastered the injection method for sonorants and vowels at the one-syllable level, any combination of sonorants and vowels may be used. From the two-syllable level on, the laryngectomee is practicing control of the injected air and learning to increase the number of syllables per air charge.

Levels VI and VII: Polysyllabic Phrases and Sentences with Sonorants and Vowels

Note that as in previous stimuli lists, no obstruents occur to assist the laryngectomee in "loading" air (injection method for obstruents). As the number of syllables in the utterance increases, the laryngectomee's ability to prolong the exiting air charge is challenged. The number of syllables that can be voiced with one air charge is limited by the capacity of the esophageal reservoir. Berlin [22] suggests that *latency* is a better indicator of proficient esophageal speech than number-of-syllables-per-air charge. *Latency* is defined two ways: (1) the amount of time between the command to inject and the injection (preparatory latency), and (2) the amount of time between the injection and voicing (production latency). According to Berlin [22], laryngectomees who are rated as good speakers have production latencies of 0.5 second or less. Therapy time is better spent developing the laryngectomee's ability to frequently and efficiently re-inflate the esophagus while maintaining smoothness and continuity of connected speech than striving to increase the number of syllables said on one injection.

TEACHING ESOPHAGEAL SPEECH: INHALATION METHOD

Both methods of injection use labial and lingual movements to inject or force air from the oral cavity through the PE segment into the esophagus. In the inhalation method, a vacuum effect is created within the esophagus and, rather than being forced, oral air is literally sucked into the esophagus through the PE segment.

The clinician should offer a variety of instructions to the laryngectomee to assist him or her in drawing air into the esophagus. Common to all instructions is the idea that the breath intake must be swift and the oropharyngeal region open. One suggestion is to have the laryngectomee, with the lips slightly apart, take in a quick breath through the stoma, as if gasping or surprised. Another instruction has the laryngectomee take in a breath through the stoma, filling the lungs approximately halfway. Then the stoma is covered with the fingers, and a quick breath is attempted. Diedrich and Youngstrom [8] use the descriptors *sniffing air, sucking air*, and *yawning* to create imagery of fast air intake with pharyngeal openness.

Salmon [14] explains the purpose of a quick inhalation accompanied by an open airway between the PE segment and the oral and nasal cavities. Short, rapid inhalation sharply increases the negative pressure within the thoracic cavity, virtually doubling the already negative pressure within the esophagus. The atmospheric air pressure within the oral and nasal cavities is positive in relation to the negative air pressure within the upper esophagus. Air under positive pressure in the oral and nasal cavities will move toward the esophagus, an area of negative pressure, to equalize the pressure in both areas. The instructions to quickly breathe in, sniff, or yawn have the benefit of relaxing the oropharyngeal and esophageal musculature and distending the passageway—all conducive to moving air from oral and nasal cavities into the upper esophagus.

As air is drawn into the esophagus through the PE segment, the SLP can feel a slight movement by placing the fingertips (or better, the laryngectomee's fingertips) against the side of the laryngectomee's neck. In quiet surroundings, the "click" produced by the suction of the air through the closed PE segment is audible. Once air is trapped in the upper esophagus, the laryngectomee reacts by producing the vowel /ɑ/. Some expiratory effort is required, including use of the abdominal muscles; however, the idea is to tighten the muscles, not to exhale forcibly. Forceful exhalation is not beneficial to expelling the air trapped in the esophagus; instead, the air in the lungs exits the stoma with a loud and distracting stoma blast.

Both the injection method for sonorants and vowels and the inhalation method move air into the upper esophagus before speech production. Neither method depends on specific consonant productions to facilitate air intake. The inhalation method differs from the injection method for sonorants and vowels in that the inhalation method does not use labial or lingual movements for air intake; in fact, during the inhalation method, the tongue is in a lowered position in the mouth to maintain oropharyngeal openness. The injection method *forces* air through the PE segment and the inhalation method *draws* air through the PE segment. Regardless of the method, once the air is within the upper esophagus, instructions for air expulsion are the same.

To avoid confusion as to whether an obstruent within the stimulus is facilitating air intake, no obstruents appear in the stimuli lists for the inhalation method. The practice stimuli for the inhalation method are restricted to sonorants and vowels. A hierarchical sequence of vowels and sonorants is used throughout the practice materials for learning the inhalation method. Only mid and low vowels are used in the first level of the activity hierarchy because in the inhalation method, a lowered tongue position facilitates the return of air into the oral cavity. The hierarchy for the length of utterance begins with one-syllable words, followed by two syllables, three and four syllables, and five- to six-syllable words and phrases.

All practice stimuli for the inhalation method are found in Appendix G. There are seven levels of stimuli arranged according to a hierarchy of restricted phonetic context and length of utterance. The practice stimuli for the inhalation method are the same stimuli used for the injection method for sonorants and vowels.

ESTABLISHING GOALS FOR TEACHING ALL METHODS OF ESOPHAGEAL SPEECH

Although the methods of moving air into the esophagus are very different, once the air is returned from the esophagus, the speech production goals and the design of practice stimuli for each method parallel one another. All three methods of air intake for esophageal speech—the injection method for obstruents, the injection method for sonorants and vowels, and the inhalation method—share mutual goals. Goals for teaching esophageal speech are divided into two categories: voicing and intelligibility. *Voicing* goals are concerned with the laryngectomee's ability to move air into the esophagus, return the air to the oral cavity, and produce esophageal quality voicing—all in a timely manner. The goals of voicing are the following: esophageal quality of voicing, consistency of voicing, and latency. Once esophageal voicing is achieved, *intelligibility* of the production is addressed in terms of articulatory precision, an appropriate rate, and attention to nonverbal behaviors associated with speaking. Each of the goals for achieving proficient esophageal speech is discussed in the following section, along with suggestions for teaching each skill, providing feedback, and solving problematic behaviors that may occur. The information provided applies to all methods of esophageal speech unless otherwise noted.

Goal One: Esophageal Quality of Voicing

The laryngectomee is asked to produce the stimulus appropriate to the method of air intake. When the air is successfully injected or inhaled into the upper esophagus, tightening of the thoracic and abdominal musculature returns the air to the oral cavity, vibrating the PE segment and creating sound. The quality of this sound is referred to as *esophageal*.

Pharyngeal Quality: Injection Methods

If the positive air pressure and accompanying compression produced by oral movements are insufficient to overcome the resistance of the PE segment, air does not move into the esophagus, and esophageal quality of voicing does not occur. Damsté [23] reports pharyngeal voice is more often the result of improper practice of the injection method for obstruents. Air is trapped in the hypopharynx (at the base of the tongue) rather than descending to the PE segment. If the air turbulence is sufficient to vibrate the surrounding pharyngeal walls, pharyngeal voicing occurs. Pharyngeal quality voicing is undesirable in that the tone is somewhat higher in pitch, shorter in duration, and lower in volume than esophageal quality speech.

Illustrations should be used to show the laryngectomee where the injected air is supposed to go. The laryngectomee should place his or her hand against the side of the neck at the approximate site of the PE segment to understand how far down the air has to be moved. Relaxation exercises (see Appendix B) should be used to reduce tension in the shoulders, neck, and jaw. The laryngectomee should visualize the openness in the throat produced during chewing or yawning. He or she should use a vowel that encourages openness of the throat (e.g., /ɑ/, /aʊ/, or /ɔ/). For the injection method for obstruents, an obstruent is used to release one of these vowels. Although the laryngectomee's lips are pressed tightly together for the production of /p/, the pharyngeal area should be open and relaxed. The laryngectomee frequently responds to the suggestion to say the vowel in a "low pitch" by lowering the chin and expanding the oropharyngeal area.

Pharyngeal Quality: Inhalation Method

Pharyngeal quality voicing is not as common an occurrence for the inhalation method because the teaching instructions encourage oropharyngeal openness. If the production is of pharyngeal quality, the laryngectomee should be reminded to breathe in quickly, sniff the air, or mimic a yawn. These techniques may assist in the reduction of tension in the muscles adjacent to the PE segment, allowing air to move easily through the PE segment into the esophagus.

Goal Two: Consistency of Voicing

Once the laryngectomee successfully moves air from the oropharyngeal area into the esophagus to vibrate the PE segment, practice is needed to perform the act consistently. Producing esophageal quality speech on demand lies at the core of successful esophageal speech.

Inconsistent or No Voicing

Using visual, auditory, and tactile stimulation, the SLP should review the instructions for the specific method of air intake with the laryngectomee. A relaxed and supportive learning environment should be provided. The clinician should use light humor. Above all, the temptation to move too quickly through the lower levels of production to get to connected speech should be resisted. Ample time should be allowed for the laryngectomee to gain control over the air-in-air-out process.

Injection Method for Obstruents If the laryngectomee is having difficulty moving air back with a certain unvoiced obstruent (e.g., /p/) other unvoiced obstruents should be tried. In the early stages of therapy, voicing of the vowel is more likely to be facilitated when preceded by the unvoiced plosive /p/ or /t/ than by any other obstruent. The laryngectomee may find voicing with some obstruents easier than with others. The specific phoneme practice lists found in Appendix F should be used and therapy activities should be focused on the laryngectomee's key sounds. The laryngectomee should practice repetitions of /pɑ/ or /pʌ/. The laryngectomee should try to facilitate oral air pressure buildup by making two or three productions of /pɑ/ before the word /pɑp/ (i.e., /pɑ-pɑ-pɑp/). If the laryngectomee has poor lingual or labial strength, oral-facial exercises should be used to strengthen and gain better control (see Appendix C). During the production of /pɑ/, the laryngectomee's fingers or a small piece of paper should be placed in front of the lips to detect the percussion. Although mirror practice is an effective tool for visualizing /p/ productions, tactile sensation provides more appropriate feedback for the other obstruents. The /t/ is made by pressing the tip of the tongue firmly against the alveolar ridge and bouncing the tongue away for the /tɑ/. The client should produce /f/ by pressing the upper teeth against lower lip and literally exploding the /fɑ/. He or she should practice /s/, /ʃ/, and /tʃ/ in isolation, using the tongue to move the oral air and create an audible hissing sound; these sounds should then be paired with a low or mid vowel. Consistency of voicing and articulatory precision are interrelated (see "Goal Four: Articulatory Precision").

Injection Method for Sonorants and Vowels The four methods for pumping or sweeping air with the tongue into the oropharynx should be reviewed. The SLP should illustrate the positioning and movements of the tongue against the hard and soft palates with his or her hands: One hand represents the tongue; the other hand represents the hard and soft palates. A very narrow straw should be placed along the length of the laryngectomee's tongue to create the perception of an air-filled groove. Moving of the air back may be likened to sucking through a straw. The laryngectomee should be instructed to hold a Cheerio against the alveolar ridge with the tongue tip while performing a pumping or wave-like action with the remainder of the tongue to facilitate air injection.

Hypotonic Pharynx

Approximately 15% of the individuals who have difficulty consistently moving air into the esophagus using injection methods have very low muscular tension in the pharyngeal walls. When air from the esophagus is returned, the low resistance of the surrounding pharyngeal musculature results in weak or no vibration of the PE segment [24]. If external digital pressure is applied to the anterior portion of the neck at the level of the PE segment, the walls of the pharynx are approximated, the PE segment is vibrated, and voicing occurs [24, 25]. Commercially produced elastic neck bands and varied pressure heads are available so the laryngectomee does not have to keep the hand to the neck during speaking (see Appendix A).

Hypertonic to Spastic Pharynx

Elevated tonicity of the PE segment after total laryngectomy is an important factor in the failure to acquire esophageal voicing [26, 27]. In a radiologic study, McIvor et al. [24] identified narrowing of the pharynx in varying degrees (i.e., hypertonic pharynx, spastic pharynx, or stricture of the pharynx) as the interfering factor in moving oral air into the esophagus in 85% of 134 poor and failed esophageal speakers. Singer et al. [25] observed that elevated pharyngeal wall tension can trap the air intake, forcing the air into the stomach. Singer and Blom [26] reported that dilations, muscle relaxants, anticholinergic drugs, and tranquilizers were ineffective in relieving the tightened PE segment. Surgical myotomy is the treatment of choice for individuals with increased PE tone [24, 25, 26]. Singer et al. [25] suggested the addition of a pharyngeal plexus neurectomy at primary laryngectomy for all laryngectomees. The procedure interrupts the motor reflex for the upper esophageal sphincter closure during esophageal distention, resulting in lower airflow resistances. Singer et al. [23] noted that the neurectomy may accelerate the rate of acquiring esophageal speech and cause a more natural vibratory quality.

Blom et al. [27] suggest routine administration of the esophageal insufflation test to identify individuals who may be at risk for alaryngeal speech failure. In particular, they advise testing laryngectomees who are having difficulty acquiring voice in the early stages of esophageal speech therapy.

Goal Three: Latency

Latency refers to the time taken by the laryngectomee to produce a target utterance. In the early stages of learning esophageal speech—before the actual intake of air—the laryngectomee may engage in extraneous oral-facial behaviors (e.g., pursing the lips, groping for tongue placement, or grimacing). These behaviors delay speech production. Ideally, the interval between the stimulus command and the production of the target behavior should be within one second, regardless of which air intake method is used. Judgments of this type of latency, or timing of productions, are more critical in the beginning phase of teaching esophageal speech when the client is learning how to take in air quickly and smoothly.

In the beginning stages of therapy, the duration of phonation is usually limited to a one-syllable utterance per air charge. With practice, the laryngectomee learns to increase the duration of a single vowel to 2 seconds or more, a behavior conducive to producing longer utterances in connected speech. According to Martin [28], "a duration of 2 seconds or better is pretty good and may be adequate for producing connected speech, especially if the speaker uses multiple methods of air charging."

Delayed Latency Related to Searching
Behaviors: Injection Methods

If the laryngectomee has difficulty finding the best articulatory placement for sound production, the process should be simplified. The clinician should focus on a specific (key) consonant or vowel, and use visual, auditory, and tactile feedback to stimulate the production. Illustrations (e.g., "Your tongue tip goes right here and then you flatten the tongue against the roof of your mouth") or a mirror (e.g., "Watch your mouth as you make the /t/. Your lips are slightly apart and your tongue tip is up.") should be used. Word lists are available that address specific obstruents (see Appendix F) or specific sonorants and vowels (see Appendix G). Once the placement is understood, the theme of the activity is to "make the contact, do the contact, and say the sound" in a smooth, continuous manner without hesitations.

Delayed Latency Related to Searching
Behaviors: Inhalation Method

When teaching the inhalation method, imagery is frequently used—for example, yawning, sucking, or covering the stoma momentarily during inhalation attempts. These techniques are facilitators and should be discarded as soon as the laryngectomee has the idea of inhalation. These behaviors can easily become habituated, resulting in exaggerated oral opening, chin jutting, or noisy or prolonged air intake. The laryngectomee is encouraged to "sniff in and say the sound" in an easy, continuous manner.

Short Latency on Vowels

Early in therapy, lack of control of the air charge usually limits voicing to a one-syllable production. Once consistent voicing of the vowel in single syllables is achieved, the laryngectomee practices elongating the vowels as a warm-up exercise. A series of short words—for example, /pɑp/, /tæp/, /kek/ (injection method for obstruents) or /ʌp/, /ɑn/, /lo/ (injection method for sonorants and vowels or inhalation method)—are used with the instruction, "hold out the vowel as long as you can." A minimum 2-second duration on the vowel is adequate and demonstrates increased control of the air charge.

Goal Four: Articulatory Precision

Vibrating the PE segment provides the voicing portion of the utterance, but the articulators shape the sound into meaningful speech. Intelligibility of esophageal speech relies on articulatory precision. This goal focuses on the accurate production of vowels and consonants with attention to known stumbling blocks in esophageal speech production. Specific target behaviors include making voiced-voiceless consonant distinctions, maintaining the velopharyngeal opening for the production of nasals, and approximating the /h/. The esophageal speaker no longer has the liberty of speaking without attention to the intelligibility of the consonants and vowels.

Using the injection method for obstruents, the lingual and labial contacts for plosives, fricatives, and affricates must be distinct and *slightly* exaggerated. Strong articulatory contacts are required during the production of obstruents to build up intraoral pressure and compression of the air within the oral cavity. With sufficient intraoral air pressure to overcome the resistance of the PE sphincter, air is moved into the esophagus and then returned to the oral cavity.

Imprecise Articulation

The clinician should investigate the laryngectomee's pre- and postoperative speech patterns for foreign accents, regional dialects, dysarthrias, or articulation disorders. As a result of surgical interruption of mandibular and lingual muscle attachments, the laryngectomee almost always experiences a dysarthric component of speech. Oral-facial exercises for the lips, tongue, and jaw (see Appendix C) and articulation drills are used to improve articulatory strength, control, and precision. The reward for the time invested in building a strong foundation of articulatory precision at the one-syllable level is realized fully in more advanced speech activities.

Ill-Fitting Dental Appliances

Ill-fitting dentures separate from the gums during esophageal speech and interfere with articulatory precision. If the use of a denture adhesive is unsuccessful, a referral to the dentist or prosthodontist for adjustment of the dentures is needed.

Hearing Loss

A high-frequency hearing loss can significantly interfere with speech intelligibility by impairing the laryngectomee's ability to receive auditory feedback during speech production. Speech proficiency is at risk, particularly for the fricatives. In the absence of auditory information, the client must rely on visual cues (e.g., mirror feedback) and sensory cues (e.g., the location of the tongue tip against the alveolar ridge for the production of /s/).

Listener Confusion for Voiced-Unvoiced Obstruents

When the injection method for obstruents is used, listeners of esophageal speech frequently perceive the initial obstruents in words as voiced, regardless of the speaker's intent. For example, /paɪ/ is heard as /baɪ/. Sacco et al. [16] found that listener confusion for voiced-unvoiced consonants is related to the length of voicing for the accompanying vowel. The esophageal speaker can enhance listener perception by learning the strategy of producing a shorter vowel with the unvoiced consonant than that produced with the voiced consonant. Obstruent contrast drills are found in Appendix E. There are lists of minimal word pairs using voiced and unvoiced cognates.

Achieving Nasal Resonance for /m/, /n/, and /ŋ/

Injection Method for Sonorants and Vowels   The injection method requires velopharyngeal closure to prevent airflow into the nasal cavity. The consequence is that the laryngectomee frequently continues to maintain velopharyngeal closure during speech, a behavior that is not problematic unless nasals are required. When produced with a closed velopharyngeal segment, the nasals /m/, /n/, and /ŋ/ are denasalized and are perceived by the listener as the plosives /b/, /d/, and /g/, respectively. Specific practice using plosive and nasal contrasts are helpful in restoring good nasal resonance (see Appendix E). The laryngectomee should place several fingers against the nose and hum or, using the injection method for sonorants and vowels, focus on the /m/ and /n/ practice lists found in Appendix G, Levels III and IV.

Inhalation Method   The laryngectomee is encouraged to keep the velopharyngeal port open during the inhalation method to draw air from the nasal as well as the oral cavities into the esophagus. For this reason, denasalization of /m/, /n/, and /ŋ/ is less likely to occur in the inhalation method. If denasalization does occur, the previous suggestions for the injector apply to the inhaler.

Compensating for the Glottal Fricative /h/

In the laryngeal speaker, /h/ is produced by adducting the vocal folds slightly (but not sufficiently to produce vocal fold vibration) and exhaling. Teaching the esophageal production of the glottal fricative /h/ is often ignored because of the loss of the needed airstream from the lungs to the oral cavity. When omitted in esophageal speech, the /h/ is frequently understood within the context of the utterance—for example, "You can 'ave my chair." Substitution of the /h/ with the plosive /k/ using a prolonged but less intense velar contact results in a sound that is similar to the German word *ich* [6]. Further reduction of the physical contact between the tongue and palate creates turbulence that closely resembles the glottal fricative /h/ [10]. (Practice lists for the /h/ at the single syllable level are found in Appendix F, Levels I and II.)

Goal Five: Rate

More important than rate to the intelligibility of esophageal speech is articulatory precision [29]. That said, studies indicate that superior esophageal speakers enjoy a faster speaking rate than do poor esophageal speakers [30, 31]. The mean speaking rate for the superior esophageal speaker is 113 words per minute [32], which is approximately two-thirds the average rate for laryngeal speakers [6]. Defining the parameters of rate for evaluation and teaching purposes is an elusive task. Intelligibility of esophageal speech is a complex mix of rate, articulatory precision, and meaningful phrasing. To selectively speed up or slow down rate without attention to articulation or phrasing almost always has a negative effect on intelligibility [28, 30, 31].

Too Fast Rate

Rate is frequently perceived as "too fast" when the pace the client is using interferes with the intelligibility of the utterance. When the speed of production exceeds the limits of the laryngectomee's muscular control of the articulators or ignores the prosodic elements of phrasing, intelligibility suffers. Articulatory control and appropriate phrasing are prerequisites to increasing one's rate. Specific practice activities for the improvement of articulation are discussed under "Goal Four: Articulation." In longer utterances—for example, four- to five-syllable phrases and sentences—appropriate pausing underscores the meaning and contributes to the listener's comprehension. The clinician or the laryngectomee can mark the target pauses in the stimuli lists before practice. Having the laryngectomee develop a mental image of the listener "taking notes" as he or she speaks may help slow the rate and increase articulatory precision.

Too Slow Rate

Esophageal speakers with too slow a rate are usually perceived as below-average in their speaking ability. In the early stages of therapy in which the laryngectomee is learning to articulate during one- and two-syllable words, rate is not an issue. The target behavior is to use precise articulation and short production latency. With increased control of articulatory precision, the laryngectomee advances into longer phrases and sentences and is expected to blend the syllables into connected speech. Again, articulatory precision and phrasing become important components in the perception of appropriate rate. If the laryngectomee is drawing out the vowels excessively, the SLP should encourage shorter duration on the vowels. If the laryngectomee is producing each syllable individually, the client should practice blending the syllables into one continuous phrase. Pausing occurs only when necessary to renew the air charge or emphasize the meaning of the utterance.

Goal Six: Attention to Nonverbal Behaviors

A goal sometimes slighted in esophageal speech training is the need for the laryngectomee to approximate, as closely as possible, the speech mannerisms of laryngeal speakers. Observation of the model laryngeal speaker quickly reveals the target behaviors: frequent eye contact with listener, accompanying hand gestures, facial expression, variations in loudness and pitch, pauses for emphasis, and interjections, such as "um" or "er." Some laryngectomees spontaneously resume their prelaryngectomy speech behaviors; other laryngectomees benefit from instruction and practice in using such mannerisms.

Not infrequently, the laryngectomee engages in behaviors that detract from or interfere with effective esophageal communication. Among these mannerisms are multiple injections or inhalations, excessive stoma noise, loss of eye contact, extraneous head movements, facial grimacing, and klunking. All of these behaviors are related to excessive tension during air injection or inhalation. Excessive muscle tension sabotages fluent, easily produced esophageal speech. The potential for these behaviors to become habitual, and thus resistant to intervention, is high. If identified and addressed early in therapy, these problems can be reduced and even eliminated by the client. When the laryngectomee appears relaxed and confident during speech production, the listener is more likely to attend to *what* the laryngectomee is saying rather than to *how* he or she is saying it.

Multiple Injections or Inhalations

During proficient use of the injection or inhalation methods, only one air charge is necessary to move the oral air into the esophagus. Sometimes the new esophageal speaker engages in multiple injections or inhalations in an effort to achieve voicing. Multiple injections or inhalations fatigue the laryngectomee, distract the listener, interfere with the smoothness of esophageal speech production, and bring extra air into the esophagus, resulting in an accumulation of gas in the stomach. The SLP should explain the futility and undesirable side effects of multiple injections or inhalations. During the therapy activity, the laryngectomee should be instructed to "Inject (or inhale) once. Say the word only once and stop." Individual trials to achieve voicing of the stimulus word have more learning value than multiple "false starts" within a single trial.

Excessive Stoma Noise

The *laryngeal* speaker relies on the controlled and prolonged exhalation of air through the vocal folds for speech production. During esophageal speech, however, forced exhalation frequently results in stoma noise—the sound of air turbulence in the trachea. The clinician and the laryngectomee must work diligently to suppress stoma noise from the onset. Hearing-impaired laryngectomees may need to rely on tactile feedback for awareness of the air escape by placing his or her fingertips in front of, but not touching, the stoma. Comparison of loud versus quiet productions may help the laryngectomee discriminate between forceful and subdued exhalations. Although the listener can use a hand signal to alert the laryngectomee of distracting stoma noise, it is more important that the client develop self-monitoring for stoma noise.

Facial Grimaces, Extraneous Head Movements, and Loss of Eye Contact

The session should begin with exercises to relax oral, facial, and shoulder muscles and promote general body relaxation (see Appendix B). Using a mirror, the laryngectomee may self-monitor for contortions of the face and lip muscles, squinting, and erratic head movements. Maintaining eye contact may be practiced by placing a brightly colored sticker on the mirror at eye level and instructing the laryngectomee to "watch the sticker" while speaking. If the laryngectomee's eyes close or roll upward, he or she should be asked to refocus on the sticker. Normal eye contact with the listener during spontaneous conversation occurs 80% of the time.

PHASES FOR PRACTICE ACTIVITIES

Practice activities for the six goals are divided into phases: initial, intermediate, and advanced. In the initial phase of teaching the injection or inhalation methods of esophageal speech, one goal is identified for practice per activity. In the intermediate phase, a combination of two goals is focused on during an activity. In the advanced phase, the laryngectomee attends to all six goals within the same activity.

A typical therapy session begins with warm-ups in the form of relaxation exercises; proceeds to oral-facial exercises, articulatory precision drills, and practice of specific goals at the appropriate levels on the hierarchy; and closes with the assignment of activities for the laryngectomee to complete at home. Each therapy session should be ended positively; the clinician should take care not to introduce a more difficult level of production toward the end of the session when the client is tired. It is unfair to the laryngectomee to introduce a challenging task and not resolve it before the close of the session.

A set of 10 stimuli is selected for the level of production in which the laryngectomee is anticipated or known to be successful 70–80% of the time. At this level of accuracy, the correct response is strengthened and the laryngectomee is motivated to continue practicing. The criterion to move to the next step on the activity hierarchy is 90% accuracy on three consecutive sets of stimuli at the current level of production. Activity score sheets are provided to assist the SLP in leading the laryngectomee through a series of exercises designed to develop proficient esophageal speech. For each therapy activity, a score sheet is used to record client responses (Figure 6.2). Score sheets are labeled according to the number of goals included within the activity—that is, initial phase, intermediate phase, and advanced phase. After determining the goal(s) for the activity, a set of stimuli are chosen according to the appropriate level of production. The stimuli are entered in the 10 blanks provided. Scores for the client's productions are entered as correct (+) or incorrect (–). A more sophisticated level of scoring can

Name_____ Date_____

Method of ❐ Injection for obstruents
air intake: ❐ Injection for sonorants/vowels
❐ Inhalation

Phase: ❐ Initial (one goal)
❐ Intermediate (two goals)
❐ Advanced (multiple goals)

Goal(s): ❐ Esophageal quality ❐ Articulation
❐ Consistency of voicing ❐ Rate
❐ Latency ❐ Nonverbal behaviors

Level of ❐ Single syllable ❐ Three- to four-syllable words/phrases
production: ❐ Two-syllable words/phrases ❐ Five- to six-syllable words/phrases

Target ❐ Unvoiced obstruents ❐ Mid and low vowels
sounds: ❐ Voiced obstruents ❐ Other vowels
❐ Obstruent blends ❐ Sonorants
❐ Specific consonant _____

Monitoring: ❐ Clinician
❐ Laryngectomee/clinician
❐ Laryngectomee

	Stimuli Appendix: Level: Set:	Trial No.	Comments
1.			
2.			
3.			
4.			
5.			
6.			
7.			
8.			
9.			
10.			
	Total correct		
	Percent correct		

Figure 6.2 Activity score sheet for teaching esophageal speech.

also be used—for example, designating whether a correct response was immediate, delayed, assisted, or self-corrected. In the initial phase, the clinician provides feedback with suggestions for improvement. The SLP should encourage the laryngectomee to make judgments about the production. The laryngectomee is invited to self-monitor before receiving the clinician's feedback in the intermediate phase. In the advanced phase, the laryngectomee is expected to self-monitor accurately for each production.

The Initial Phase

The starting point for learning any of the methods of air intake is the initial phase. Within the first several sessions, activities are designed to address each of the six goals. The level of production begins with single syllables. To ensure the laryngectomee experiences 70–80% accuracy during the activity, the SLP must define a "correct" production. For example, if a newly laryngectomized client is learning to move the air back and return it consistently, the goal is identified as "consistency of voicing." The beginning level of production is single syllables. Because the client is learning the injection method for obstruents, the target sounds are unvoiced obstruents combined with mid and low vowels. Set 1 of the one-syllable words listed in Appendix F, Level I (/p/ words) is selected. The stimulus items may be printed on individual cards, presented as a list, or modeled (if the client cannot read). During the first few sessions—and before the client's speech attempts—the SLP should model the /p/, popping the lips firmly together. If the client produces the /p/ word with voicing, the scoring is a correct, but assisted, response and entered in the comments section of the form. The secondary consistency of voicing goal becomes "The client will achieve 80% consistency of voicing with cueing." As quickly as possible, the SLP should lessen his or her input as the client is observed making the target productions. Another example of a correct response qualifier addresses time delays—for example, the secondary latency goal might be "The client will initiate and produce esophageal voicing within 3 seconds." These secondary goals are considered half steps leading up to the desired "immediate and correct response." Once the client has achieved 90% accuracy over three consecutive sets of stimuli at Level I, the intermediate phase is introduced.

All laryngectomees begin esophageal speech training at the initial phase; the focus is on one goal per activity using the one-syllable level of production. Within one session, esophageal quality, consistency of voicing, latency, articulation, and nonverbal behaviors are addressed during separate activities. When the laryngectomee is working on esophageal quality, feedback addresses esophageal quality *only*; errors related to consistency of voicing, articulation, latency, and nonverbal behaviors are not mentioned. During articulation practice, feedback is limited to information about articulatory movements and precision. In the early stages of therapy, the laryngectomee is vulnerable to information overload. Keeping the components of esophageal speech separate allows the laryngectomee to concentrate on one area at a time.

Intermediate Phase

In the intermediate phase, the laryngectomee monitors for two goals during the same activity—for example, esophageal quality *and* articulation at the one-syllable level. Throughout the intermediate level, the clinician alternately pairs the six goals of esophageal speech with one another until the laryngectomee achieves 90% overall accuracy for the paired goals over three consecutive sessions at that level of production.

As an example, in the first activity of a session, the client is asked to monitor for esophageal quality *and* consistency of voicing. In the second activity, the client is asked to evaluate latency *and* articulation. This cycle is continued until the client demonstrates the ability to perform a variety of paired goals per activity with 90% accuracy over three consecutive sessions.

Advanced Phase

In the advanced phase, the client continues to produce Level I stimuli but now must self-monitor for all six goals of esophageal speech within a single activity. After each production, the client informs the clinician about the quality and consistency of voicing, the latency of response, the precision of the articulation, the appropriateness of rate, and the occurrence of any distracting nonverbal behaviors. All six goals must be achieved before that response is scored as correct. When all six goals are met with 90% accuracy or better for three consecutive sets of stimuli, the client is ready to begin Level II of the hierarchy and cycle through the three phases at Level II. The same pattern of cycling through phases occurs at each level of production until the final level of production is successfully completed for each method of air intake.

Feedback and Self-Monitoring Skills

In the beginning therapy interactions with the laryngectomee, it is especially important for the laryngectomee to receive clinician feedback after each production. The clinician does not need to be able to produce esophageal speech to model target as well as error behavior. A glottal fry is a fairly close approximation of esophageal speech and is adequate for teaching purposes. Demonstration is a valuable learning tool for the laryngectomee. When the target behavior is successful, the laryngectomee needs to know how success was achieved—for example, "That was esophageal quality. You moved the air into the esophagus." If the production is in error, the SLP should identify the error and provide a suggestion for improvement. An example of clinician feedback during the injection method for obstruents might be the following: "That was pharyngeal sound. That means the air did not go all the way down to the esophagus. Try saying 'pop' again, and this time, press your lips firmly together as you make the /p/. Like this. [The laryngectomee's fingertips are held in front of the clinician's mouth while the clinician explodes the /p/.]"

The development of self-monitoring skills is an important component of alaryngeal speech rehabilitation. Laryngectomees who are able to self-monitor and self-correct have the potential to manage and perfect their speech at all times, not just during the scheduled therapy session. The ability to self-monitor accurately is a giant step in the direction of becoming one's own therapist.

PROFICIENT ESOPHAGEAL SPEECH

The therapy activity hierarchies for the three methods of air intake in esophageal speech—injection method for obstruents, injection method for sonorants and vowels, and the inhalation method—are kept separate up to and including the five- to six-syllable phrases and sentences level of production. The laryngectomee practices each of the methods in separate activities that use the appropriate phonetic context. Frequently, the laryngectomee experiences differential success among the methods of air intake. The ultimate goal of esophageal speech is for the laryngectomee to be able to produce every utterance as desired, regardless of phonetic context or syllable length. The use of combined methods of esophageal speech allows the laryngectomee freedom to do just that.

Combining the Injection and Inhalation Methods

The criterion for combining the various methods of esophageal speech is that the laryngectomee must demonstrate 90% or better performance for all six goals at the five- to six-syllable phrases and sentences level of production using the following:

- The injection method for obstruents (Appendix F, Level X) *and*
- The injection method for sonorants and vowels *or* the inhalation method (Appendix G, Level VII).

Such a performance protocol suggests that, entering this stage of the therapy hierarchy, the laryngectomee reliably produces esophageal quality speech with less than a 1-second latency, uses good articulation and an appropriate rate, and has few, if any, nonverbal behaviors that are distracting to the listener.

Advanced Goals

With the basic skills for esophageal speech accomplished, the laryngectomee is ready to address the goals of combined esophageal speech—all pertinent to intelligibility—including meaningful phrasing, pitch control via intonation and stress, and increased loudness. Articulation precision and appropriate rate are retained as goals because these two factors are inextricably tied into the intelligibility of speech. Attention to nonverbal behaviors that add to, or distract from, the listener's understanding of the message continues.

Goal One: Improving Articulatory Precision

The SLP should continue to emphasize practice for specific sounds that need attention in the laryngectomee's articulatory repertoire—for example, fricatives, nasals, the approximation of /h/, and voiced-unvoiced obstruent contrasts. Practice lists for obstruent contrasts in the initial and final positions of words appear in Appendix E.

Goal Two: Approaching Appropriate Rate

A successful increase in the laryngectomee's rate of speech depends on his or her articulatory control and the ability to move air in and out of the esophagus quickly and effectively (see "Goal Five: Rate," discussed earlier in this chapter).

Goal Three: Meaningful Phrasing

When practicing the injection method for sonorants and vowels or the inhalation method, the laryngectomee elongates vowels and says two or more syllables on one air intake to increase the duration of phonation. Now, under the conditions of an unrestricted phonetic context, the laryngectomee has the opportunity to take advantage of the occurrence of obstruents in the stimuli to prolong the utterance. The SLP should preview the stimulus phrase, sentence, or reading passage and predict the places at which air intake is needed using either inhalation or the injection method for sonorants and vowels. These places should be marked for air intake with a red slash. The obstruents should be circled in red in the releasing position of syllables to highlight their importance in injecting air for the continuation of speech.

Berlin [22] observed that laryngectomees who are rated as good speakers have production latencies of one-half second or less. The laryngectomee's ability to frequently and efficiently re-inflate the esophagus while maintaining smoothness and continuity of connected speech is a better indicator of proficient esophageal speech than the number of syllables spoken per air charge. To achieve appropriate phrasing, the laryngectomee attends to the grouping of syllables and words into meaningful phrases. Sometimes it is helpful if the clinician suggests pausing, injecting, or inhaling where a comma or period is placed in the written text.

Goal Four: Pitch Control Via Intonation and Stress

Pitch variation and inflection are practiced using contrastive stress drills and emotionally charged utterances. Through the use of a prepared utterance—for example, "Betty likes to read books"—the SLP asks a variety of questions that require differentiated stress or intonation in the laryngectomee's response. An example of an exchange between the SLP and the laryngectomee is as follows:

SLP:	*Brenda* likes to read books?
Laryngectomee:	*Betty* likes to read books.
SLP:	Betty *hates* to read books?

Laryngectomee:	Betty *likes* to read books.
SLP:	Betty likes to *write* books?
Laryngectomee:	Betty likes to *read* books.
SLP:	Betty likes to read *letters*?
Laryngectomee:	Betty likes to read *books*.

Role play is an activity that improves pitch control via intonation and stress. The laryngectomee chooses one of several emotions (e.g., happiness, sadness, anger, or fear) and attempts to portray the emotion in a prepared utterance. Fellow laryngectomees, family members, or the clinician identify the emotion being depicted. For example, the statement "I knew that would happen" takes on various connotations based on the underlying intonation and stress used by the speaker.

Hyman [10] reports that the esophageal speaker is capable of pitch inflection by as much as two octaves. He suggests intoning the vowel /ɑ/ from lowest to highest pitch range, gliding the /ɑ/ from low to high pitch and back to low pitch, and asking questions with an upward inflection at the end (e.g., How are you?). Nursery rhymes, limericks, and poetry may assist the laryngectomee in pitch flexibility due to their prosodic nature.

Goal Five: Increasing Loudness

In the final stages of therapy, loudness is addressed. The intensity of esophageal speech is approximately 6–10 dB less than the intensity of laryngeal speech [33]. The range of loudness for the esophageal speaker is 20 dB, as compared with a 45-dB range for the laryngeal speaker [28]. Digital pressure against the neck (at the level of the PE segment), increased oral opening, and contraction of the abdominal muscles have the potential to assist loudness; however, the clinician and the client must guard against the development of inappropriate secondary behaviors—for example, stoma noise, increased bodily tension, and exaggerated articulation. During the production of the stimulus sets, the laryngectomee can alternate saying the phrase with increased or decreased loudness—that is, the speaking voice versus the confidential voice. The SLP may sit at varying distances from the client during the speech activity so the laryngectomee responds "naturally" to the situation with increased or decreased loudness levels. The practice statements used in "Goal Four: Pitch Control via Intonation and Stress" are helpful because loudness, intonation, and stress are interrelated. The emotion of sadness usually conjures up the image of decreased loudness; anger or excitement may have the opposite effect by suggesting increased loudness.

Compensatory measures for loss of loudness also involve manipulation of the environment—for example, choosing a quiet place to converse, sitting or standing opposite the listener to facilitate lipreading, informing the listener of the topic before initiating the discussion, using gestures to complement speaking, and supplementing esophageal speech with the artificial larynx or writing. Another option for the laryngectomee who desires increased loudness is the use of a personal amplifier with microphone (see Appendix A).

Goal Six: Nonverbal Behaviors

The laryngectomee who has reduced or eliminated distracting nonverbal behaviors while working at the lower levels of the therapy hierarchy continues to monitor for negative behaviors—for example, stoma noise, klunking, repetitive oral movements, and facial grimacing. With these behaviors under control, the emphasis for this goal turns to enhancing the communicative effectiveness of the esophageal speaker. Attention to positive behaviors—for example, eye contact, facial expressions, hand gestures congruent to the message, and judicious use of interjections "um," "er," and "hmm"—increase the naturalness of communication. When the laryngectomee is at the structured or spontaneous levels of production, pragmatic issues sometimes arise. The laryngectomee, like any good communicator, must be sensitive to the listener's needs, observe the rules of taking turns, stay within the limits of the conversational situation, and check frequently to make sure the message has been understood by the listener.

Activity Hierarchy and Combined Methods of Esophageal Speech

The activity hierarchy for combined methods of esophageal speech (Figure 6.3) are divided into phases. In the initial phase, one goal is identified for practice per activity. Two goals are focused on during each activity in the intermediate phase, and all six goals are addressed within each activity in the advanced phase. Six levels of production for practicing the combined methods of esophageal speech are identified in Appendix D:

- Level I: two- to four-syllable phrases and sentences
- Level II: five- to seven-syllable phrases and sentences
- Level III: eight-syllable or more phrases and sentences
- Level IV: oral reading of paragraphs
- Level V: structured conversation
- Level VI: spontaneous and extended conversation

The laryngectomee has proved the ability to produce five to six syllables using a specific method of air intake within a restricted phonetic context. Because the esophageal speaker now has access to multiple air intake methods to articulate obstruents, sonorants, and vowels, the stimuli are drawn from an unrestricted phonetic context of consonants and vowels. To facilitate early success in combining the esophageal speech methods, the therapy hierarchy drops back one level of production, to the two- to four-syllable level. The laryngectomee progresses through each of the three phases at each level of production before advancing to the next level.

The esophageal speaker who is using the combined methods of air intake is encouraged to self-monitor and self-correct productions. Home activities are assigned based on the laryngectomee's ability to perform the behavior within the therapy session with at least 80% accuracy.

Name_____ Date_____

Phase:
    ❏ Initial (one goal)
    ❏ Intermediate (two goals)
    ❏ Advanced (multiple goals)

Goal(s):
    ❏ Articulation   ❏ Intonation and stress
    ❏ Rate   ❏ Loudness
    ❏ Phrasing   ❏ Nonverbal behaviors

Level of production: Unrestricted phonetic context:
    ❏ I. Two- to four-syllable words/phrases   ❏ IV. Oral reading of paragraphs
    ❏ II. Five- to seven-syllable words/phrases   ❏ V. Structured conversation
    ❏ III. Eight-syllable or more   ❏ VI. Spontaneous
            phrases/sentences   conversation

Monitoring:
    ❏ Clinician
    ❏ Laryngectomee/clinician
    ❏ Laryngectomee

	Stimuli Appendix: Level: Set:	Trial No.	Comments
1.			
2.			
3.			
4.			
5.			
6.			
7.			
8.			
9.			
10.			
	Total correct		
	Percent correct		

Figure 6.3 Activity score sheet for teaching combined methods of esophageal speech.

CONCLUSION

The proficient esophageal speaker

- Consistently and effectively produces esophageal quality of voicing using combined methods of air intake
- Is able to self-monitor and self-correct his or her speech with attention to articulatory precision and appropriate rate, phrasing, intonation and stress, and loudness to achieve a high level of intelligibility
- Practices the rules of communication etiquette conscientiously.

REFERENCES

1. Salmon SJ. Artificial Larynx Speech: A Viable Means of Alaryngeal Communication. In Y Edels (ed), Laryngectomy: Diagnosis to Rehabilitation. Rockville, MD: Aspen, 1983;143.
2. King PS, Fowlks EW, Pierson GA. Rehabilitation and adaptation of laryngectomy patients. Am J Phys Med 1968;47:192.
3. Gilmore SI. Failure in Acquiring Esophageal Speech. In SJ Salmon, KH Mount (eds), Alaryngeal Speech Rehabilitation for Clinicians by Clinicians. Austin, TX: PRO-ED, 1991;194.
4. Doyle PC. Foundations of Voice and Speech Rehabilitation Following Laryngeal Cancer. San Diego: Singular, 1994;121, 144.
5. Casper JK, Colton RH. Clinical Manual for Laryngectomy and Head and Neck Cancer Rehabilitation. San Diego: Singular, 1993;56.
6. Shanks JC. Developing Esophageal Communication. In RL Keith, FL Darley (eds), Laryngectomee Rehabilitation (3rd ed). Austin, TX: PRO-ED, 1994;205.
7. Snidecor JC. Speech Rehabilitation of the Laryngectomized (2nd ed). Springfield, IL: Thomas, 1974;147, 182.
8. Diedrich WM, Youngstrom KA. Alaryngeal Speech. Springfield, IL: Thomas, 1966;37, 59, 91.
9. Gardner WH. Laryngectomee Speech and Rehabilitation. Springfield, IL: Thomas, 1971;94.
10. Hyman M. The Intermediate Stage of Teaching Alaryngeal Speech. In RL Keith, FL Darley (eds), Laryngectomee Rehabilitation (3rd ed). Austin, TX: PRO-ED, 1994;309.
11. Shanks JC. Evoking esophageal voice. Semin Speech Lang 1986;7:1.
12. Diedrich WM. Anatomy and Physiology of Esophageal Speech. In SJ Salmon, KH Mount (eds), Alaryngeal Speech Rehabilitation for Clinicians by Clinicians. Austin, TX: PRO-ED, 1991;18.
13. Duguay MJ. Esophageal Speech Training: The Initial Phase. In SJ Salmon, KH Mount (eds), Alaryngeal Speech Rehabilitation for Clinicians by Clinicians. Austin, TX: PRO-ED, 1991;48.
14. Salmon SJ. Methods of Air Intake and Associated Problems. In RL Keith, FL Darley (eds), Laryngectomee Rehabilitation (3rd ed). Austin, TX: PRO-ED, 1994;221.
15. Moolenaar-Bijl A. Connection between consonant articulation and the intake of air in oesophageal speech. Folia Phoniatr 1953;5:212.
16. Sacco PR, Mann MB, Schulz MC. Perceptual confusions among selected phonemes in esophageal speech. J Indian Speech Hear Assoc 1967;26:19.

17. Horii Y, Weinberg B. Intelligibility characteristics of superior esophageal speech presented under various levels of masking noise. J Speech Hear Res 1975;18;413.
18. Nicolosi L, Harryman E, Kresheck J. Terminology of Communication Disorders: Speech-Language-Hearing (2nd ed). Baltimore: Williams & Wilkins, 1983;259.
19. Edels Y. Pseudo-Voice—Its Theory and Practice. In Y Edels (ed), Laryngectomy: Diagnosis to Rehabilitation. Rockville, MD: Aspen, 1983;112.
20. Shanks JC. Esophageal Speech, A Yardstick. Stockton, CA: California Association of Laryngectomees 1996 Annual Meeting.
21. McDonald ET. Articulation Testing and Treatment: A Sensory-Motor Approach. Pittsburgh: Stanwix House, 1964;115.
22. Berlin CI. Clinical measurement of esophageal speech: I. methodology and curves of skill acquisition. J Speech Hear Disord 1963;28:42.
23. Damsté PH. Some Obstacles in Learning Esophageal Speech. In RL Keith, FL Darley (eds), Laryngectomee Rehabilitation (3rd ed). Austin, TX: PRO-ED, 1994;236.
24. McIvor J, Evans PF, Perry A, Cheesman AD. Radiological assessment of post laryngectomy speech. Clin Radiol 1990;41:312.
25. Singer MI, Blom ED, Hamaker RC. Pharyngeal plexus neurectomy for alaryngeal speech rehabilitation. Laryngoscope 1986;96(1):50.
26. Singer MI, Blom ED. Selective myotomy for voice restoration after total laryngectomy. Arch Otolaryngol 1981;107:670.
27. Blom ED, Singer MI, Hamaker RC. An improved esophageal insufflation test. Arch Otolaryngol 1985;111:211.
28. Martin DE. Evaluation Esophageal Speech Development and Proficiency. In RL Keith, FL Darley (eds), Laryngectomee Rehabilitation (3rd ed). Austin, TX: PRO-ED, 1994;331.
29. Hyman M. Factors Influencing the Intelligibility of Alaryngeal Speech. In RL Keith, FL Darley (eds), Laryngectomee Rehabilitation (3rd ed). Austin, TX: PRO-ED, 1994;259.
30. Hoops HR, Noll JD. Relationship of selected acoustic variables to judgment of esophageal speech. J Commun Disord 1969;2:1.
31. Shipp T. Frequency, duration and perceptual measures in relation to judgments of alaryngeal speech acceptability. J Speech Hear Res 1967;10:417.
32. Snidecor JC, Curry ET. Temporal and pitch aspects of superior esophageal speech. Ann Otol Rhinol Laryngol 1959;68:623.
33. Robbins J, Fisher HB, Blom ED, Singer MI. A comparative acoustic study of normal, esophageal, and tracheoesophageal speech production. J Speech Hear Disord 1984;49:202.

7

Teaching Tracheoesophageal Speech

Tracheoesophageal (TE) speech is facilitated by a surgical procedure that creates an airway between the lungs and the oral cavity. The fistula, an opening in the posterior wall of the trachea leading into an opening in the anterior wall of the esophagus, allows air to pass from the lungs through the trachea, into the upper esophagus, and into the oropharyngeal cavity for the purposes of speech. Respiration continues to occur through the surgically created stoma in the anterior neck. The fistula can close; therefore, a prosthetic device, called a TE prosthesis (TEP), is inserted into the fistula to maintain the opening. The prosthesis acts as a one-way valve: When the stoma is occluded, lung air is directed through the prosthesis into the esophagus. However, food and liquids are prevented from entering the trachea [1].

To produce voicing, the laryngectomee takes a breath and occludes the stoma with a finger or a tracheostoma valve. Lung air is redirected into the voice prosthesis and into the esophagus. The air moves up toward the oropharyngeal cavity, setting the pharyngoesophageal (PE) segment into vibration. The vibrated air is resonated in the pharyngeal, oral, and nasal cavities, where the articulators form the sound into meaningful speech.

PATIENT SELECTION CRITERIA

Although the literature is replete with success stories of TE speech, the rehabilitation team must select TEP candidates carefully [2–4]. Bosone [1] cites physical, mental, and social conditions that influence the use of the TEP:

- The laryngectomee elects to use the TEP based on personal motivation and not as an act of succumbing to the pressures of the surgeon, speech clinician, family members, or fellow laryngectomees.
- The laryngectomee is mentally alert and capable of understanding and following the rehabilitation team's instructions. The laryngectomee carries TEP supplies for routine maintenance of the TEP and for emergency situations (Table 7.1). In the event of an emergency, the

Table 7.1   Suggested items for a voice prosthesis maintenance kit

---

Emergency identification card

American Cancer Society's *First Aid for Laryngectomees* booklet

Spare voice prosthesis and insertion device (not required for the individual who has an indwelling low-pressure voice prosthesis)

Hand mirror

Pen light

Cotton swabs, cotton balls, gauze, tissue

Half-inch surgical tape

Tweezers

Alcohol packets

No. 16 French catheter (or size suggested by physician) or tracheoesophageal puncture stent

Disposable saline tube, needle-less syringe, or flushing pipet

Pipe cleaners

Spare tracheostoma valve and valve housing (if used)

Silicone adhesive (if used)

Electrolarynx and spare batteries

Names, addresses, and phone numbers of physicians, hospital, family members, and medical insurance company

---

laryngectomee is able to seek medical care and reinsert either the prosthesis or a catheter as appropriate. (Alcoholism or drug addiction often prevent the responsible use of the TEP [2].)

- The laryngectomee demonstrates manual dexterity and visual acuity sufficient to take care of the prosthesis and the stoma. In the case of the indwelling prosthesis, this requirement may not be as crucial to the success of using a TEP.
- The laryngectomee has adequate pulmonary support for speech production. (Negative factors include emphysema, chronic pulmonary obstructive disease, and asthma.)
- The laryngectomee accepts that one hand is needed to manually occlude the stoma during speaking. Use of a tracheostoma valve has a limited rate of success among current TEP speakers.
- There is no evidence of cancer recurrence.
- The trachea and the proposed site of the fistula (i.e., the posterior tracheal wall and the anterior esophageal wall) are healthy.
- The diameter of the stoma is no smaller than a No. 8 French laryngectomy tube (approximately 1.5–2.0 cm).
- The PE segment has been determined functional after evaluation by esophageal air insufflation testing [5, 6].

Insufflation testing, a reliable guide to patient selection, is used to determine the functional adequacy of the PE segment for TE speech before fistulization [6]. Blom et al. [5] suggest routine administration of the esophageal insufflation test to identify individuals who may be at risk for alaryngeal speech failure. The speech-language pathologist (SLP) who has received training in insufflation testing is an appropriate administrator of the test. According to the procedure described by Blom and his colleagues [5], air is introduced transnasally through a No. 14 French catheter into the esophagus in an attempt to produce esophageal sound. On one end of the catheter is a tracheostoma adapter and flexible housing that is attached to the laryngectomee's stoma. When the laryngectomee exhales through the stomal adapter, air is introduced into the esophagus. The laryngectomee is instructed to prolong the vowel /ɑ/ and count from one to 15. A favorable result, indicating a functional PE segment for TE speech, is prolongation of the vowel for 10–15 seconds and an easily vocalized count from one to 15. If the laryngectomee is unable to attain voicing during the procedure, a referral to the otolaryngologist is appropriate.

TRACHEOESOPHAGEAL VOICING: A PREREQUISITE TO THERAPY

Before the initiation of speech therapy, the TEP is fitted by the laryngectomee's physician or an SLP who has been trained in the procedure. The depth of the TE puncture tract is measured at the time of fitting. Correct sizing is important because if the prosthesis is too short, the esophageal end of the puncture tract can close; if the prosthesis is too long, leaking, aspiration, and loss of voicing can occur [7]. Over time, changes in the configuration of the TE puncture tract may necessitate resizing of the prosthesis. The most common reasons for downsizing the length of the prosthesis are edema or scar contraction of the common wall between the trachea and the esophagus, leakage of a duckbill prosthesis when pressed against the posterior esophageal wall, leakage resulting from the piston-like action of the low-pressure prosthesis within the TE puncture tract, and loss of voicing due to esophageal mucosa obstructing the prosthesis [7].

TE voicing is a prerequisite to the initiation of TE speech training. The expectation of the rehabilitation team is that TE voicing will occur immediately after successful insertion of the TEP. Failure to produce TE sounds, however, may occur for a variety of reasons. The observations and recommendations offered by Bosone [1] and Blom et al. [8] are summarized in the following sections discussing troubleshooting procedures for the TEP and in Table 7.2.

Poor or No Sound at the Time of Fitting

If the laryngectomee experiences poor or no sound at the time of the TEP fitting, several problem-solving procedures should be investigated:

- If the new TEP is a duckbill type (see Figure 3.6), the slit valve in the duckbill tip may not be completely separated. After the prosthesis is

Table 7.2 Troubleshooting procedures related to care and maintenance of the tracheoesophageal tract and prosthesis

Problem	Cause	Solution
There is poor or no sound *at the time of fitting.*	Slit in duckbill-type prosthesis is stuck together.	Remove prosthesis and gently separate duckbill.
	Valved end of prosthesis is stuck due to mucus.	Flush prosthesis with water-filled syringe or pipet.
	Prosthesis is too long; duckbill tip is contacting posterior esophageal wall.	Recheck depth of TE tract; replace with shorter prosthesis.
	Prosthesis is too short; tip is occluding fistula.	Recheck depth of TE tract; replace with longer prosthesis.
	There is too much digital valving pressure.	Lighten digital valving pressure.
	The PE segment is hypertonic.	Reduce oropharyngeal tension, loudness, and rate of speech.
		Perform insufflation test.
		Perform pharyngeal plexus nerve block.
		Perform surgical myotomy or pharyngeal plexus neurectomy.
	The PE segment is hypotonic.	Apply digital pressure to external neck (anteriorly).
There is poor or no sound *after voicing is established.*	Slit in duckbill-type prosthesis is stuck together.	Remove prosthesis and gently separate duckbill.
	Interior of prosthesis is occluded with mucus.	Flush prosthesis with water-filled syringe or pipet.
	The fistula has closed.	Remove prosthesis and try voicing with "open" fistula. If there is no sound, the fistula may be closed.
		With prosthesis removed, take a sip of water. Observe fistula; if there is no leakage, fistula may be closed.
		With prosthesis removed, try to gently insert catheter into fistula.
There is leakage *through* the prosthesis.	Prosthesis is too long; duckbill tip is contacting posterior esophageal wall.	Replace with shorter prosthesis or switch to low-pressure type.
	Prosthesis has deteriorated.	Replace prosthesis.
	There are *Candida* deposits on or in valve.	Replace prosthesis.
		Soak prosthesis in nystatin or hydrogen peroxide.
		Use nystatin (Nystatin Oral Suspension) mouthwash.

Problem	Cause	Solution
There is leakage *around* the prosthesis.	Prosthesis is too long; piston-like action has dilated TE tract.	Replace with shorter prosthesis; use retention collar design.
	Common TE wall is weak.	Surgically reconstruct common TE wall.
	Tissue is irradiated.	Remove prosthesis at night and insert smaller-diameter catheter.
		Surgically reconstruct area surrounding fistula.
A macrostoma is present.	Trachea may be naturally large, or there may be the presence of tracheomalacia.	Use tracheostoma vent, tube, or button.
A microstoma is present.	There is stenosis of the trachea.	Use tracheostoma vent, tube, or button.
		Surgically revise the tracheostoma.
There is loss of an airtight seal for the tracheostoma valve.	Skin has been inadequately prepared.	Follow valve directions carefully.
		Remove old adhesive and apply new adhesive with each application.
	Housing has been improperly applied.	Center housing over stoma; avoid occluding stoma.
		Allow adhesive to become tacky before applying housing.
	There is excessive back pressure behind the valve.	Assess pressure with insufflation test using manometer or pressure gauge.
		Reduce oropharyngeal tension, loudness, and rate of speech.
		Remove valve before coughing.
		Switch to low-pressure prosthesis.
		Perform pharyngeal plexus nerve block.
		Perform surgical myotomy or pharyngeal plexus neurectomy.

TE = tracheoesophageal; PE = pharyngoesophageal.
Source: Data from ZT Bosone. Tracheoesophageal Fistulization/Puncture for Voice Restoration: Presurgical Considerations and Troubleshooting Procedures. In RL Keith, FL Darley (eds), Laryngectomee Rehabilitation (3rd ed). Austin, TX: PRO-ED, 1994;359; and ED Blom, RC Hamaker, SB Freeman. Postlaryngectomy Voice Restoration. In FE Lucente (ed), Highlights of the Instructional Courses. St. Louis: Mosby, 1994;7, 9.

removed, the sides of the duckbill tip should be squeezed gently. Then the prosthesis is reinserted.

- Occlusion of the prosthesis with mucus or saliva prevents air from passing into the esophagus. Flushing the prosthesis with a water-filled syringe or pipet should clear the obstruction.

- If the prosthesis is too long, the tip of the prosthesis contacts the posterior esophageal wall, interfering with sound production. The depth of the TE tract should be rechecked using a voice prosthesis sizer, and, if necessary, the TEP should be replaced with a shorter prosthesis.
- If the prosthesis is too short, the tip of the prosthesis lodges in the fistula and interferes with the transfer of air from the trachea to the esophagus. The depth of the TE tract should be rechecked using a voice prosthesis sizer, and, if necessary, the TEP should be replaced with a longer prosthesis.
- If the laryngectomee applies too much digital pressure to the stomal end of the prosthesis, the prosthesis is forced posteriorly into the esophageal wall and sound is interrupted. The laryngectomee should be instructed to use lighter finger pressure but still cover the stoma completely.
- Elevated tonicity of the PE segment after total laryngectomy is an important factor in the failure to acquire TE voicing [5, 9]. When there is excessive tension in the PE segment (e.g., hypertonicity or spasm), the air entering the esophagus is unable to overcome the muscular resistance to vibrate the PE segment. A relaxed hypopharynx, PE musculature, and upper esophagus are prerequisites for easy passage of air through the region. A relaxed approach to speech attempts and a reduction in loudness and rate of speech should be encouraged. An insufflation test is a reliable method for determining the functionality of the PE segment for TE speech. Pharyngeal plexus nerve block, a temporary procedure, allows the physician and the SLP to predict the effectiveness of a pharyngeal plexus neurectomy [10]. Myotomy, the dissection of selected pharyngeal musculature, is another surgical option [9, 10].
- In a hypotonic PE segment, there is insufficient resistance to the air passing through the musculature and little or no vibration occurs. The laryngectomee should be instructed to apply digital pressure to the neck immediately anterior to the level of the PE segment during phonation attempts. External pressure has the effect of narrowing the walls of the pharynx, increasing the likelihood of vibration. If external digital pressure assists voicing, commercially produced elastic neck bands and varied pressure heads are available so the laryngectomee does not have to keep the hand to the neck during speaking (see Appendix A).

Poor or No Sound After Voicing Has Been Established

If the laryngectomee experiences poor or no sound after having successfully produced TE speech for a period of time, several causes need investigation before a referral is made to the physician:

- If the loss of voicing occurs immediately after replacement of the old prosthesis with a new prosthesis, some of the same causes for no voicing at the time of initial fitting may be present. The slit in the duckbill prosthesis should be checked and the prosthesis should be flushed with a water-filled syringe or pipet. The depth of the TE tract should be rechecked with a voice prosthesis sizer; it is not uncommon for physical changes to occur within the TE tract over time.

- Closure of the fistula between the trachea and the esophagus means air can no longer pass through the prosthesis into the esophagus. With the prosthesis removed, the laryngectomee should try voicing. An open fistula offers little resistance to the pulmonary air; if there is no voicing, the fistula may have closed. With the prosthesis removed, the laryngectomee should take a small sip of water. The SLP should observe the fistula with a pen light; an open fistula permits liquid into the trachea. The SLP should attempt to insert a catheter (lubricated tip) into the fistula; the catheter cannot pass through a closed fistula.

Leakage Through *the Prosthesis*

Leakage may occur through the TEP for a variety of reasons:

- If the prosthesis is too long for the TE tract, the tip of the prosthesis contacts the posterior esophageal wall. The slit in the duckbill-type prosthesis is forced open, allowing liquids to enter the prosthesis and spill into the trachea. The solution is to refit the laryngectomee with a shorter prosthesis or switch to the low-pressure prosthesis with a beveled tip.
- The breakdown of the one-way valving properties of the prosthesis is signaled by gradual aspiration of liquids from the esophagus through the prosthesis into the trachea. The prosthesis should be replaced.
- *Candida*, a yeastlike fungi, may compromise the one-way valving properties of the prosthesis by separating the slit of a duckbill prosthesis. An increase in the growth of *Candida* has been observed in laryngectomees who have undergone radiation therapy or chemotherapy [1]. Blom and Singer [11, 12] recommend soaking the prosthesis overnight in nystatin or hydrogen peroxide as well as the daily use of nystatin (Nystatin Oral Suspension) mouthwash.

Leakage Around *the Prosthesis*

Leakage around the prosthesis indicates that the prosthesis is not fitting snugly within the fistula. Troubleshooting procedures include the following:

- If the prosthesis is too long, its tip touches the posterior esophageal wall. During valving, the prosthesis is pushed inward; during swallowing, the prosthesis is moved outward. Over time, this piston-like action results in dilation of the fistula and leakage occurs. A shorter prosthesis may solve the problem. A prosthesis with a retention collar design may form a better seal at the fistula site (see Figure 3.6).

- Weakness of the common wall between the trachea and the esophagus permits dilation of the fistula. Surgical reconstruction of the wall with a muscle flap may be needed.
- Radiation may affect the elastic properties of the tissue comprising the fistula. The SLP should suggest that the laryngectomee remove the prosthesis at bedtime and insert a catheter of smaller diameter overnight. Surgical reconstruction is another option.

Macrostoma or Microstoma

The diameter of the stoma, whether too large or too small, has the potential to interfere with the proper fitting of the tracheostoma prosthesis. A tracheostoma vent, tube, or button may facilitate the use of the TEP. In more severe cases, surgical revision of the tracheostoma in terms of reduction or enlargement is necessary.

Loss of Airtight Seal for Tracheostoma Valve

A tracheostoma valve eliminates the need to cover the stoma with a finger during speech production. The valve and housing are worn in addition to the voice prosthesis (see Figures 3.8 and 3.9). TEP users vary in their ability to successfully use a tracheostoma valve. Establishing and maintaining an airtight seal with the outer housing of the TE valve can be problematic because of the following reasons:

- The housing is attached to the skin surrounding the stoma with silicone adhesive. Improper preparation of the skin and application of the adhesive result in poor adherence of the housing to the skin. The skin must be free of previous adhesive. Some laryngectomees are allergic to the adhesive and are unable to wear the valve.
- The housing must be centered directly over the stoma so that the stoma is not occluded. The housing must be positioned so that the inferior portion of the housing does not occlude the lower portion of the stoma and serve as a collection point for mucus. Mucus collection can loosen the seal. The adhesive should be tacky before the housing is applied to the skin.
- For a number of reasons, increased air pressure within the PE area can create "back pressure" behind the valve and interfere with voicing. An insufflation test modified by an attachment to a manometer or a pressure gauge is used to assess the presence of excess air pressure. The

laryngectomee is encouraged to voice with relaxed oropharyngo-esophageal musculature, reducing the rate of speech and loudness. If the sensation of coughing occurs, the valve should be removed first. If the laryngectomee is using the duckbill prosthesis, a switch to the low-pressure prosthesis may help reduce the need to push air through the prosthesis. As previously discussed, if the excess air pressure is the result of a hypertonic PE segment, surgical intervention—that is, myotomy or pharyngeal plexus neurectomy—may be needed.

ESTABLISHING GOALS FOR TEACHING TRACHEOESOPHAGEAL SPEECH

The laryngectomee who has been fitted with a TEP and has established voicing is now ready to address the goals for intelligibility of TE speech.

According to Amster and Amster [3], "readily available pulmonary air supply and immediate voice production do not ensure fluent speech or communication adequacy. Factors of quality of voice, pitch, rate, loudness, and articulation require refinement during the advanced stage for TE speakers, just as they do for esophageal speakers and for those using artificial larynges."

Five target behaviors are basic to successful TE speech: valving, articulation, rate, phrasing, and attention to nonverbal behaviors. Each of the goals for achieving proficient TE speech is discussed in the remainder of this chapter, along with suggestions for teaching each skill, providing feedback, and troubleshooting for certain problems that may arise.

Goal One: Valving

An airtight seal must occur at the stoma so that all exiting pulmonary air is redirected through the prosthesis into the esophagus for TE speech. The laryngectomee has two options for occluding the stoma during TE speech production: digital placement or the use of a tracheostoma valve. The first option is to place the thumb, a finger, or a combination of fingers over the stoma during exhalation to redirect pulmonary air into the prosthesis and into the esophagus (Figures 7.1 and 7.2). The dimensions of the stoma as well as the fingers determine the best arrangement. The objective is to place the nondominant hand on the neck and occlude the stoma with the most comfortable finger position possible. The laryngectomee should vary the finger pressure over the stoma until optimal voicing is achieved. Air should not escape around the edges of the finger(s). The laryngectomee should practice coordinating inhalation and exhalation with the movement of the fingers on and off the stoma. Contraction of abdominal muscles during exhalation is also important for proper timing.

The second option for valving—use of a tracheostoma valve—requires careful attention to the application of the valve housing to the neck area. The area surrounding the stoma must be clean and dry. The prosthesis is inserted

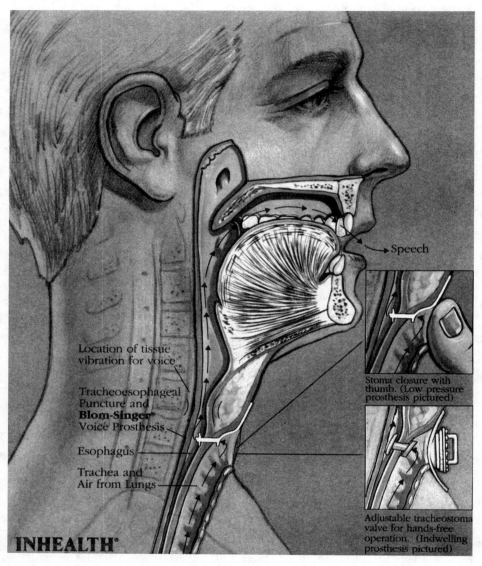

Figure 7.1 The Blom-Singer (InHealth Technologies [Carpenteria, CA]) tracheo-esophageal voice prosthesis. Air from the trachea is shunted through the voice prosthesis into the esophagus. The pharyngoesophageal segment is vibrated, producing voice. The articulators shape the tone into speech. (Reprinted with permission of InHealth Technologies. Postlaryngectomy Training Aid Set. Carpinteria, CA: InHealth Technologies, 1995.)

Figure 7.2
This laryngectomee is using a combination of fingers to redirect air from the trachea into the esophagus for tracheoesophageal speech production.

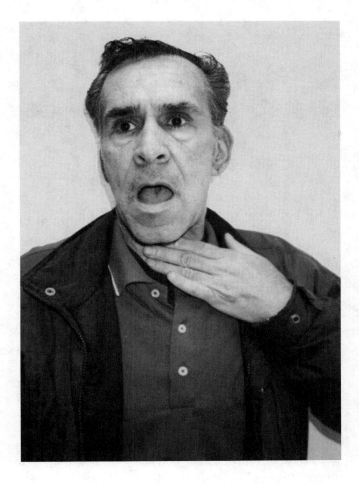

(see Figures 7.1 and 7.3), and silicone adhesive for securing the valve housing is brushed onto the area around the stoma and allowed to air dry for a few minutes. In the meantime, the tracheostoma valve housing is prepared using an adhesive foam disc. When the silicone adhesive feels tacky, the housing is pressed into place around the stoma. Care must be taken to smooth out any air bubbles so that an airtight seal is made. The valve is then snapped into place within the housing assembly. Once the valve and housing are in place, the laryngectomee is able to breathe normally and speak on demand without touching the tracheostoma valve (see Figure 7.1).

More often than not, improper valving results in loss of voicing or stoma noise. The problems related to loss of voicing due to inadequate valving are addressed earlier in "Patient Selection Criteria" and are summarized in Table 7.1. Stoma noise, the sound of air escaping the stoma under tension, occurs in

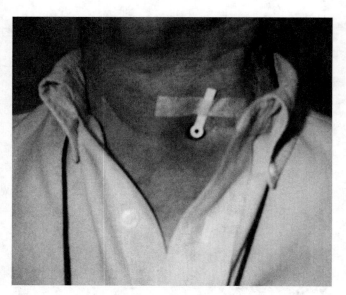

Figure 7.3
The Blom-Singer voice prosthesis (InHealth Technologies [Carpenteria, CA]) in place with tape to secure the strap.

TE speech in the absence of an airtight seal at the stoma. The laryngectomee's finger position against the stoma should be checked. There are a variety of ways to accomplish full coverage of the stoma—that is, index finger, middle finger, two or more fingers, or the thumb. If possible, the nondominant hand should be held against the stoma, freeing the dominant hand for other activities (e.g., writing, holding the telephone, or shaking hands).

If stoma noise occurs while the laryngectomee is wearing a TE valve, it is the result of an improper seal of the housing against the skin. The clinician should review the discussion under "Loss of Airtight Seal for Tracheostoma Valve." A therapy session (or two) spent in instructing the laryngectomee how to properly apply the TE housing and valve may be beneficial.

Goal Two: Articulation

Like esophageal speech and artificial larynx speech, TE speech is most intelligible when the articulation of consonants and vowels is distinct. TE speech is subject to the same listener confusion factors discussed in Chapter 6, "Teaching Esophageal Speech." The listener tends to confuse unvoiced-voiced consonants because of the loss of the vocal folds and their valving abilities during connected speech. The PE segment does not have these valving capabilities; air passed through the PE segment sets the musculature into vibration. The TE speaker learns that unvoiced consonants appearing at the beginning or ends of phrases must be made with labial or lingual movements only. In addition, unvoiced-voiced distinctions are made by the listener according to the length of the accompanying vowel. When the vowel following one of the consonant cognates is shortened, the consonant is perceived as unvoiced. To assist the TE speaker in making unvoiced-voiced consonant contrasts, word-list drills are presented in Appendix E.

Intelligibility Factors

The factors that influence intelligibility of esophageal speech also influence TE speech: foreign accent, regional dialect, dysarthria, articulation disorders, ill-fitting dental appliances, hearing loss, and loss of standard /h/ production. See Chapter 6, "Goal Four: Articulatory Precision," for the discussion of these factors and suggestions for remediation.

Wet or Gurgling Sound During Voicing

In radiographic studies, Simpson et al. [13] identified pouches (diverticula) at the base of the tongue and at the level of the PE segment in some laryngectomees. These bulges represent constrictions and may interfere with the movement of air through the pharyngeal region on the way to the oral cavity. Air, mucus, saliva, and other liquids may become trapped in the pouches and affect the quality of the TE voice. During phonation, the liquid within the pouches vibrates causing the perception of a wet or gurgling voice. The laryngectomee can swallow hard several times, turn the head from side to side, or lean the head and upper torso forward while in a sitting position. These are short-term remedies that flatten the pouches so that the liquid is squeezed from the area or allow gravity to drain the fluid from the pouches.

Hard Attack

The laryngectomee who uses too much tension to force air through the prosthesis into the esophagus frequently produces a "hard attack" on the initial phoneme or syllable of the utterance. The laryngectomee should practice the sequence of taking in air through the stoma, covering the stoma, and steadily but smoothly exhaling to begin speaking. Practice words beginning with /h/—for example, *honey*—may help the laryngectomee visualize the idea of a gentle rather than a harsh attack on the initiation of speaking.

Goal Three: Phrasing

The third objective is to produce normal prosody—that is, phrase speech into meaningful units. Even though the TE speaker has a large supply of pulmonary air available, that does not mean he or she speaks during the entire breath without pausing. Successful phrasing requires the laryngectomee to coordinate respiration, valving, and articulation with meaningful pauses.

One of two types of phrasing errors can occur. The laryngectomee may not phrase at all and simply take a breath, begin speaking, and cease only when the lung air has been exhausted. This type of run-on speech lacks the natural rhythm of the laryngeal speaker. The client should practice breaking longer utterances into shorter phrases—for example, "Go to the store and buy milk, eggs, and butter" becomes "Go to the store / and buy milk / eggs / and butter." A facilitating technique is to have the laryngectomee indicate the pauses before actual production. The clinician (or laryngectomee) can draw a vertical line to indicate pauses between the words in practice phrases or sentences.

Goal Four: Rate

At 127 words per minute (wpm), the average speaking rate for the TE speaker falls between that of the esophageal speaker (99 wpm) and that of the laryngeal speaker (173 wpm) [14, 15]. Even though the TE speaker has access to the pulmonary air supply, he or she is required to maintain high air flow rates through the PE segment to produce voicing [16]. The resistance offered by the PE segment translates to the TE speaker's need for more frequent air intakes than the laryngeal speaker.

Defining the rate parameters for evaluation and teaching purposes is an elusive task. Intelligibility of TE speech is a complex mix of rate, articulatory precision, and meaningful phrasing. To selectively speed up or slow down rate without attention to articulation or phrasing almost always has a negative affect on intelligibility [17–19].

Too Fast Rate

Intelligibility suffers when the speed of production exceeds the limits of the laryngectomee's muscular control of the articulators or ignores the prosodic elements of phrasing. Articulatory control and appropriate phrasing are prerequisites to increasing one's rate. Specific practice activities for the improvement of articulation were discussed under "Goal Two: Articulation." In longer utterances—for example, five- to seven-syllable phrases and sentences—appropriate pausing underscores the meaning and contributes to listener comprehension. The clinician or the laryngectomee can mark the target pauses in the stimulus list before practice. A suggestion that may help slow the rate and increase articulatory precision is the mental image of the listener "taking notes" as the laryngectomee speaks.

Too Slow Rate

TE speakers who use an excessively slow rate are usually perceived as below average in their speaking ability. Provided the laryngectomee demonstrates good articulatory control, the suggestion to step up the pace may increase intelligibility. Again, articulatory precision and phrasing become important components in the perception of an appropriate rate. If the laryngectomee is drawing out the vowels excessively, the SLP should encourage shorter duration on the vowels. If the laryngectomee is producing each syllable individually, he or she should practice blending the syllables into one continuous phrase. Pausing occurs only when necessary to inhale or to emphasize the meaning of the utterance.

Goal Five: Attention to Nonverbal Behaviors

The fifth goal of TE speech training pertains to the need for the laryngectomee to approximate, as closely as possible, the speech mannerisms of laryngeal speakers. Demonstration of good communication skills in the laryngeal speaker includes frequent eye contact with listener; complementary hand gestures and facial expressions; variations in loudness and pitch; pausing for emphasis; and interjections, such as "um" or "er." Some TE speakers spontaneously resume their prelaryngectomy speech behaviors; other TEP users benefit from the instruction and practice in using such mannerisms.

The TEP speaker is subject to many of the same extraneous behaviors experienced by the esophageal speaker and the user of the artificial larynx. Not infrequently, the laryngectomee engages in behaviors that detract from, or interfere with, effective TE communication. Among these mannerisms are excessive loss of eye contact, extraneous head movements, and facial grimacing. All of these behaviors are related, in some way, to excessive tension during the speaking process. Excessive muscle tension sabotages fluent, easily produced TE speech. The potential for these behaviors to become habitual, and thus resistant to intervention, is high. If identified and addressed early in therapy, these problems can be reduced and even eliminated by the laryngectomee.

ACTIVITY HIERARCHY AND TRACHEOESOPHAGEAL SPEECH

An activity hierarchy for the five goals is provided to guide the laryngectomee through a series of exercises designed to develop proficient use of the TEP. Practice activities are divided into three phases: initial, intermediate, and advanced. In the initial phase of teaching TE speech, *one* goal is identified for practice per activity. In the intermediate phase, a combination of *two* goals is focused on during an activity. In the advanced phase, the laryngectomee monitors for all *five* goals within the same activity.

In Appendix D, six levels of production for practicing TE speech are identified:

- Level I: two- to four-syllable phrases and sentences
- Level II: five- to seven-syllable phrases and sentences
- Level III: eight-syllable-or-more phrases and sentences
- Level IV: oral reading of paragraphs
- Level V: structured conversation
- Level VI: spontaneous and extended conversation

The stimuli represent vocabulary and topics common to the laryngectomee's experience. Because the TE speaker does not rely on specific consonants to assist air intake, the stimuli are drawn from an unrestricted phonetic context of consonants and vowels. The basic level of production for practicing TE speech is two- to four-syllable phrases. At the lower levels of production, the use of rote or common phrases frees the laryngectomee to concentrate on valving, articulation, phrasing, rate, and nonverbal behaviors.

The laryngectomee successfully completes each of the three phases at each level of production before advancing to the next level. For example, a set of 10 stimuli is selected for the level of production in which the TE speaker is known to be successful 70–80% of the time. The TE speaker monitors for one of the five goals per activity (initial phase) until 90% accuracy for each goal has been achieved over three consecutive sets of stimuli. Then, the intermediate phase is introduced, still at the same level, and the laryngectomee must monitor for com-binations of two goals within the same activity. After maintaining 90% accuracy for alternating paired goals over three consecutive sets of stimuli, the TE speaker is ready for the advanced phase at the same level. Within the same activity, the laryngectomee monitors for all five goals of TE speech. Activities are based on this premise until the laryngectomee scores 90% or better accuracy for three consecutive trials. Now the laryngectomee is ready to cycle through the next level beginning with the initial phase—that is, one goal is addressed per activity.

A therapy session for the TE speaker typically begins with warm-ups in the form of relaxation exercises, proceeds to oral-facial exercises and articulatory precision drills, and then moves to practice of specific goals at the appropriate level of production. The session closes with the assignment of activities for the laryngectomee to complete at home. The therapy session is ended on a positive note; care is taken not to introduce the next phase or a more difficult level of production at the close of the session when the laryngectomee is fatigued.

Activity score sheets are provided to assist the SLP in leading the laryngec-tomee through a series of exercises designed to develop proficient TE speech. For each therapy activity, a score sheet is used to record client responses (Figure 7.4). Score sheets are labeled according to the number of goals included within the activity—that is, initial phase, intermediate phase, and advanced phase. After determining the goal(s) for the activity, a set of stimuli are chosen according to the appropriate level of production. The stimuli are entered in the 10 blanks pro-vided. Scores for the laryngectomee's productions are entered as correct (+) or incorrect (–). A more sophisticated level of scoring can be used—for example, designating whether a correct response was immediate, delayed, assisted, or self-corrected. In the initial phase, the clinician provides feedback with suggestions for improvement. The TE speaker should be encouraged to make judgments about the production. The laryngectomee should be encouraged to self-monitor before receiving the clinician's feedback in the intermediate phase. In the advanced phase, the laryngectomee is expected to self-monitor accurately for each production. The development of self-monitoring skills is an important com-ponent of alaryngeal speech rehabilitation. Laryngectomees who are able to self-monitor and self-correct have the potential to manage and perfect their speech at all times, not just during the scheduled therapy session.

Name_____ Date _____

Phase: ❒ Initial (one goal)
            ❒ Intermediate (two goals)
            ❒ Advanced (multiple goals)

Goal(s): ❒ Valving   ❒ Rate
            ❒ Articulation   ❒ Nonverbal behaviors
            ❒ Phrasing

Level of Unrestricted phonetic context:
production: ❒ I. Two- to four-syllable phrases   ❒ IV. Oral reading of paragraphs
            ❒ II. Five- to seven-syllable phrases   ❒ V. Structured conversation
            ❒ III. Eight-syllable phrases or more   ❒ VI. Spontaneous conversation

Monitoring: ❒ Clinician
              ❒ Laryngectomee/clinician
              ❒ Laryngectomee

	Stimuli Appendix: Level: Set:	Trial No.	Comments
1.			
2.			
3.			
4.			
5.			
6.			
7.			
8.			
9.			
10.			
	Total correct		
	Percent correct		

Figure 7.4 Activity score sheet for tracheoesophageal speech.

REFERENCES

1. Bosone ZT. Tracheoesophageal Fistulization/Puncture for Voice Restoration: Presurgical Considerations and Troubleshooting Procedures. In RL Keith, FL Darley (eds), Laryngectomee Rehabilitation (3rd ed). Austin, TX: PRO-ED, 1994;359.
2. Donegan JO, Gluckman JL, Singh J. Limitations of the Blom-Singer technique for voice restoration. Ann Otol Rhinol Laryngol 1981;90:495.
3. Amster WW, Amster JB. Developing Effective Communication After Laryngectomy. In RL Keith, FL Darley (eds), Laryngectomee Rehabilitation (3rd ed). Austin, TX: PRO-ED, 1994;263.
4. Sanders AD, Blom ED, Singer MI, Hamaker RC. Reconstructive and rehabilitative aspects of head and neck cancer in the elderly. Head Neck Dis Elderly 1990;23:1159.
5. Blom ED, Singer MI, Hamaker RC. An improved esophageal insufflation test. Arch Otolaryngol 1985;111:211.
6. Singer MI, Blom ED. An endoscopic technique for restoration of voice after laryngectomy. Ann Otol Rhinol Laryngol 1980;89:529.
7. Leder SB, Sasaki CT. Incidence, timing, and importance of tracheoesophageal prosthesis resizing for successful tracheoesophageal speech production. Laryngoscope 1995;105;827.
8. Blom ED, Hamaker RC, Freeman SB. Postlaryngectomy Voice Restoration. In FE Lucente (ed), Highlights of the Instructional Courses. St. Louis: Mosby, 1994;7, 9.
9. Singer MI, Blom ED. Selective myotomy for voice restoration after total laryngectomy. Arch Otolaryngol 1981;107:670.
10. Singer MI, Blom ED, Hamaker RC. Pharyngeal plexus neurectomy for alaryngeal speech rehabilitation. Laryngoscope 1986;96:50.
11. Blom ED (ed). Correct use of nystatin. Clin Insights 1995;1:1.
12. Blom ED, Singer MI. Disinfection of silicone voice prostheses. Arch Otolaryngol Head Neck Surg 1986;112:1303.
13. Simpson IC, Smith JCS, Gordon MT. Laryngectomy: the influence of muscle reconstruction on the mechanism of oesophageal voice production. J Laryngol Otol 1972;86:961.
14. Robbins J. Acoustic differentiation of laryngeal, esophageal, and tracheoesophageal speech. J Speech Hear Res 1984;27:577.
15. Robbins J, Fisher HB, Blom ED, Singer ML. A comparative acoustic study of normal, esophageal, and tracheoesophageal speech production. J Speech Hear Disord 1984;49:202.
16. Doyle PC. Foundations of Voice and Speech Rehabilitation Following Laryngeal Cancer. San Diego: Singular, 1994;230.
17. Martin DE. Evaluation Esophageal Speech Development and Proficiency. In RL Keith, FL Darley (eds), Laryngectomee Rehabilitation (3rd ed). Austin, TX: PRO-ED, 1994;331.
18. Shipp T. Frequency, duration and perceptual measures in relation to judgments of alaryngeal speech acceptability. J Speech Hear Res 1967;10:417.
19. Hoops HR, Noll JD. Relationship of selected acoustic variables to judgment of esophageal speech. J Comm Disord 1969;2:1.

8

Group Therapy

One-on-one therapy offers the laryngectomee the attention necessary for instruction and practice of the alaryngeal speech method(s) as well as counseling about topics specific to his or her situation—for example, physical, psychological, social, and economic [1]. The group situation expands the laryngectomee's perspective of alaryngeal speech rehabilitation by permitting observation of other laryngectomees (and sometimes their families) at various stages of rehabilitation. Laryngectomees have the potential to be excellent role models and sources of information for one another. Stone and Hamilton [2] refer to group therapy as "a 'social learning laboratory' in which patients can develop attending behavior, listening skills, turn-taking rather than interrupting a speaker, augmentation of body language, and alternative ways of expressing unpopular or threatening ideas."

Group therapy has been used for many years to facilitate individual member's abilities to learn to recognize and cope with personal stress [2]. For the laryngectomee, group therapy is a sheltered environment in which to practice communication skills learned during one-on-one therapy. On a continuum, group therapy is the transition stage between individual therapy and the outside world in terms of the demands of communication. Many times, the group environment allows laryngectomees to learn from each other about being a laryngectomee. The alaryngeal speech group is homogenous in the sense that the members are there for a common purpose, to learn more about coping with "being a laryngectomee." In another sense, the group is heterogenous—that is, differing in age, gender, medical history, educational background, and social status. Becoming a laryngectomee is a great equalizer. The laryngectomees bond with each other and develop friendships that might not have occurred under different circumstances. When the members come to think of each other as an extended family, the group is considered *cohesive*. Through the years, the cohesiveness of our alaryngeal group has waxed and waned as membership changed, altering the group dynamics. Most of the time, the laryngectomees in the group become supportive of each other. Newcomers are received with almost too much affection in the sense that everyone wants to share their experience, offer support and advice, and reassure the new laryngectomee and family about the future.

The group environment serves different functions through a variety of themes—educational, speech activities, social interaction, and support-counseling. Although these functions are not mutually exclusive and are, more often than not, combined goals of any one group session, an attempt is made in the following sections to separate out the components for academic clarity.

EDUCATIONAL THEMES

During educational sessions, topics vary widely, but the discussion pertains in some way to the process of understanding the facets of alaryngeal speech rehabilitation. Topics include, but are not limited to, anatomic and physiologic changes, medical conditions and procedures, alternative communication methods, alaryngeal speech products and services, diet, rules of etiquette for the laryngectomee, decreased visual or hearing acuity, and selection of therapy goals.

Anatomic and Physiologic Changes

Among the anatomic and physiologic changes resulting from laryngectomy are altered breathing, vulnerability of the airway to foreign substances and water, limitations of lifting and bearing down, reduced smell and taste, altered eating patterns, and limited neck and shoulder movements (see Chapter 2, "The New Laryngectomee," for an in-depth discussion of the adjustments the laryngectomee faces after surgery). When possible, photographs, drawings, and models are used to illustrate the anatomic changes. The laryngectomees in the group are encouraged to relate their personal experiences as a result of the surgery.

Medical Conditions and Procedures

Medical conditions—for example gastroesophageal reflux, hyper- and hypotonic pharyngoesophageal segments, *Candida* growth, and altered pharyngeal anatomy—and their interaction with various communication methods are good topics for group discussion. Not infrequently, laryngectomees experience these conditions and are scheduled to undergo medical tests or procedures. Using illustrations and simplistic descriptions, procedures such as esophageal insufflation, myotomy, and neurectomy are explained when the laryngectomees have questions.

Knowledge is power. A recent experience in our group illustrates the need to understand the purpose of procedures. One of the laryngectomees had difficulty attaining tracheoesophageal (TE) voicing with his TE prosthesis (TEP). After a referral and a phone call to the laryngectomee's otolaryngologist, a series of appointments was scheduled, and subsequently canceled, by the laryngectomee. When the laryngectomee was questioned about the canceled appointments, his first response was related to reluctance to undergo any more invasive procedures. Further questioning revealed that his underlying fear was that the surgeon was looking for more cancer. Once the misperception was cleared, the laryngectomee called the physician's office and rescheduled the appointments.

Methods of Alternative Communication

When there are new laryngectomees in the group, a presentation of the various speech options is appropriate. On occasion, manufacturers will loan new devices to our group for educational purposes. Demonstration videos—for example, Ultra Voice (Health Concepts [Malvern, PA]; see Appendix A) or the Blom-Singer Adjustable Tracheostoma Valve (InHealth Technologies [Carpinteria, CA]; Figure 8.1)—are well received by the group. When possible, individuals who work in alaryngeal speech rehabilitation visit our group. For example, a speech-language pathologist who specializes in alaryngeal speech rehabilitation may visit a group to share information about the TEP and its care.

Alaryngeal Speech Products and Services

In addition to artificial larynges and TEPs, a host of alaryngeal speech products and services are available to the laryngectomee. New information can often be shared with the laryngectomees from manufacturer catalogs and samples. Among the products available are stoma covers, shower shields, personal amplifiers, neck bands, medical identification, and even swimming devices (see Appendix A).

Diet and Alaryngeal Speech

After surgery, a well-balanced diet is needed to maintain appropriate body weight, regain strength, and rebuild normal tissues. The laryngectomee does not always have a large appetite. Eating smaller but more frequent meals throughout the day may be helpful. Milk and milk products (e.g., cheese, yogurt, and ice cream) sometimes thicken mucus and saliva, interfering with respiration and alaryngeal speech. The reduction (or absence) of smell and taste are related to appetite. The laryngectomees share the ways they stimulate air flow within the nasal cavity to arouse the unimpaired olfactory sensors.

Rules of Etiquette for the Laryngectomee

Although not a sterile area, the stoma must be kept meticulously clean. Information regarding the care and maintenance of the stoma is always appropriate for group discussion. Regardless of the alaryngeal speech method, the laryngectomee should carry the supplies necessary for cleaning and care of the stoma. Contents of the TEP maintenance kit are listed in Table 7.1. The laryngectomee should wash his or her hands frequently to avoid contaminating the stoma and to reduce the transfer of bacteria from the stoma to objects and other people. If at all possible, the laryngectomee should touch the stoma with the nondominant hand and shake hands with the dominant hand. *Never* does the laryngectomee care for the stoma or the TEP at the table or in public; a retreat to the lavatory is appropriate.

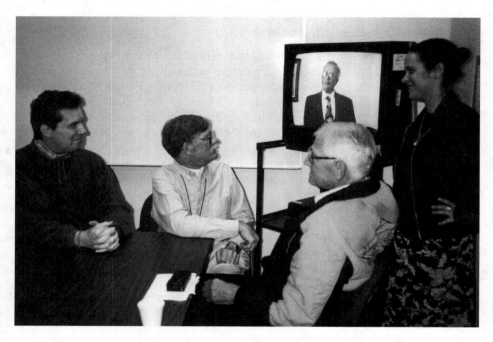

Figure 8.1 Members of our alaryngeal speech group view an educational video, "Blom-Singer Adjustable Tracheostoma Valve" by Richard Crum (1996). (VHS image reprinted with permission of InHealth Technologies, Carpinteria, CA.)

Personal hygiene—for example, daily bathing, use of deodorant, hair washing, tooth brushing, denture cleaning, fresh change of clothing and stoma cover—is vital. Reduction or loss of sense of smell may make the laryngectomee unaware of body odors. The laryngectomee must be sensitive to the potential reactions of others to behaviors related to having a stoma. The stoma should be kept covered at all times. When the need to cough arises, a handkerchief or tissue is placed discretely under the stoma cover. If the cough is serious or mucus removal is needed, the laryngectomee should excuse himself or herself from the room and take care of matters in private. When tissues, stoma covers, and other paraphernalia are soiled, they should be quietly and quickly tucked away from sight.

Decreased Visual or Hearing Acuity

When a laryngectomee has reduced visual or hearing acuity, he or she receives preferred seating in the group. The laryngectomee is asked periodically if the glasses or hearing aid are adequate for his or her needs, and, of course, the laryngectomee is encouraged to wear the glasses or hearing aid to therapy. If a vision problem or hearing loss is suspected, a referral to an ophthalmologist or an audiologist is appropriate.

Choosing Goals for Alaryngeal Speech

The reasons behind the selection of goals for the various alaryngeal speech methods are not always clear to the laryngectomee. The two dominating factors in speech rehabilitation involve getting voicing and intelligibility. Careful explanation of the activity hierarchy with comparisons to the learning of other skilled behaviors often convinces the laryngectomee of the need to take speech one step at a time.

SPEECH ACTIVITIES THEME: ENHANCEMENT AND GENERALIZATION OF FUNCTIONAL COMMUNICATION SKILLS

The primary purpose of an alaryngeal speech group is to offer the laryngectomees an opportunity to interact with one another in a somewhat contrived but more transitional communication situation than that occurring in one-on-one therapy. The group session takes different directions at times but is always based on the methods of communication, the levels of production, and the needs of the individual laryngectomees within the group. The laryngectomees in the group may differ widely in their methods of communication and levels of production. Activities can be adjusted to fit the individual needs of the members; an advanced speaker can read a question aloud to the group or respond in two to three sentences. The beginning esophageal speaker may be limited to a one-word response and is encouraged to use the artificial larynx for conversational tasks. The laryngectomee should not be asked to perform at a higher level of production than he or she does in individual therapy. Conversational attempts that result in loss of voicing, increased stoma noise, facial grimacing, and loss of eye contact are nonproductive and foster the habituation of poor speaking skills.

Warm-Ups

At the beginning of the group session, the laryngectomees may want to engage in a relaxation exercise, oral-facial exercises, or consonant-vowel combinations (depending on the speech method). Examples of relaxation exercises are found in Appendix B; oral-facial exercises are found in Appendix C.

Consonant Contrast Drills

As a carryover activity from individual therapy, 3-in. × 5-in. cards with stimulus words are prepared. The cards are passed around the group, and each laryngectomee takes one and says the stimulus word or phrase. The other laryngectomees identify what they hear. Carrier phrases are used so contextual cues are not available to the listener—for example, "I can say _____" or "The word is _____." Word lists for obstruent contrast drills are found in Appendix E. Depending on the group's preference, these drills can be used as a game with team members and played for points.

Contrastive Stress Drills

To generalize the practice of contrastive stress in individual therapy, a list of sentences is presented to the group. Although the question varies, the answer for round one is always the same—for example, "Walter ran to catch the bus." The clinician asks the question, "Did *Frank* run to catch the bus?" and the first laryngectomee responds with "No, *Walter* ran to catch the bus," with the emphasis on *Walter*. The clinician then asks, "Did Walter *walk* to catch the bus?" and the second laryngectomee responds by saying "No, Walter *ran* to catch the bus." Turn-taking continues around the table with each laryngectomee emphasizing the key word appropriate to the question. This activity can be used with the artificial larynx, intermediate to advanced levels of esophageal speech, and TE speech. As discussed in Chapters 5–7, emphasis is a function of increased loudness, pausing, or pitch inflection, depending on the method of alaryngeal speech used.

SOCIAL INTERACTION THEME

The foundation of alaryngeal speech group interactions is for participants to learn perceptive and efficient communication. A good communicator is sensitive to the listener's needs, observes the rules of taking turns, stays within the time limits of the conversational situation, and checks frequently to make sure the message has been understood by the listener. Teaching and reminding the laryngectomee about the habits of a considerate communicator from the early stages of alaryngeal speech therapy adds to the laryngectomee's desirability as a communication partner.

Within the sheltered environment of group therapy, the competition for the "communication floor" is relatively low. When one of the laryngectomees attempts to monopolize the conversation, threatening the goal of interactive communication, several tactics are used. First, the clinician leading the group gently brings closure to the laryngectomee's statements by making a comment such as "Thank you for sharing that information. The next thing we want to do is _____." Or the clinician can call on another laryngectomee by saying "What kind of stoma cover do *you* use, Frank?" The offending laryngectomee can be approached before therapy with the clinician's request to "help make sure the other laryngectomees are participating by asking them questions or encouraging them to talk." When all else fails, directness, done in private, is in order.

A variety of topics may be introduced to generate conversation among the laryngectomees, using trivia questions, newspaper advice columns, situational dilemmas, current events, carefully selected adult aphasia materials, and family photographs. These topics allow the laryngectomee to answer questions from experience. Questions about who, what, where, when, why, how many, and how much stimulate conversation. Information regarding speech strategies used by superior alaryngeal speakers is shared—for example, face the listener, announce the topic, increase loudness, increase visual cues, decrease rate of speech, increase articulatory precision, and, when all else fails, write it down.

Nonverbal cues that complement communication—for example, hand gestures, facial expression, body posture, and eye contact—are also used. Fellow laryngectomees are asked to comment on the use of these facilitating behaviors by each laryngectomee during turn-taking exercises.

The group should be asked to assist in listening and providing feedback for individuals' productions. The advice offered by fellow laryngectomees is often very powerful for the laryngectomee on the receiving end. The speech-language pathologist (SLP) should emphasize feedback regarding intelligibility by asking group members, "Did you understand what Joe said?" Natural reinforcement occurs when the laryngectomee asks a question or makes a statement and the group responds to the question/response appropriately. Gentle but honest feedback, tempered with praise and support, should include suggestions for improvement.

SUPPORT-COUNSELING THEME

In the adjustment process after laryngectomy, the laryngectomee must address and learn to cope with problems that block recovery of presurgical lifestyle and attitude. The supportive-counseling theme of group therapy is to help the laryngectomee and family resume effective functional activities of daily living. Group therapy offers a protective and supportive environment in which the clinician, the laryngectomees, and the families can examine and explore issues such as problem-solving abilities, reality testing, psychological fears, and sense of loss.

Enhancement of Problem-Solving Abilities

The clinician should design therapy activities for the group that encourage independence as well as independent thinking. A number of texts are available for working with adult aphasics and head-injured individuals who need practice with thinking, reasoning, and organizing skills. Of particular value in this area are the workbooks offered by Susan Howell Brubaker (Wayne State University Press) (see Appendix A). Newspaper advice columns are another source of problem-solving stimuli—the problem is read to the group and the group members are invited to answer.

Reality Testing

The clinician should devise questions that encourage group members to honestly assess where they are in the rehabilitation process. Questions should be asked in a turn-taking fashion so that each laryngectomee answers questions such as "What alaryngeal speech methods do you plan to use?"; "What are your speech goals?"; "What are you doing to get there?"; "What if you don't make it?"; "What are your options?"; and "How long will you try before trying the alternate plan?" The clinician should ask the hard question: "Are you a victim or a survivor of laryngeal cancer?" The laryngectomee's response gives insight into his or her view of the situation and opens the door to further discussion.

Role Playing and Role Reversal

Role play and role reversal allow the laryngectomee to practice using alaryngeal speech in a protected environment and to learn communication strategies—for example, when using the telephone, the laryngectomee should announce his or her speech style so the listener won't hang up. The laryngectomees should practice making telephone calls to each other. In groups, the laryngectomees should place mock telephone calls. The laryngectomees can be paired as phone buddies and then call each other and pretend to make reservations or ask informational questions. The phone buddies can make actual calls to each other during the week. Problem-solving situations should be offered—for example, "What to do when someone else doesn't understand you, rushes you, finishes your statement for you, appears uncomfortable, or shouts at you?" The laryngectomees should take turns "being the speaker" and "being the listener" so they have the opportunity to see the laryngectomee from the perspective of the listener. Throughout these activities, the emphasis should be on delivery and intelligibility of the message.

Addressing Psychological Issues

Group therapy offers the opportunity for the laryngectomee to share the range of emotions about the laryngectomized condition with others who are experiencing the same condition. Opening up to others with the same problem is less risky than sharing with someone who has not had the experience. The group setting has the potential of providing the laryngectomee a sense of security and camaraderie, as well as the ability to express opinions. A simultaneous spousal support group may be of benefit in helping family members understand and work through their own fears and concerns about living with a laryngectomee. An individual's inability to cope with and make adjustments to being a laryngectomee may be complicated further by alcoholism, poor cognition, physical limitations, depression, hearing loss, or poor or no family or external support. A referral to a professional counselor or psychologist is appropriate for the client whose needs are not being met by the group therapy interaction.

Addressing Fears

Facing cancer tends to heighten one's sense of mortality and frequently causes fear and a sense of loss [3]. Preoperatively, many laryngectomees are already dealing with issues associated with aging—for example, hearing loss, dentures, memory loss, and decreased stamina. Now, the fear of aging may take on greater proportions. Certainly, the fear of recurrence of cancer looms large on the laryngectomee's mind. Group discussions can center around the ability to take charge of one's diet, physical exercise, and health care. Many laryngectomees are faced with the fear of being rejected by family, friends, and the community. Being a member of the alaryngeal speech group may give laryngectomees a sense of belonging and dispel the feeling that they are "going through this alone." The ability to see other laryngectomees and hear their experiences may help alleviate some fears. The laryngectomee who witnesses another individual with greater physical or communication difficulties may become more thankful than critical of his or her own condition.

Addressing Losses

Loss is experienced by cancer patients in a number of areas. Rohe [3] offers five categories of loss associated with laryngectomy: physical, sensory, behavioral, psychological, and social. Physical losses include loss of the larynx and surrounding tissue, reduced neck and shoulder flexibility, and reduced stamina. Reduction or absence of smell, taste, and sensation in the neck and shoulder areas are sensory losses. Verbal and nonverbal communication behaviors are permanently altered, and the laryngectomee may no longer be able to whistle, sigh, cry, or laugh out loud. Certain behaviors, taken for granted preoperatively, are difficult for the laryngectomee: sneezing, blowing the nose, blowing, and sucking. Psychologically, the laryngectomee may experience loss of self-esteem as a result of disfiguration (e.g., stoma and scarring) and the loss of voice. Among the potential social losses are the loss of control, independence, role within the family and community, and financial security. The clinician must learn to recognize and acknowledge normal grief reactions to these losses but at the same time watch for symptoms of a more major depression. The need for referral may be indicated by behaviors such as resistance to or refusal to comply with the physician's treatment recommendations, poor follow-through in speech therapy, confusion and difficulty making decisions, changes in behavior, and verbalized suicide thoughts [4].

AN EXAMPLE: OUR ALARYNGEAL SPEECH GROUP

In our university clinic setting, the laryngectomee receives individual therapy for 50 minutes followed by a 30-minute small-group interaction. Whenever new laryngectomees visit our clinic, we invite them and their families to observe the individual sessions and then join the group session afterwards. If the laryngectomee returns the following session, intake procedures are initiated. In this way, the laryngectomee is able to preview a variety of alaryngeal speech methods being taught, observe the way we conduct the clinic, and meet the clinicians and the laryngectomees without feeling pressured to make a commitment. Naturally, we make an effort to make the laryngectomee and family feel welcome and to answer their questions. The laryngectomee who returns to the following session is saying, "I want to be part of the group" and is more likely to be a motivated, involved member of the group than a person who was coerced into joining. If the laryngectomee does not come back the next week, a courtesy inquiry call is made, the referring physician is notified, and then contact is suspended.

In the group meeting room, chairs are arranged around a large table so that all the laryngectomees are sitting in a circle and are able to see all other members of the group. The student clinicians sit next to their client during the session, so the seating arrangement alternates SLPs and clients. During the session, each clinician is accessible to his or her client to provide input, support, and feedback to the laryngectomee. The clinicians take turns leading the group discussion. Although the topic varies from session to session, the primary purpose of the group is generalization of communication skills: The laryngectomees are encouraged to talk, share, and interact with one another and the clinicians. Following the protocol for group therapy, a variety of themes are used—that is, education, speech activities, social interaction, and supportive counseling. These categories are not mutually exclusive. In fact, it is not unusual for the session to begin with an educational topic that evolves into a support issue. Family members are encouraged to attend the group sessions and participate in the discussions.

LARYNGECTOMEE CLUBS

Laryngectomee clubs are similar in purpose to the laryngectomee group. The primary difference is that the club is usually run by the laryngectomees. The club offers a protected environment, a transition place between structured therapy and the outside world. Minear and Lucente [5] surveyed 60 laryngectomees and reported that 92% of them rated membership in a laryngectomee club as "beneficial." Although the laryngectomees organize and run the club, a member of the alaryngeal rehabilitation team (e.g., a surgeon or an SLP) frequently serves as the club's advisor. For a listing of laryngectomee clubs, contact the local American Cancer Society or the International Association of Laryngectomees. For laryngectomees interested in starting their own club, an excellent booklet, *Building A Successful Laryngectomee Club*, is available from the American Cancer Society and details the procedures for getting started (see Appendix A).

REFERENCES

1. Edels Y. Pseudo-Voice—Its Theory and Practice. In Y Edels (ed), Laryngectomy: Diagnosis to Rehabilitation. Rockville, MD: Aspen, 1983;140.
2. Stone RE, Hamilton R. Laryngectomee rehabilitation in a group setting. Semin Speech Lang 1986;7:53.
3. Rohe DE. Loss, Grief, and Depression after Laryngectomy. In RL Keith, FL Darley (eds), Laryngectomee Rehabilitation (3rd ed). Austin, TX: PRO-ED, 1994;487.
4. Renner MJ. Counseling laryngectomees and families. Semin Speech Lang 1995;16:215.
5. Minear D, Lucente F. Current attitudes of laryngectomy patients. Laryngoscope 1979;89:1061.

9

Accountability

From the first interaction with the laryngectomee and the family, the speech-language pathologist (SLP) should document the alaryngeal speech rehabilitation. Although many of us view paperwork as a never-ending battle, the truth is that intake and progress evaluations, initial and final reports, lesson plans, and therapy logs are the tangible manifestations of our efforts to provide efficient, productive alaryngeal speech therapy. Without a structured approach to record keeping, the objectivity of the rehabilitation effort may be lost. As integral members of the rehabilitation team, we are held accountable for our role. In Chapter 2, "The New Laryngectomee," the procedures and paperwork involved for the intake interview, oral examination, and audiologic evaluation are presented. This chapter details and demonstrates evaluation procedures for the laryngectomee-in-training, goal setting, lesson planning, and report writing.

EVALUATION OF ALARYNGEAL SPEECH

Periodic evaluation of the laryngectomee's alaryngeal speech is performed for a variety of reasons, the most obvious being for the purpose of giving direction to future therapy. Depending on the work setting, the laryngectomee's speech productions are assessed at various intervals. Our alaryngeal speech clinic at San Francisco State University operates on a semester schedule; evaluation of the laryngectomee's speech productions occurs approximately every 3 months. Periodic evaluation is necessary to document the status of a new laryngectomee who transfers into an SLP's practice from another setting, to obtain insurance or Medicare benefits, or simply for the purposes of record keeping and accountability.

After a specified period of therapy (or when a laryngectomee seeking speech therapy first enters an SLP's practice), the laryngectomee's speech method is evaluated. To ensure consistency of measurement, structured assessment measures are used. The stimuli for evaluating the artificial larynx, esophageal speech, and tracheoesophageal (TE) speech appear in Appendix H. Goals specific to teaching the artificial larynx, esophageal speech, and TE speech are listed separately. On completion of the evaluation, results are transferred to the appropriate summary sheet(s) (Figures 9.1–9.5).

163

Client name _____

Clinician _____

Type of artificial larynx used _____

Percent of time used _____

Placement: ☐ Neck ☐ Cheek ☐ Intraoral ☐ Stoma

Situations used _____

Date _____

Level of production	Placement	"On" control	Articulation	Phrasing	Rate	Nonverbal
			Goals			
I. Two- to four-syllable phrases and sentences	%	%	%	%	%	%
II. Five- to seven-syllable phrases and sentences	%	%	%	%	%	%
III. Eight-syllable or more phrases and sentences	%	%	%	%	%	%
IV. Oral reading of paragraphs	%	%	%	%	%	%
V. Structured conversation	%	%	%	%	%	%
VI. Spontaneous and extended conversation	%	%	%	%	%	%

Description of error behaviors _____

Note: Percentages are transferred from the "Stimuli for Evaluation of the Artificial Larynx" forms found in Appendix H.

Figure 9.1 Summary sheet for the evaluation of the artificial larynx.

Client name _____
Clinician _____   Date _____

Level of Production	Esophageal Quality	Consistency of Voicing	Latency	Articulation	Nonverbal Behaviors
			Goals		
One-syllable words					
I. Unvoiced obstruents plus mid and low vowels	%	%	%	%	%
II. Unvoiced obstruents plus other vowels	%	%	%	%	%
III. Voiced obstruents plus mid and low vowels	%	%	%	%	%
IV. Voiced obstruents plus other vowels	%	%	%	%	%
V. Unvoiced and voiced obstruent blends	%	%	%	%	%
Two-syllable words and phrases					
VI. Unvoiced obstruents	%	%	%	%	%
VII. Unvoiced and voiced obstruents	%	%	%	%	%
VIII. Voiced obstruents	%	%	%		%
Three- to four-syllable phrases and sentences					
IX. Unvoiced and voiced obstruents	%	%	%	%	%
Five- to six-syllable phrases and sentences					
X. Unvoiced and voiced obstruents	%	%	%	%	%

Description of error behaviors _____

Note: Percentages are transferred from the "Stimuli for Evaluation of the Injection Method for Obstruents" forms found in Appendix H.

Figure 9.2 Summary sheet for the evaluation of the injection method for obstruents in esophageal speech.

Client name _____

Clinician _____

Date _____

Level of Production	Goals				
	Esophageal Quality	Consistency of Voicing	Latency	Articulation	Nonverbal Behaviors
One-syllable words					
I. Mid and low vowels	%	%	%	%	%
II. Other vowels	%	%	%	%	%
III. Sonorants plus mid and low vowels	%	%	%	%	%
IV. Sonorants plus other vowels	%	%	%	%	%
Two-syllable words and phrases					
V. Sonorants and vowels	%	%	%	%	%
Three- to four-syllable phrases and sentences					
VI. Sonorants and vowels	%		%	%	%
Five- to six-syllable phrases and sentences					
VII. Sonorants and vowels	%	%	%	%	%

Description of error behaviors _____

Note: Percentages are transferred from the "Stimuli for Evaluation of the Injection Method for Sonorants and Vowels and Evaluation on the Inhalation Method" forms found in Appendix H.

Figure 9.3 Summary sheet for the evaluation of the injection method for sonorants and vowels and the evaluation of the inhalation method in esophageal speech.

Client name _____

Clinician _____ Date _____

Level of Production	Goals						
	Articulation	Rate	Phrasing	Intonation	Loudness	Nonverbal
I. Two- to four-syllable phrases and sentences	%	%	%	%	%	%
II. Five- to seven-syllable phrases and sentences	%	%	%	%	%	%
III. Eight-syllable or more phrases and sentences	%	%	%	%	%	%
IV. Oral reading of paragraphs	%	%	%	%	%	%
V. Structured conversation	%	%	%	%	%	%
VI. Spontaneous and extended conversation	%	%	%	%	%	%

Description of error behaviors _____

Note: Percentages are transferred from the "Stimuli for Evaluation of Combined Methods of Esophageal Speech" forms found in Appendix H.

Figure 9.4 Summary sheet for the evaluation of combined methods of esophageal speech.

Client name _____

Clinician _____   Date _____

Level of Production	Goals				
	Valving	Articulation	Phrasing	Rate	Nonverbal
I. Two- to four-syllable phrases and sentences	%	%	%	%	%
II. Five- to seven-syllable phrases and sentences	%	%	%	%	%
III. Eight-syllable or more phrases and sentences	%	%	%	%	%
IV. Oral reading of paragraphs	%	%	%	%	%
V. Structured conversation	%	%	%	%	%
VI. Spontaneous and extended conversation	%	%	%	%	%

Description of error behaviors _____

Note: Percentages are transferred from the "Stimuli for Evaluation of Tracheoesophageal Speech" forms found in Appendix H.

Figure 9.5 Summary sheet for the evaluation of tracheoesophageal speech.

To determine the level of production to begin testing, the clinician should review the results of the laryngectomee's previous therapy sessions. The clinician should begin testing at the level of production immediately preceding the performance level. For example, if the laryngectomee is using the artificial larynx and is performing at the 80% level during eight-syllable or more phrases and sentences, testing should begin one level of production below that (i.e., five- to seven-syllable phrases and sentences). If the clinician is uncertain as to which level to begin testing, he or she should begin at the two- to four-syllable phrase and sentence level. The consequence of starting with a level of production considerably below the laryngectomee's abilities is that it takes additional time to produce the stimuli, and the laryngectomee may tire by the time the appropriate level of production is reached.

In Appendix H, stimuli are grouped into sets of 10 for each level of production according to the method of alaryngeal speech. The hierarchy for teaching individual alaryngeal speech methods is presented in Chapters 5–7. A restricted phonetic context is used during the teaching of esophageal speech. The stimuli for each of the esophageal speech methods have been selected based on the phonetic context included at that level of the hierarchy. In artificial larynx speech, advanced esophageal speech, and TE speech, the phonetic context is unrestricted—that is, any consonant or vowel combination is used. Thus, the stimuli used to evaluate progress with these methods are representative of all the consonant and vowel combinations that appear in English. Because the goals for these alaryngeal speech methods differ from one another, separate evaluation forms are used.

Stimuli to assess the injection method for obstruents begin with one-syllable words using the restricted phonetic context of unvoiced obstruents and mid- to low-back vowels. The level of production advances to five- to six-syllable phrases and sentences that contain both unvoiced and voiced obstruents in the releasing position of syllables. Production of esophageal speech using the injection method for sonorants and vowels and the inhalation method requires a phonetic context restricted to sonorant and vowel combinations. The lowest level of production is one-syllable words beginning with mid- to low-back vowels; the highest level of production is five- to six-syllable phrases using sonorants and vowels in the releasing positions in syllables.

The stimuli are presented (e.g., orally, on 3-in. × 5-in. cards, or as a list) and the accuracy of production is determined based on the goals for that method. Scoring is binary; each production is either correct or incorrect. The SLP may elect to use a more complex method of scoring, but the binary method is the choice of the author for simplicity. The laryngectomee is asked to say each stimulus item twice, if needed, to determine accuracy for all listed goals. After the laryngectomee has completed the 10 stimulus productions, each column is totaled and percentages determined. If the overall accuracy of production is 70% or greater, he or she should move up to the next level of production. The SLP should continue up the hierarchy of stimuli until the laryngectomee fails to maintain at least a 60% average across the goals. The clinician should discontinue testing at that level.

The results of the evaluation (see Appendix H) are determined and transferred to the summary forms shown in Figures 9.1–9.5. This information is useful for preparing the therapy report, educating the laryngectomee and family about progress, and providing future direction of therapy.

GOAL SETTING

Evaluating alaryngeal speech methods provides the clinician with information to design goals specific to the needs of the individual. The stimuli used in the instruction of artificial larynx speech differ from those used to teach beginning esophageal speech. In Chapters 5–7 regarding instruction for the alaryngeal speech methods, an explanation is given for each of the goals used along with discussion of potential problems that may arise during therapy. The purpose of this section is to assist the clinician in determining goals from a technical standpoint.

Putting goals into behavioral terms is an excellent way to maintain accountability. Being able to describe behaviors at certain levels of the hierarchy by providing percentages or ratios allows the SLP to objectify the laryngectomee's behaviors and readily chart his or her progress or lack of progress. There are three parts to writing a goal in behavioral terms. The client must *do something* under *certain conditions* with a predetermined *level of accuracy*. For example, a goal for the new user of the artificial larynx would read, "The laryngectomee will use appropriate placement during the production of two- to four-syllable phrases and sentences with 80% accuracy." The *do* portion of the goal defines the behavior—for example, the laryngectomee will use appropriate placement. The *conditions* under which the behavior is to be performed are given—for example, during two- to four-syllable phrases and sentences. Third, the *level of accuracy* identifies the minimum performance expected—for example, 80%.

Behavioral goals may be written from several perspectives. Long-term behavioral goals are frequently written for the therapy report. These goals usually describe the terminal behavior of the laryngectomee, the behaviors expected by the termination of therapy. Short-term goals are used to define target behaviors within a shorter period of time—for example, within a single therapy session. These secondary goals, also called subgoals, represent sequential steps in the hierarchy of behaviors needed to reach the final goals. They are found in lesson plans and in the daily therapy log, a record of the laryngectomee's performance.

LESSON PLANNING

Lesson planning for alaryngeal speech therapy gives the clinician time to determine which goals to address within the session and to prepare materials. A well-designed lesson plan has several components (see sample in Table 9.1). For each activity within the session, the following items are identified: (1) the goal, (2) the

Table 9.1 Sample lesson plan for artificial larynx speech

Goal 1: P.R. will use appropriate placement during two- to four-syllable phrases and sentences with 80% accuracy.

Rationale: Appropriate placement reduces extraneous buzzing and enhances intelligibility of speech.

Baseline: None. This is P.R.'s first therapy session.

Procedure: The clinician will model each of the 10 stimuli from Appendix D, Level I, Set 1.

Performance summary: P.R. used appropriate placement during two- to four-syllable phrases and sentences with 80% accuracy with clinician guidance of the hand.

Goal 2: P.R. will coordinate use of the "on" control with speaking during two- to four-syllable phrases and sentences with 80% accuracy.

Rationale: When the "on" control is operated in synchrony with speech, voiced and unvoiced sounds are perceived correctly by the listener. Unnecessary buzzing is eliminated.

Baseline: None. This is P.R.'s first therapy session.

Procedure: The clinician will model each of the 10 stimuli from Appendix D, Level I, Set 2.

Performance summary: P.R. coordinated use of the "on" control with speaking during two- to four-syllable phrases and sentences with 50% accuracy. He tends to turn the artificial larynx on too soon.

Goal 3: P.R. will use precise articulation during two- to four-syllable phrases and sentences with 80% accuracy.

Rationale: Clear, well-articulated sounds boost intelligibility of speech.

Baseline: None. This is P.R.'s first therapy session.

Procedure: The clinician will model each of the 10 stimuli from Appendix D, Level I, Set 3.

Performance summary: P.R. used precise articulation during two- to four-syllable phrases and sentences with 70% accuracy. Mild dysarthric movements responsible for errors.

rationale explaining the goal, (3) baseline performance, (4) procedures to enact the activity, and (5) space to summarize the laryngectomee's performance.

Goals

The purpose of lesson planning is to select short-term goals and design therapy activities to implement those goals. Goals are always written in behavioral terms.

Rationale

For each goal, a brief rationale is prepared and shared with the laryngectomee. The informed client is more likely to cooperate and follow through with the activity when he or she understands the reason for the activity.

Baseline

Baseline represents the laryngectomee's performance in a previous therapy session and is used as a reference point to predict behavior and performance for the current session. The performance in the current session becomes the baseline for the next therapy session.

Materials and Therapy Procedure

The selection of materials is based on the alaryngeal speech method, the level of production, and the phonetic context. The stimuli can be presented orally by the SLP, printed on 3-in. × 5-in. cards, or printed as a list. The clinician describes the method of presentation—that is, auditory, visual, or tactile. Any facilitating cues are written under *procedures*. A score sheet is prepared for each activity within the session (see score sheets for the appropriate alaryngeal speech method in Chapters 5–7).

Performance Summary

After the session is completed, the clinician summarizes and records the laryngectomee's performance on the lesson plan (see Table 9.1). This information is used to write therapy log notes in the laryngectomee's file. The performance summary also becomes the baseline for the next therapy session.

Clinical Example 1: P.R.

An example of a lesson plan for a beginning user of the artificial larynx, P.R., is shown in Table 9.1. Using the artificial larynx successfully means the laryngectomee is able to quickly locate the appropriate placement of the artificial larynx, coordinate the "on" control with speaking, articulate the sounds precisely, observe natural pauses, use a rate that is appropriate to the speaking situation, and monitor for accompanying nonverbal mannerisms. Selection of the therapy goals for the beginning artificial larynx user is relatively straightforward: The goals are separated into individual activities and the level of production for each goal begins at the two- to four-syllable phrase and sentence level.

Goals

This lesson plan represents P.R.'s first therapy session. Activities for three of the goals for artificial larynx speech have been planned. Note that the goals are addressed individually so that within each activity, the clinician does not monitor for any of the other goals.

Rationale

For each goal, a brief explanation of why this activity is being performed is included. This rationale was shared with P.R. at the beginning of each activity. Understanding the reason behind the expected behavior gives the laryngectomee control of, and insight into, alaryngeal speech production.

Baseline

In the example, P.R. had not undergone previous therapy, so there was no baseline. His performance in the current session becomes the baseline for the next therapy session. The SLP has recorded information about facilitating cues that will be helpful in the upcoming sessions as well.

Materials and Therapy Procedure

In this example, the SLP chose stimuli sets from Appendix D, Level I: two- to four-syllable phrases and sentences. The appropriate stimuli were entered on a score sheet for each of the three activities (see Figure 5.4). The clinician modeled the 10 stimuli in each therapy activity, so there were no materials to prepare.

Performance Summary

The clinician anticipated 80% accuracy for each of the goals. Immediately after the session, the clinician tallied the three score sheets representing the three activities and entered the results under *Performance summary* on the lesson plan. This information was used to write therapy log notes in the laryngectomee's file. The performance summary also becomes the baseline for the activities in P.R.'s next therapy session.

Clinical Example 2: A.S.

In this example, A.S. is a laryngectomee who is learning to use the injection methods for esophageal speech. The completed lesson plan appears in Table 9.2. The goals for efficient esophageal speech include the ability to consistently voice after injection, attain esophageal quality, inject and produce the utterance with brief latency, articulate precisely, and attend to nonverbal mannerisms that accompany speech.

Goals

Selection of the therapy goals for A.S. is based on previous therapeutic performance. An example of two activities are provided for this session. The first activity addresses the injection method for obstruents, and the second activity focuses on the injection method for sonorants and vowels. In the first activity, A.S. is expected to attend to two goals: consistency of voicing and esophageal quality of voicing during the injection method for obstruents. In the second activity—the injection method for sonorants and vowels—A.S. is asked to attend to the one goal of articulation.

Rationale

Before initiating each activity, the SLP explains the goal and the reason for the procedure. A.S. should understand that he is practicing at the one-syllable level

Table 9.2 Sample lesson plan for esophageal speech methods

Goal 1: Using the injection method for obstruents, A.S. will achieve consistency of voicing and esophageal quality of voicing during one-syllable words beginning with voiced obstruents plus mid and low vowels 80% of the time.

Rationale: Pairing mid and low vowels with voiced obstruents facilitates production.

Baseline: In separate activities, consistency of voicing and esophageal quality of voicing were achieved 90% of the time during one-syllable words beginning with voiced obstruents plus mid and low vowels over three consecutive trials.

Procedure: The clinician will model each of the 10 stimuli from Appendix F, Level III, Set 1. A.S. will monitor for both consistency of voicing and esophageal quality of voicing after each production.

Performance summary: A.S. achieved consistency of voicing and esophageal quality of voicing during one-syllable words beginning with voiced obstruents plus mid and low vowels with 80% accuracy.

Goal 2: Using the injection method for sonorants and vowels, A.S. will articulate precisely 90% of the time during the production of one-syllable words beginning with sonorants and other vowels.

Rationale: Clear articulation is essential to good intelligibility.

Baseline: Articulatory precision achieved 90% of the time during one-syllable words beginning with sonorants and other vowels over two consecutive trials.

Procedure: The clinician will model each of the 10 stimuli from Appendix G, Level IV, Set 7.

Performance summary: A.S. achieved articulatory precision during one-syllable words beginning with sonorants and other vowels with 90% accuracy. He is ready to move to the next step on the hierarchy, the intermediate phase at Level IV.

---

during esophageal speech to gain control of the air charge and to be understood by his listeners.

Baseline

The SLP based the goals for the current session on A.S.'s productions in the previous session (baseline). For the first activity, the baseline indicates that during the last session, A.S. achieved 90% accuracy over three consecutive trials for consistency of voicing and esophageal quality (in separate activities). A.S.'s performance met the criteria for moving to the next step on the hierarchy, from the initial phase to the intermediate phase at the same level of production. For the current session, the two goals are combined into one activity.

For the second activity, A.S. has achieved articulatory precision 90% of the time during the last two consecutive trials. If he maintains 90% accuracy in the activity during the current session, he will meet the criteria to move to the intermediate phase at Level IV.

Table 9.3 Sample lesson plan for tracheoesophageal speech method

Goal: C.C. will use appropriate rate and phrasing during eight-syllable or more phrases and sentences 80% of the time with clinician cues.

Rationale: Inappropriate rate and phrasing interfere with intelligibility.

Baseline: C.C. has used appropriate rate and phrasing during eight-syllable or more phrases and sentences 80% of the time during one activity. All responses were cued by the clinician.

Procedure: The clinician will present 3-in. × 5-in. cards with stimuli taken from Appendix D, Level III, Set 4. The clinician will cue C.C. regarding phrasing by marking the pause on the stimulus card with a red pen. C.C. uses an appropriate rate.

Performance Summary: C.C. achieved appropriate rate and phrasing 90% of the time during eight-syllable or more phrases and sentences. Will try dropping red-pen cue next time.

Materials and Therapy Procedure

Appropriate stimuli were selected from the appendices according to the method of alaryngeal speech. The appropriate stimuli were entered on a score sheet for each of the three activities (see score sheets in Chapter 6). The SLP modeled the 10 stimuli in each therapy activity, so there were no materials to prepare.

Performance Summary

The target behavior for goal one was met. The clinician will continue with this goal at this level of production next session. For goal two, A.S. achieved articulatory precision for this specific task with 90% accuracy for the third consecutive trial. A.S. has met the criteria to move to the next step on the hierarchy: the intermediate phase at Level IV. The results of the session are entered into the therapy log notes of the laryngectomee's file.

Clinical Example 3: C.C.

C.C. is a laryngectomee who is learning how to use her TE prosthesis (TEP). A portion of the lesson plan appears in Table 9.3. The goals for TE speech address valving the stoma to redirect air into the esophagus, precise articulation, appropriate phrasing and rate, and attention to nonverbal behaviors.

Goals

Selection of the therapy goals for C.C. is based on previous therapeutic performance. Because C.C. is in the intermediate phase at Level III of the therapy hierarchy, C.C. is expected to attend to two goals within the same activity: rate and phrasing.

Rationale

Before the speech activity, the clinician explains the goal and the reason for the procedure. C.C. should understand that she is learning to control the air exhaled through the TEP by using brief but effectively placed pauses.

Baseline

During the last session, C.C. performed the same activity planned for the current session with 80% accuracy. All responses were cued by the clinician in terms of marking the pause on the stimulus card with a red pen.

Materials and Therapy Procedure

Stimuli appropriate to TE speech practice were selected from Appendix F. The stimuli were entered on a score sheet (see Figure 7.4). One eight-syllable or more phrase or sentence was written on each of ten 3-in. × 5-in. cards for the activity. In the previous session, the clinician cued C.C. before each production. In the current session, the clinician plans to repeat the activity, with cueing, by marking the appropriate pause with a red pen.

Performance Summary

The target behavior for the activity was measured at 90% accuracy with cueing. According to the clinician's note, the cue will be dropped the next session to see if C.C. is able to maintain her level of performance. The results of the session will be entered into the therapy log notes of the laryngectomee's file.

THERAPY LOGS

After every therapy session or significant interaction with the laryngectomee, the family, or a member of the rehabilitation team, an entry should be made into the laryngectomee's file. The performance summary is transferred from the lesson plan to the therapy log. The entry is written in behavioral terms. In addition to the laryngectomee's performance, the clinician may choose to make notes in terms of the direction of future therapy—for example, "will try dropping red-pen cue next time," or "ready to move to five- to seven-syllable phrases with emphasis on articulation." The entry is written in ink and includes the date and the clinician's signature. Telephone calls or conferences with the laryngectomee, family members, or members of the rehabilitation team are noted. The minimum information required is the date of the call, the person's name, and a brief summary of the contact.

The therapy log should be considered a legal record of interactions with the laryngectomee in the rehabilitation process. Careful documentation of dates, people's names, therapeutic procedures, and recommendations eliminates the frustration of trying to remember such information in the future.

REPORT WRITING

Report writing varies considerably among professional settings. A few of my colleagues do no more than periodically evaluate the laryngectomee's alaryngeal speech productions, record the responses on the score sheet, and place the form in the client's file. Most SLPs engage in some level of report writing. In the alaryngeal speech clinic at San Francisco State University, the laryngectomee's speech is evaluated at the beginning of the semester, and a therapy report, outlining the goals for the semester, is generated. At the close of the semester, the laryngectomee is evaluated again and a progress report is written.

An example of the report outline used in our clinic is illustrated in Figure 9.6. Arrangement of the data may differ according to the requirements in other work settings. Not every method of communication may be used by the laryngectomee; the methods irrelevant to the individual laryngectomee are omitted.

Name: _____   Physician: _____
Address: _____   Address: _____
Telephone: _____   Telephone: _____
Date of birth: _____   Date of surgery: _____
Date of clinic entrance: _____   Clinician: _____
Date of report: _____

  I. Background information
 II. Results of evaluation
     A. Artificial larynx
       1. Type of artificial larynx used; percent of time used; situations used
       2. Placement
       3. Coordination of the "on" control with speaking
       4. Articulation
       5. Rate and phrasing
       6. Nonverbal behaviors
     B. Esophageal speech
       1. Method(s) of air intake used
       2. Voicing
          a. Consistency of voicing
          b. Esophageal quality
          c. Latency
       3. Intelligibility
          a. Articulation
          b. Nonverbal behaviors
          c. Rate and phrasing
          d. Intonation
          e. Loudness
     C. Tracheoesophageal speech
       1. Valving
       2. Articulation
       3. Phrasing
       4. Rate
       5. Nonverbal behaviors
III. Goals
     A. Artificial larynx
     B. Esophageal speech
     C. Tracheoesophageal speech
IV. Progress
     A. Artificial larynx
     B. Esophageal speech
     C. Tracheoesophageal speech
  V. Recommendations

Figure 9.6 Therapy report outline.

10

Saying Good-Bye

In every practice, the therapeutic relationship with the client eventually ends. The termination of therapy occurs in various ways. In alaryngeal speech rehabilitation, the laryngectomee and clinician can agree that the goals of therapy have been met; that the time, effort, and money needed to continue therapy do not merit continuance; or that the therapeutic relationship is no longer viable. The laryngectomee may choose to transfer to another speech therapy program; join a laryngectomee club; or, without the consent of the clinician, discontinue therapy services. In some cases, the laryngectomee has a recurrence of cancer or a coexisting condition that precludes continuing rehabilitation, or the laryngectomee may die.

The most favorable condition is that the laryngectomee works diligently on his or her efforts to achieve functional alaryngeal speech communication and satisfies the goals of the rehabilitation team. The preparation for the discontinuation of therapy begins several sessions before termination. The clinician evaluates the laryngectomee's speech and meets with the laryngectomee and family to discuss the progress report. Everyone is usually in agreement that the laryngectomee is successfully communicating needs, opinions, and information. The laryngectomee is aware of good speech habits and is able to self-monitor consistently and accurately. In essence, the laryngectomee has become his or her own therapist. In our clinic, there is an end-of-the-semester farewell party, complete with a computer-generated "graduation" certificate, and fellow laryngectomees wish the graduate well. Several follow-up telephone calls are made by the speech-language pathologist (SLP) to the laryngectomee or family over the next 3–6 months.

In less than ideal situations, the laryngectomee fails to achieve functional communication skills using one or more of the alaryngeal speech methods. As previously discussed in Chapter 4, a host of reasons are responsible, including medical, surgical, motivational, situational, cognitive, and psychological factors. The clinician has a responsibility to assess the laryngectomee's speech progress periodically and confer with the laryngectomee and the family. When it becomes apparent that the laryngectomee has reached a plateau, the SLP needs to openly discuss the situation with the laryngectomee and family. After a period of time, if the laryngectomee is not making steady progress toward functional communication, the time and money invested in future sessions may not be warranted. If the laryngectomee is making progress but is unable to pay for services or has had insurance coverage terminated, the clinician may consider referring the laryngectomee to a university-run alaryngeal speech clinic or to a local American Cancer Society or International Association of Laryngectomees (IAL) Club. Another consideration is to schedule several laryngectomees for group rather than individual therapy, enabling the laryngectomees to share the cost of the therapy hour.

For various reasons, the learning of an alaryngeal speech method does not take top priority in some laryngectomees' lives. The laryngectomee may lack motivation to follow through on home practice assignments, or the family may not offer support in the learning of a new method. There may be no family or network of close friends to encourage communication skills. One of our laryngectomees lived in a large apartment complex downtown, had no relatives living nearby, and professed to having few friends. His limited communication needs centered around his daily outing. In the afternoon, he walked from his apartment several blocks to a small restaurant where he had an early dinner. On his way back to his apartment, he stopped by the corner market to buy a small carton of milk and a package of rolls for the next morning's breakfast. This gentleman talked more during the once-a-week session at our speech clinic than he did in the entire interim period! He appeared motivated to learn to use the artificial larynx "just in case I need to talk," but he was not particularly interested in learning esophageal speech or pursuing tracheoesophageal (TE) speech. Within the first semester in our clinic, he gained good placement of the artificial larynx, learned to coordinate the "on" control with speaking, and paced himself so he was quite intelligible to the listener. We were not surprised when he declined to return to the clinic the following semester. His communication needs had been met.

Because most SLPs are avid communicators, it is sometimes difficult for them to accept that not everyone is a talker. Sam, one of our more reserved laryngectomees, failed to follow through with speech practice week after week, even after the clinician's explanations of how important carryover into the home environment is to the acquisition of successful alaryngeal speech. Knowing Sam was married, the clinician inquired what Sam thought about his TE speech when he was conversing with his wife. With a wry smile, Sam positioned his finger against his stoma, and, in effortful TE speech, replied "We don't talk. We've been married for 37 years so she already *knows* what I want."

Most of the laryngectomees who attend our alaryngeal speech clinic also frequent one of the area laryngectomee clubs or support groups such as offered by the IAL. We encourage socialization and the opportunity for "our" laryngectomees to interact and communicate with other laryngectomees and their families. In turn, the laryngectomees often bring a friend back to our group. Occasionally, because a laryngectomee prefers the structure offered in another group, the teaching style or personality of another SLP, the convenience of location, or the members in another group, he or she transfers out of our group. With the laryngectomee's permission, therapy records are shared with the new SLP.

Infrequently, one of the laryngectomees moves out of commuting distance. The American Cancer Society or the IAL national listing is an excellent source for assisting the laryngectomee and family in locating contacts in their new area of residence (see Appendix A).

On every laryngectomee's mind is the threat of recurring cancer. The laryngectomees frequently talk about their fears with each other and do occasionally express their concern to the clinician. Sometimes cancer does return. Our alaryngeal speech clinic has lost laryngectomees to cancer and related illnesses. During the writing of this book, two of the laryngectomees in our group passed away, and a third suffered a recurrence. It is never easy to hear the laryngectomee's words: "I went to the doctor and she says the cancer has spread to my lungs."

It is rewarding to work with laryngectomees and their families, and dealing with the loss of one of these special individuals is never a commonplace event for me. And yet, the circle of life in the alaryngeal speech group continues. With the passing of current members of the group, new members come into the group. Recently, I was sitting at my desk, feeling sorrowful after just learning of a client's death. The telephone rang. A physician was calling to refer a recently laryngectomized woman to our alaryngeal speech group—would I mind calling her son to assist them in obtaining an artificial larynx? Within minutes, I had contacted the son and was sharing information with him about the device and making arrangements for the two of them to visit our clinic.

In a moment of reflection, it became clear to me what it means to be part of alaryngeal speech rehabilitation. As SLPs, we are there when the laryngectomee emerges from surgery. Our role is to provide information, comfort and support, and the methods by which to communicate again. In the process, we continually seek ways to serve the laryngectomee's and the family's needs and answer their questions. Because we view the laryngectomee as an individual who needs communication to maintain control of his or her life, we strive to provide therapy that results in efficient, productive, and successful alaryngeal speech. And, when all is said and done, we can say we met the laryngectomee halfway.

It occurred to me that an analogy could be drawn between the reading of a novel and the performance of alaryngeal speech rehabilitation. In a well-written novel, the story does not have to end happily ever after for the reader to say, "That was a good book!" Because no two stories are ever alike, the enjoyment of a novel occurs in the *reading* of the passages and in the anticipation of the story's outcome. Page by page, the reader gains insight into the strengths and weaknesses of the characters as they face life's challenges. The completion of an excellent novel does not dampen the reader's thirst for further reading. Instead, the reader's desire to repeat the experience with a new story is heightened.

If pleasure is derived from the reading of a novel, then satisfaction in alaryngeal speech therapy lies within the *ongoing therapeutic interactions* between the clinician and the laryngectomee. Naturally, the desire to have a happy ending is always present; the essence of motivation is eternal hope. The events that occur *during* the rehabilitation process are of utmost importance. Because no two clients are exactly alike, no two therapies are ever exactly alike. In the process of meeting the challenges of alaryngeal speech, both the clinician and the laryngectomee must give their best performance. When the therapeutic relationship with the laryngectomee ends, the clinician, inspired by the experience, readily begins the rehabilitation process with a new individual and family.

To be proficient clinicians, we bear the responsibility of being knowledgeable of alaryngeal speech rehabilitation, determined in our efforts, deeply caring in our relationships, and constant in our desire to help the laryngectomee and the family. To the laryngectomee and family, to our profession, and to ourselves, we owe nothing less.

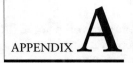

APPENDIX **A**

Guide to Suppliers of Alaryngeal Speech Products and Services

ARTIFICIAL LARYNGES, BATTERIES, AND AMPLIFIERS

Anchor Audio, Inc.
913 West 223rd Street
Torrance, CA 90502
(800) 262-4671

MINI-VOX Amplifier with CM-1000 collar microphone

A. S. Telecom, Inc.
9915 Saint Vital Street
Montreal, Quebec H1H 4S5 Canada
(514) 326-5423
Fax: (514) 326-6576

Service for all artificial larynges
ROMET Speech Aid
Cooper-Rand Electronic Speech Aid
Voice amplifiers
Nu-Vois Artificial Larynx
PO Vox Companion

AT&T Repair Center
Attention: DSR, 5885
Fulton Industrial Boulevard, SW
Atlanta, GA 30378

Repair for AT&T Model Type 5E and 5C Electronic Larynx

Audiphone Company of South Texas
711 Navarro, Suite 204
San Antonio, TX 78205
(210) 223-2033
(800) 683-3277

Servox Inton Electronic Speech Aid

Band K Prescription Shop
601 East Iron
Salina, KS 67401
(913) 827-4455
(800) 432-0224

Servox Inton Electronic Speech Aid
AT&T Electronic Larynx

Beneventine, Tom
58 Woodstock Drive
Wayne, NJ 07470-3548
(201) 694-8417
Fax: (201) 694-0626

Servox Inton Electronic Speech Aid
"Using a Speech Aid" booklet
available in English and Spanish

Bio Support Systems, Inc.
P.O. Box 97
Old Bethpage, NY 11804-0097
(516) 755-3030
(800) 426-9041

Batteries for electronic speech aids

Bivona Medical Technologies
5700 West 23rd Avenue
Gary, IN 46406
(219) 989-9150
(800) 424-8662
Fax: (219) 844-9031
Customer service: (800) 348-6064

OptiVox Artificial Larynx
Nu-Vois Artificial Larynx, charger,
oral adapter and batteries

Brenkert & Deming
P.O. Box 75
Royal Oak, MI 48068
(313) 588-9655

Macrovox Amplifiers (½- and ⅓-watt
versions)
Combination artificial larynx and
amplifier with neck bracket (holds
microphone for hands-free operation)

Brooklyn Respiratory Home Care
7903 17th Avenue
Brooklyn, NY 11214
(718) 331-7769

Servox Inton Electronic Speech Aid
AT&T Electronic Larynx
Jedcom Artificial Larynx
Speech amplifier w/microphone
and headset

Bruce Medical Supply
411 Waverly Oaks Road
P.O. Box 9166
Waltham, MA 02254
(800) 225-8446
Fax: (617) 894-9519

Servox Inton Electronic Speech Aid
BRUCE Lectro Larynx, oral adapter
and replacement batteries

California Speech and Hearing Instruments
1930 Wilshire Boulevard #810
Los Angeles, CA 90057
(213) 483-4481
Fax: (213) 483-0527

Cooper-Rand Electronic Speech Aid
Neovox Artificial Larynx
Servox Inton Electronic Speech Aid
Macrovox
Voicette
ROMET Speech Aid
Nu-Vois Artificial Larynx
Accessories, batteries
Repairs
Hearing aids

Care Medical Supply
2 Harvey Street
Rome, GA 30161
(706) 232-2001
(800) 273-1763

Servox Inton Electronic Speech Aid
Batteries, dual and single charging units
Speech amplifiers
Oral connectors

Chatterbox Club of Santa Cruz
c/o O. C. Eldridge
76 Sincero Drive
Watsonville, CA 95706
(408) 728-4704

Cooper-Rand and AT&T operating instructions in Spanish
Esophageal speech instruction audio-cassette in Spanish (76 mins)

Communicative Medical, Inc.
P.O. Box 8241
2518 South Grand Boulevard
Spokane, WA 99203-0241
(509) 838-1060
(800) 944-6801

Servox Inton Electronic Speech Aid
ROMET Speech Aid
TruTone Electronic Speech Aid
Nu-Vois Artificial Larynx
Chargers, batteries
Servox Inton Electronic Speech Aid and ROMET Speech Aid
FLEX-MIKE Personal Amplifier
MINI-VOX Amplifier
Piper-1 Personal Amplifier and adapter
Repairs
Reconditioned artificial larynxes

Earphonics, Inc.
22777 Kelly Road
Eastpointe, MI 48021
(810) 773-3300

Servox Inton Electronic Speech Aid

EZ Speech, Inc.
P.O. Box 31
11300 Ironbridge Road, Suite D
Chester, VA 23831
(804) 796-1917
(800) 758-8255
Fax: (804) 796-9332

Servox Inton Electronic Speech Aid
Nu-Vois Artificial Larynx
ROMET Speech Aid
PO Vox Companion
SPKR Artificial Larynx
Jedcom Artificial Larynx
MINI-VOX Amplifier
Batteries and accessories
Servox Inton Electronic Speech Aid or
    Nu-Vois Artificial Larynx

Freeman's Hearing Aid Center
2230 East Pikes Peak Avenue
Colorado Springs, CO 80909
(719) 632-2376

Servox Inton Electronic Speech Aid
Nu-Vois Artificial Larynx

Hart, Jessie
1750 Avenue East
Grand Prairie, TX 75051
(214) 264-3129

Servox Inton Electronic Speech Aid
ROMET Speech Aid
Nu-Vois Artificial Larynx
SPKR Artificial Larynx
Batteries

Health Concepts, Inc.
279-B Great Valley Parkway
Malvern, PA 19355
(215) 889-7363
(800) 721-4848 or (800) 673-7881

Ultra Voice

InHealth Technologies
1110 Mark Avenue
Carpinteria, CA 93013-2918
(805) 684-9337
(800) 477-5969
Fax: (805) 684-8594
http://www.inhealth.com

Servox Inton Electronic Speech Aid

International Medical Resource
    Industries (IMRI)
P.O. Box 120
Brookfield, CT 06804-0120
(203) 775-6336
Fax: (203) 775-0522

Batteries for Servox Inton Electronic
    Speech Aid, ROMET Speech Aid,
    Western Electric Artificial Larynx,
    and Cooper-Rand Electronic
    Speech Aid

Janssen, Kenneth W.
9407 Catalina Drive
Bradenton, FL 34210
(813) 792-4251

Servox Inton Electronic Speech Aid
ROMET Speech Aid
Oral connector and replacement parts

Kemp, Jack
44547 Woodrow Way
Hemet, CA 92544
(909) 927-7534

TruTone Electronic Speech Aid

Lakewood Hearing and Speech Center
3110 S. Wadsworth, Suite 107
Lakewood, CO 80227
(303) 988-7299

Servox Inton Electronic Speech Aid
Oral connectors
Batteries
Chargers
Repair

Lauder Enterprises
11115 Whisper Hollow
San Antonio, TX 78230-3609
(210) 492-1984
(800) 388-8642
Fax: (210) 492-0864

Servox Inton Electronic Speech Aid
Nu-Vois Artificial Larynx
TruTone Electronic Speech Aid
Denrick Speech Aid
Servox holsters
Batteries and chargers
FLEX-MIKE and MINI-VOX amplifiers
The Vocal Assistant
Repair

Luminaud, Inc.
8688 Tyler Boulevard
Mentor, OH 44060
(216) 255-9082
(800) 255-3408
Fax: (216) 255-2250

Servox Inton Electronic Speech Aid
Nu-Vois Artificial Larynx
Denrick Speech Aid
Cooper-Rand Electronic Speech Aid
   (regular and 9-V versions; no
   hands; amplifier)
TruTone Electronic Speech Aid
Voicette Amplifier
MINI-VOX Amplifier
Texas Instruments Vocaid
Accessories
Repair

Main Street Pharmacy
2121 Main Street
Buffalo, NY 14214
(716) 835-2118

Servox Inton Electronic Speech Aid

MedMart, Inc.
P.O. Box 724
Glendora, CA 91740
(818) 963-0620
(800) 725-1414

Servox Inton Electronic Speech Aid
Batteries

Medical West
444 South Brentwood
Clayton, MO 63105
(800) 489-1888

Servox Inton Electronic Speech Aid

Park Surgical Company, Inc.
5001 New Utrecht Avenue
Brooklyn, NY 11219
(718) 436-9200
(800) 633-7878
Fax: (718) 854-2431

BRUCE Lectro Larynx
Servox Inton Electronic Speech Aid
Park Speech Amplifier with headset
  or throat microphone
Extension speaker
Park Pausaid

**Professional Hearing and
  Speech Aids Service**
30 Salem Marketplace (Jct Rt 82 and 85)
Salem, CT 06420
(203) 525-2131 or (203) 859-2807
(800) 454-7778
Fax: (203) 859-3102

Servox Inton Electronic Speech Aid
ROMET Speech Aid
Cooper-Rand Electronic Speech Aid
Nu-Vois Artificial Larynx
FLEX-MIKE Amplifier
Rand Amplifier
Texas Instruments Vocaid
Voicette Amplifier
Speechmaker Amplifier

**Radio Shack. A Division of the
  Tandy Corporation**
Check distributors listed in the
  white pages of the local telephone
  directory.

Amplifiers

ROMET, Inc.
929 SW Higgins Avenue
Missoula, MT 59803
(406) 721-7150
(406) 721-7442
Fax: (406) 721-7261

ROMET Speech Aid, batteries,
  charger and oral adapter

ROMET-West
15525 6th Avenue, SW, #12
Seattle, WA 98166
(206) 242-5009

ROMET Speech Aid, batteries,
  and charger

Rosencrans, Dean
P.O. Box 310
Nampa, ID 83653-0128
(208) 467-4790
(800) 522-4425 or (800) 237-3699

Varta battery (fits Servox Inton
Electonic Speech Aid, ROMET
Speech Aid, Jedcome/Bruce Lectro
Larynx)
SPKR Artificial Larynx

Siemens Hearing Instruments, Inc.
16 East Piper Lane, Suite 128
Prospect Heights, IL 60070-1799
(708) 808-1200
(800) 333-9083
Fax: (708) 808-1299

Servox Inton Electronic Speech Aid
Batteries
Oral connectors
Charging units

Slobodian Enterprises
345 Millpond Drive
San Jose, CA 95126
(408) 297-3469

Servox Inton Electronic Speech Aid
ROMET Speech Aid
Nu-Vois Artificial Larynx
SPKR Artificial Larynx
Batteries

Synergistic Batteries, Inc.
3760 Lower Roswell Road
Marietta, GA 30068
(404) 973-2220
(800) 634-6000

Batteries for Servox Inton Electronic
Speech Aid and ROMET Speech Aid

UNI Mfg. Co.
P.O. Box 607
Ontario, OR 97914 Canada
(503) 889-6567
(800) GET-SPKR

SPKR Artificial Larynx and charging
unit

Unipower
1216 West 96th Street
Minneapolis, MN 55431
(612) 884-2933
(800) 542-6998
Fax: (612) 884-1726

Batteries for Servox Inton Electronic
Speech Aid

Welch, Clyde
2027 Read Street #53
Omaha, NE 68112
(402) 453-6320

Tokyo Artificial Larynx

MEDICAL EMERGENCY INFORMATION

Bruce Medical Supply
411 Waverly Oaks Road
P.O. Box 9166
Waltham, MA 02254
(718) 894-6262
(800) 225-8446
Fax: (617) 894-9519

Medical identification jewelry bracelets and pendants

CareCard Corporation
P.O. Box 6555
Denver, CO 80206
(303) 321-8583

Laminated medical data cards with immediate, individual, and in-depth information in two styles: CareCard (wallet) and SportshoeCard

IAL National Office
c/o American Cancer Society
1599 Clifton Road, NE
Atlanta, GA 30329
(404) 320-3333

Pocket emergency identification cards for "Total Neck Breather" (Code #4520), "TEP Laryngectomees" (Code #4525), and "Total Neck Breather" (Spanish version, Code #4513)

IAL Treasurer
c/o American Cancer Society
1599 Clifton Road, NE
Atlanta, GA 30329
(404) 320-3333

Emergency windshield stickers (English or Spanish), $0.25 each
IAL Lapel Pins $3.00 each

Medic Alert Foundation International
2323 Colorado Avenue
Turlock, CA 95380
(800) 432-5378

Bracelet or necklace engraved with identification
Wallet card
24-hour hotline: (800) 432-5378

Stoma Button Company, Inc.
P.O. Box 985
Baker, OR 97814-0984
(503) 894-2367

Emergency information kit (key tag with ring, engraved pocket information card, and free window sticker)

WORLD WIDE WEB SITES ABOUT LARYNGEAL CANCER

http://www.inhealth.com

Product catalog
Updates and resources
Featured products
Troubleshooting
Related web sites

http://cancer.med.upenn.edu/
  disease/larynx/index

http://oncolink.upenn.edu/
  disease/larynx

PUBLICATIONS

American Cancer Society
1599 Clifton Road NE
Atlanta, GA 30329-4251

Pamphlets available free of charge:
Advanced Cancer: Living Each Day
*Building a Successful Laryngectomee
  Club*
*California Cancer Facts & Figures—
  1996*
Cancer Facts & Figures—1996
*Chemotherapy and You: A Guide to
  Self-Help During Treatment*
Eating Hints for Cancer Patients
*Facing Forward: A Guide for Cancer
  Survivors*
Facts on Cancer of the Larynx
*First Aid for Laryngectomees (Neck
  Breathers)*
*First Steps: Helping Words for the
  Laryngectomee*
*IAL: Directory of Instructors of
  Alaryngeal Speech*
IAL Club Directory
*IAL Directory of Instructors of
  Alaryngeal Speech*
IAL News Mailing List Request Card
IAL Newsletter
IAL: Rehabilitating Laryngectomees
Laryngectomized Speakers' Source Book
Neckwear Pattern Book

*Radiation Therapy and You: A Guide
to Self-Help During Treatment
Rescue Breathing for Laryngectomees
and Other Neck Breathers
Taking Time: Support for People with
Cancer and the People Who Care
About Them
What You Need to Know About
Cancer of the Larynx
When Cancer Returns: Meeting the
Challenge Again
When Someone in Your Family Has
Cancer
Your New Voice*

**The Bill Wilkerson Hearing and
Speech Center**
1114-19th Avenue South
Nashville, TN 37213
(615) 320-5353

Progressive Steps to a New Voice

Bradford Publications
5805 Fox Chapel Drive
Austin, TX 78746-6209
(800) 354-2760

Say That Again Please by Tom Bradford

Butterworth–Heinemann
313 Washington Street
Newton, MA 02158-1626
(617) 928-2500
Fax: (617) 928-2620

Take Time to Talk (2nd ed) by
Patricia F. White

Communicative Medical, Inc.
P.O. Box 8241
Spokane, WA 99203-0241
(509) 838-1060
(800) 944-6801

Why Didn't They Tell Me? by
Donald G. Moss
The Non-Chew Cookbook by
Randy Wilson

Grune & Stratton, Inc.
111 Fifth Avenue
New York, NY 10003

The Artificial Larynx Handbook by
Shirley J. Salmon and Lewis P.
Goldstein

Keller, Margot
654 West Northern Avenue
Lima, OH 45801-2508

Speech Without Vocal Chords by
Margot Keller

Lauder Enterprises
11115 Whisper Hollow
San Antonio, TX 78230-3609
(210) 492-1984
(800) 388-8642
Fax: (210) 492-0864

Self-Help for the Laryngectomee by
  Edmund Lauder
Why Didn't They Tell Me? by
  Donald G. Moss

LWT Enterprises
8900 Thorton Road
Box 99030
Stockton, CA 95209
(209) 473-3480

*Look Who's Talking...A Guide to
  Esophageal Speech* by Jack E.
  Henslee

Pelican Publishing Company
1101 Monroe Street
P.O. Box 3110, Gretna, LA 70054
(504) 368-1175
(800) 843-1724

The Magic Box by Olga Cossi

PRO-ED, Inc.
8700 Shoal Creek Boulevard
Austin, TX 78757
(512) 451-3276
Fax: (512) 451-8542

*A Guide to Instruction in the Use of
  an Artificial Larynx* by Marilyn B.
  Rogers
*A Handbook for the Laryngectomee
  (3rd ed)* by Robert L. Keith and
  Jack E. Thomas
*After the Laryngectomy: A Post-
  Operative Orientation* by John
  Wilshaw
*Alaryngeal Speech Rehabilitation for
  Clinicians by Clinicians* by Shirley
  J. Salmon and Kay H. Mount
Laryngectomee Rehabilitation (3rd ed)
  edited by Robert Keith and Frederic
  L. Darley
*The Laryngectomee: A Booklet for
  Family and Friends (3rd ed)* by
  Barbara Dabul

Singular Publishing Group, Inc.
4284 41st Street
San Diego, CA 92105-1197
(800) 521-8545

*Clinical Manual for Laryngectomy
  and Head and Neck Cancer Rehab-
  ilitation* by Janina K. Casper and
  Raymond H. Colton
*Voice and Speech Rehabilitation
  Following Laryngeal Cancer* by
  Philip C. Doyle

Thieme Medical Publishers
381 Park Avenue S, Suite 1501
New York, NY 10157-0208
(212) 683-5088
(800) 782-3488

*Looking Forward...A Guidebook for
the Laryngectomee (3rd ed)* by
Robert L. Keith

Wayne State University Press
The Leonard N. Simons Building
4809 Woodward Avenue
Detroit, MI 48201-1309
(800) 978-7323

Workbook for Reasoning Skills by
Susan Howell Brubaker
Workbook for Cognitive Skills by
Susan Howell Brubaker
Workbook for Aphasia by Susan
Howell Brubaker
Workbook for Language Skills by
Susan Howell Brubaker
*Sourcebook for Speech, Language,
and Cognition, Books 1 and 2* by
Susan Howell Brubaker

STOMA COVERS AND NECKWEAR, AIR FILTERS, SHOWER COLLARS

A. S. Telecom, Inc.
9915 Saint Vital Street
Montreal, Quebec H1H 4S5 Canada
(514) 326-5423
Fax: (514) 326-6576

Shower protectors
Buchanan laryngectomy protectors
Foam filters

Band K Prescription Shop
601 East Iron
Salina, KS 67401
(913) 827-4455
(800) 432-0224

Shower shields
Stoma shields
Cardinal E-Z Breathe Filters
Cloth stoma covers

Becker, Sylvia
6020 Nevada Avenue #17
Woodland Hills, CA 91367
(818) 702-0562

Beaded neck pieces for women (send
SASE for price list)

Beneventine, Tom
58 Woodstock Drive
Wayne, NJ 07470-3548
(201) 694-8417

Velcro shower guard

Bivens, Norma
1614 East Myrtle #D
Canton, IL 61520
(309) 647-3299

Handmade neckwear

Bivona Medical Technologies
5700 West 23rd Avenue
Gary, IN 46406
(219) 989-9150
(800) 424-8662
Fax: (219) 844-9031
Customer service: (800) 348-6064

Stoma cover/protectors
STOM-VENT/STOM-VENT 2 heat
  and moisture exchanger
Artificial saliva
Lubricants

Brooklyn Respiratory Home Care
7903 17th Avenue
Brooklyn, NY 11214
(718) 331-7769

Shower protectors
Ultrasonic humidifiers
Suction machines
Trachea and laryngectomy tubes
Stoma scarves
Turtlenecks

Bruce Medical Supply
411 Waverly Oaks Road
P.O. Box 9166
Waltham, MA 02254
(718) 894-6262
(800) 225-8446
Fax: (617) 894-9519

Latex shower collars
Stoma covers
Foam stoma filters
Turtleneck stoma covers
Trach tube strap
Fashion stoma scarves
Ascots

Byram Healthcare Center
75 Holly Hill Lane
Greenwich, CT 06830
(800) 354-4054

Shower cover
Cotton stoma bibs
Trachea and laryngectomy brushes
Plastic and metal trachea and laryn-
  gectomy tubes
Gauze products

Cardinal Manufacturing Company
1055 East 52nd Street
Indianapolis, IN 46205
(317) 283-4175
Fax: (317) 283-1336

E-Z Breathe Filter, frame, and chain

Communicative Medical, Inc.
P.O. Box 8241
Spokane, WA 99203-0241
(509) 838-1060
(800) 944-6801

Stoma shower covers
Foam stoma filters
Artificial saliva
Cloth stoma covers
Skin barrier and adhesive remover
   products

Dietrich, Gene
1012 Townplace,
Houston, TX 77057
Telephone/Fax: (713) 789-1656
e-mail: flyer@hal-pc.org

Classic and custom-made necklaces
   and pendants for women

EZ Speech, Inc.
P.O. Box 31
11300 Ironbridge Road, Suite D
Chester, VA 23831
(804) 796-1917
(800) 758-8255
Fax: (804) 796-9332

Shower shields
Foam filters
Knit stoma covers
Stoma scarves and neckerchieves

Freeman's Hearing Aid Center
2230 East Pikes Peak Avenue
Colorado Springs, CO 80909
(719) 632-2376

Shower shield
Foam filters
Protection bibs
Polyester and knot scarves

Gibeck-Dryden Corporation
10640 East 59th Street
P.O. Box 36038
Indianapolis, IN 46236
(317) 823-6866
Customer service: (800) 428-5321

STOM-VENT
Trach-Vent

Hart, Jessie
1750 Avenue East
Grand Prairie, TX 75051
(214) 264-3129

Foam stoma protection covers
Rubber shower collar

Hegyi, Maida
IAL Auxiliary
13129 Thraves Avenue
Garfield Heights, OH 44125
(216) 662-3766

*Neckwear Pattern Book for Laryn-
gectomees* (one copy available free
of charge)

Hettrich, Joyce
8712 Livingston Lane
Eden Prairie, MN 55347
(612) 949-6534

Handmade beaded necklaces

InHealth Technologies
1110 Mark Avenue
Carpinteria, CA 93013-2918
(805) 684-9337
(800) 477-5969
Fax: (805) 684-8594
http://www.inhealth.com

Shower guard

Janssen, Kenneth W.
9407 Catalina Drive
Bradenton, FL 34210
(813) 792-4251

ROMET Filter Collars
Stoma covers
Stoma filters

Jockey International Inc.
Consumer Relations
2300 60th Street
Kenosha, WI 53140
(414) 658-8111

Mock turtleneck T-shirt, short sleeve, white (S, M, L, XL #8351; $6.00 postage paid)

Lakewood Hearing and Speech Center
3110 South Wadsworth, Suite 107
Lakewood, CO 80227
(303) 988-7299

Shower protectors
Larynx protection bibs
Stoma filters
Knit scarves and neckerchieves

Laryngectomee Fashions
Route 1, Box 88
Big Cabin, OK 74332
(918) 783-5424

Cloth stoma covers (four styles in a variety of colors and prints; special orders)

Lauder Enterprises
11115 Whisper Hollow
San Antonio, TX 78230-3609
(210) 492-1984
(800) 388-8642
Fax: (210) 492-0864

Buchanan stoma covers
Shower shields
Foam filters
Mesh stoma covers

Luminaud, Inc.
8688 Tyler Boulevard
Mentor, OH 44060
(216) 255-9082
(800) 255-3408
Fax: (216) 255-2250

Shower stoma collar
ROMET Filter Collars
Buchanan Stoma Covers
Breathe-Easy Stoma Covers
Stomafoam squares
Stoma Cover Sampler Kit
Ladies lace collars
Designer necklaces

Marx, Betty
510 East 77th Street, Suite 1008
New York, NY 10162
(212) 734-2552

Beaded necklaces
Open-back dog collars
Coordinating bracelets
Ascots

MedMart, Inc.
P.O. Box 724
Glendora, CA 91740
(818) 963-0620
(800) 725-1414

Rubber collar shower shield
StomaGuard I shower shield
Foam filter stoma covers
StomaShield Cover and Band
ReadyMade stoma shields

Park Surgical Company
5001 New Utrecht Avenue
Brooklyn, NY 11219
(718) 436-9200
(800) 633-7878

Trachea shower bib
Cotton and nylon trach bibs

**Professional Hearing and Speech
  Aids Service**
30 Salem Marketplace (Jct Rt 82 and 85)
Salem, CT 06103
(203) 525-2131
(203) 859-2807
Fax: (203) 859-3102

Shower stoma protection
ROMET Filter Collars
Breathe-Easy Stoma Filters
Foam stoma filters

ROMET, Inc.
929 SW Higgins Avenue
Missoula, MT 59803
(406) 721-7150; (406) 721-7442
Fax: (406) 721-7261

ROMET Filter Collars
Ascots

Rosencrans, Dean
P.O. Box 128
Nampa, ID 83653-0128
(208) 467-4790
(800) 522-4425 or (800) 237-3699

Contour fitting shower cover
Cloth stoma covers
Foam stoma covers
Foam filters
Beaded stoma covers for women

Shield Health Care Center
2 Armonk Street
Greenwich, CT 06830
(800) 354-4054

Cotton stoma covers

Siemens Hearing Instruments, Inc.
16 East Piper Lane, Suite 128
Prospect Heights, IL 60070
(708) 808-1200
(800) 333-9083
Fax: (708) 808-1299

Rubber shower protector
Larynx protection bibs
Knit scarves and neckerchieves
Tracheofix foam filters

Stoma Button Company, Inc.
P.O. Box 985
Baker, OR 97814-0984
(503) 894-2367

Laryngectomy tube/tracheostoma
    vent (custom sizes available)
Stoma filter button set

Thomas, Alma P.
102 Cedar Ridge Way
Niceville, FL 32578
(904) 678-9036

Crochet stoma covers (assorted
    colors and styles)

SWIMMING DEVICES

Brooklyn Respiratory Home Care
7903 17th Avenue
Brooklyn, NY 11214
(718) 331-7769

LARKEL snorkel

**H. Lee Moffitt Cancer Center &
    Research Institute**
12902 Magnolia Drive
Tampa, FL 33612-9497

LARKEL snorkel

TRACHEOESOPHAGEAL PROSTHESES AND SUPPLIES

Bivona Medical Technologies
5700 West 23rd Avenue
Gary, IN 46406
(219) 989-9150
(800) 424-8662
Fax: (219) 844-9031
Customer service: (800) 348-6064

Barton-Mayo Tracheostoma Button
Bivona-Colorado Voice Restoration
  Systems
Bivona Duckbill Prosthesis
Bivona UltraLow Resistance Voice
  Prosthesis
Bivona Tracheostoma Vents
PROVOX Voice Restoration System
Tracheostoma Valve I and II and kits

Bruce Medical Supply
411 Waverly Oaks Road
P.O. Box 9166
Waltham, MA 02254
(718) 894-6262
(800) 225-8446
Fax: (617) 894-9519

Double-sided adhesive foam discs for
  Bivona and Blom-Singer tracheostoma valves

E. Benson Hood Laboratories, Inc.
5757 Washington Street
Pembroke, MA 02359
(617) 826-7573
(800) 942-5227
Fax: (617) 826-3899

Panje Voice Prosthesis
Tracheostoma valves

Gauthier Medical, Inc.
3105 NW 22nd Street
Rochester, MN 55901
(507) 289-0761
(800) 348-6064
Fax: (507) 289-6883

Barton-Mayo Tracheostoma Button
  and Sizing Kit

InHealth Technologies
1110 Mark Avenue
Carpinteria, CA 93013-2918
(805) 684-9337
(800) 477-5969
Fax: (805) 684-8594
http://www.inhealth.com

Blom-Singer Indwelling Low Pressure
  Voice Prosthesis
Blom-Singer Voice Restoration
  Systems
Blom-Singer Adjustable Tracheo-
  stoma Valve with Humidifier
Tracheostoma accessories
Blom-Singer HumidiFilter Heat/
  Moisture Exchanger (HME)
Professional products and training aids

VIDEOTAPES

American Cancer Society
Local Unit or State Division (see white
    pages of the local telephone directory)

*Rescue Breathing for Laryngecto-
mees and Other Neck Breathers*
(16 mins)
It's Not a Walk in the Park (16 mins;
#4523.05)
Speech After Laryngectomy (21 mins;
#4536.05)
Three Critical Minutes (17 mins;
#4539.05)
The Laryngectomee Visitor (17 mins;
#4561.05)
Check the Neck (17 mins; #4534.05)

EZ Speech, Inc.
P.O. Box 31
11300 Ironbridge Road, Suite D
Chester, VA 23831
(804) 796-1917
(800) 758-8255
Fax: (804) 796-9332

EZ Speech Video (13 mins) (illustrates product line of artificial
larynges)

HarMar Enterprises, Inc.
Harvey P. Hite
P.O. Box 4056
3004 Plum Street
Parkersburg, WV 26104
(304) 428-5081

Life and Voice After Laryngectomy
Everyday Living as a Laryngectomee
Keep Smoking and Talk Like Me
Printed scripts available

InHealth Technologies
1110 Mark Avenue
Carpinteria, CA 93013-2918
(805) 684-9337
(800) 477-5969
Fax: (805) 684-8594
http://www.inhealth.com

*Blom-Singer Low-Pressure Voice
Prosthesis Kit with GEL-CAP
Insertion* (17 mins)
*Blom-Singer Tracheoesophageal
Voice Restoration* (30 mins)
Endoscopic Voice Restoration (9 mins)
Primary Voice Restoration (14 mins)
*Blom-Singer Adjustable Tracheostoma
Valve* (17 mins)

**National Clearing House of
Rehabilitation Training Materials**
Oklahoma State University
826 West 6th Avenue
Stillwater, OK 74078-0435
(405) 624-7650
(800) 223-5219
Fax: (405) 624-0695

17 videotaped sessions (e.g., esophageal speech training, use of artificial larynx, peer support, employment after laryngectomee)
A pamphlet is available for each topic

Orange County Lost Chord Club
c/o Jim Choate
American Cancer Society
3631 S. Harbor Bouelvard, Suite 200
Santa Ana, CA 92704
(714) 751-0441

It's Not a Walk in the Park (16 mins)

Rosencrans, Dean
P.O. Box 310
Nampa, ID 83653-0128
(208) 467-4790
(800) 522-4425 or (800) 237-3699

Secrets of Esophageal Speech (30 mins)

TDL Instructional Communications
60 Watervliet Avenue
Dayton, OH 45420
(513) 298-6583 or (513) 226-7877

Laryngectomy: Preoperative Counseling (25 mins)
Laryngectomy: Postoperative Care I (25 mins)
Laryngectomy: Postoperative Care II (25 mins)

Welch, Clyde
2027 Read Street, #53
Omaha, NE 68112

Two videocassettes demonstrating the Tokyo artificial larynx are available for short-term loan at no cost to the speech-language pathologist

IAL = International Association of Laryngectomees; TEP = tracheoesophageal prosthesis.

APPENDIX B

Relaxation Exercise

Directions: *The clinician may choose to read the following passage aloud to the laryngectomee or record the exercise on audiotape. The passage should be read slowly, using a soothing, low-pitched voice. Give the individual time to perform the procedures.*

Allow your muscles to become loose and heavy. Settle back quietly and comfortably in your chair. Wrinkle your forehead. Smooth it out. Picture your entire forehead and scalp becoming smoother as the relaxation increases. Now frown and crease your brows and study the tension. Let go of the tension again. Smooth out your forehead once more.

Focus on your eyes. Close your eyes tighter and tighter. Feel the tension. Relax your eyes. Keep your eyes closed, gently and comfortably, and notice the relaxation.

Clench your jaw. Bite your teeth together. Study the tightness throughout your jaw. Loosen your jaw and allow your mouth to fall open.

Part your lips slightly. Appreciate the relaxation. Keeping your mouth slightly open, press your tongue hard against the roof of your mouth. Look for the tension. Let your tongue return to a comfortable and relaxed position.

Now purse your lips and press your lips together tighter and tighter. Relax your lips. Note the contrast between tension and relaxation. Feel the relaxation all over your face—your forehead, scalp, eyes, jaws, lips, tongue, and neck muscles.

Lean your head to the right as far as you can and observe the tightness on the left side of your neck. Roll your head to the left and feel the tension shift to the right side of your neck. Straighten your head and bring it forward. Try to press your chin against your chest. Return your head to a comfortable position, and experience the relaxation.

203

Shrug your shoulders high against your neck. Hold the muscle tension. Drop your shoulders and allow them to become heavy. Shrug your shoulders again and move them around. Bring your shoulders upward and forward and then upward and backward. Feel the tightness in your shoulders and in your upper back. Drop your shoulders once more and relax. Let the relaxation spread deep into your shoulders and into your back muscles. Release the muscles of your neck and throat, your jaw, and other facial areas as complete relaxation takes over and grows deeper and deeper . . . ever deeper.

Oral-Facial Exercises

Directions:

- *The exercises are divided into sections to emphasize certain speech organs.*
- *Perform each of these exercises in a slow, smooth manner. Speed is not important unless otherwise noted.*
- *If a particular exercise is uncomfortable, do not continue it. Go on to the next exercise.*
- *Repeat each exercise five times each, twice per day. Build to 10 times each, twice per day.*

LIP EXERCISES

1. Close your lips and slowly fill your cheeks with air. When your cheeks are full of air, hold the air for 5 seconds and release. Try not to let air escape through your lips.
2. Repeat exercise 1, except this time, puff up one cheek and move the air from one cheek to the other. Release.
3. Close your lips and suck in your cheeks as tightly as you can. Hold for 5 seconds and release.
4. Form a tight circle with your lips as if to say "oh" (as in "oat"). Hold for 5 seconds and release.
5. Purse your lips as if to say "ooh" (as in "you"). Retract your lips as if to say "eee" (as in "eat"). Alternate pursing and retracting your lips. Think "ooh-eee, ooh-eee." Do your repetitions slowly at first, then build for speed.
6. Make popping sounds with your lips for the production of "pa-pa-pa." Build for speed. See how many sets you can do in 5 seconds.
7. Place a tongue blade between your lips and hold it tightly for 5 seconds. Gently tug on the tongue blade as you resist with your lips.

TONGUE EXERCISES

1. Protrude your tongue as far from your mouth as possible. Draw your tongue as far back in your mouth as possible.
2. Protrude your tongue from your mouth. Move your tongue from side to side without touching your lips (your jaw must be open).
3. Protrude your tongue from your mouth. With your tongue tip, lift your tongue toward your nose.
4. Protrude your tongue from your mouth. With your tongue tip, draw your tongue downward toward your chin.
5. Rotate your tongue around the outside of your mouth clockwise (left to right).
6. Rotate your tongue around the outside of your mouth counterclockwise (right to left).
7. With your mouth closed, rotate your tongue inside your lips clockwise (left to right).
8. With your mouth closed, rotate your tongue inside your lips counterclockwise (right to left).
9. With your mouth closed, press your tongue against the inside of your left cheek. Then press your tongue against the inside of your right cheek.
10. Click your tongue against the roof of your mouth. Imitate movements for "la-la-la."
11. Press your tongue tip against the back of your front teeth and produce "ta-ta-ta." Build for speed. See how many sets you can do in 5 seconds.
12. Pull your tongue upward and backward against the roof of your mouth and produce "ka-ka-ka." Build for speed. See how many sets you can do in 5 seconds.

JAW EXERCISES

1. Open and close your mouth. Do three repetitions slowly.
2. Open your mouth widely, as if to yawn. Hold for 5 seconds and close.
3. Open your jaw, sliding your jaw to the right. Close.
4. Open your jaw, sliding your jaw to the left. Close.
5. Imitate the way a cow chews its cud. Rotate your jaw in a circular direction, first one way, then the other.
6. Clench your jaw and hold it for 5 seconds. Relax your jaw, allowing your mouth to fall open for 5 seconds. Close your jaw gently.

Practice Stimuli, Unrestricted Phonetic Context

APPENDIX D. PRACTICE STIMULI, UNRESTRICTED PHONETIC CONTEXT

For use during
- Artificial larynx speech
- Combined methods of esophageal speech
- Tracheoesophageal speech

LEVEL I: TWO- TO FOUR-SYLLABLE PHRASES AND SENTENCES

Set 1
1. Act your age.
2. Do a good job.
3. quick and easy
4. Hurry up!
5. no parking
6. Skip lunch.
7. Come as you are.
8. Let's get started.
9. Forget it.
10. What did you say?

Set 2
1. It's a small world.
2. for the record
3. left or right
4. Put out the cat.
5. because of you
6. ten years ago
7. saved by the bell
8. Start the car.
9. happy birthday
10. bird in the bush

Set 3
1. afternoon nap
2. Check the mail.
3. young at heart
4. Three's a crowd.
5. first to know
6. in the kitchen
7. out of town
8. More coffee, please.
9. Starve a cold.
10. Boy, am I tired!

Set 4
1. near the exit
2. Pack a lunch.
3. Keep off the grass.
4. zebra's stripes
5. Move over.
6. throughout the day
7. of mice and men
8. railroad crossing
9. smile ear to ear
10. Buy a used car.

Set 5
1. I'll write a check.
2. Find it!
3. mom and pop
4. just a minute
5. Are you with me?
6. He's got cold feet.
7. quite a few
8. bacon and eggs
9. Scratch my back.
10. forty winks

Set 6
1. fresh strawberries
2. last to know
3. medium-well
4. Pay the rent.
5. no thank you
6. Ask for help.
7. Yes, I see it.
8. through thick and thin
9. Stop the paper.
10. Call the police.

Set 7
1. black and white
2. Come with me.
3. Everyone knows.
4. years from now
5. vegetable soup
6. Take two aspirin.
7. in front of me
8. Keep it simple.
9. queen mother
10. Smell the roses.

Set 8
1. soup and sandwich
2. I'm cold.
3. Good afternoon.
4. from now on
5. restful sleep
6. Oops! I dropped it.
7. Bill me later.
8. dime a dozen
9. zest for living
10. The car won't start.

APPENDIX D. PRACTICE STIMULI, UNRESTRICTED PHONETIC CONTEXT

For use during
- Artificial larynx speech
- Combined methods of esophageal speech
- Tracheoesophageal speech

LEVEL I: TWO- TO FOUR-SYLLABLE PHRASES AND SENTENCES *(continued)*

Set 9
1. Look at me.
2. Neatness counts.
3. one good reason
4. Haste makes waste.
5. Foot the bill.
6. You asked for it.
7. all together
8. up to no good
9. Phone long distance.
10. I need a ride.

Set 10
1. Give him a hand.
2. How much is it?
3. Pace yourself.
4. smart as a fox
5. at the movies
6. Close the door.
7. your turn to pay
8. too hot for me
9. busy day
10. Meet me at eight.

Set 11
1. Aim for the stars.
2. Who knows?
3. late again
4. Grand Canyon
5. raining outside
6. soap and water
7. Fight fire with fire.
8. zoo on Monday
9. Pick a time.
10. on the edge

Set 12
1. Call the doctor.
2. Figure it out.
3. bottom line
4. the more you know
5. Yankee Doodle
6. zero in
7. sunny weather
8. Mention my name.
9. glass of milk
10. off his rocker

Set 13
1. Pass the salt.
2. Kick the habit.
3. Stop for gas.
4. got the flu
5. Comb your hair.
6. Yield to pressure.
7. Answer the phone.
8. flashing red lights
9. roll of stamps
10. top of the world

Set 14
1. I want to win.
2. just between us
3. out to lunch
4. See you later.
5. back to school
6. Clap your hands.
7. Write a check.
8. too tired to move
9. button up
10. mashed potatoes

Set 15
1. easy does it
2. with a smile
3. Learn your lesson.
4. head in the clouds
5. ought to know
6. Pull my leg.
7. anything goes
8. What time is it?
9. Read a book.
10. Take a chance.

Set 16
1. by tomorrow
2. Flip a coin.
3. Catch the next bus.
4. Take it easy.
5. without a clue
6. Work it out.
7. Greet the day.
8. Have a nice time.
9. kind to others
10. Save your money.

APPENDIX D. PRACTICE STIMULI, UNRESTRICTED PHONETIC CONTEXT
For use during
- Artificial larynx speech
- Combined methods of esophageal speech
- Tracheoesophageal speech

LEVEL I: TWO- TO FOUR-SYLLABLE PHRASES AND SENTENCES (continued)

Set 17
1. Shake a leg.
2. nearly finished
3. Print your name.
4. Gain two pounds.
5. jump the gun
6. Teach a class.
7. Wait and see.
8. Visit often.
9. bed and breakfast
10. Deal me in.

Set 18
1. Feed the dog.
2. Am I clear?
3. Did you see that?
4. weekend guests
5. up and down
6. Take the day off.
7. Leave it to me.
8. I'll vote for that!
9. from me
10. Slow down.

Set 19
1. New Year's Eve
2. on the money
3. pots and pans
4. I need help.
5. my favorite
6. thank you
7. Zip it up.
8. Third floor, please.
9. What's done is done.
10. after you leave

Set 20
1. Beat the clock.
2. Call back later.
3. Eat your dinner.
4. That's news to me.
5. under the bed
6. vitamin B
7. while you're gone
8. Give to the poor.
9. heart to heart talk
10. Live and learn.

Set 21
1. past my bedtime
2. oath of office
3. pleasure trip
4. in a minute
5. milk and cookies
6. Use both hands.
7. zero in
8. Won't you be there?
9. before you go
10. Dial 9-1-1!

Set 22
1. for rent
2. almost there
3. Don't look back.
4. Watch your step.
5. United States
6. Sweep it up.
7. if you need it
8. Guide the way.
9. hid the money
10. Shop for new clothes.

Set 23
1. next in line
2. only a dollar
3. point of view
4. lose your seat
5. Yawn to relax.
6. Tell the truth.
7. world peace
8. thirty minutes
9. What's new with you?
10. day is done

Set 24
1. a good bargain
2. Can we talk?
3. Face the music.
4. The car won't start.
5. up and away
6. Wait until dark.
7. get to know you
8. Head for safety.
9. I was first.
10. Lock the door.

APPENDIX D. PRACTICE STIMULI, UNRESTRICTED PHONETIC CONTEXT

For use during
- Artificial larynx speech
- Combined methods of esophageal speech
- Tracheoesophageal speech

LEVEL I: TWO- TO FOUR-SYLLABLE PHRASES AND SENTENCES *(continued)*

Set 25
1. May I help you?
2. Greet the day.
3. It's cold outside.
4. next to nothing
5. out of coffee
6. Pay your taxes.
7. Raise the flag.
8. salt and pepper
9. time to talk
10. Wash your face.

Set 26
1. bought out the store
2. common sense
3. for you
4. down the street
5. no shade in sight
6. public servant
7. red as a beet
8. Go to bed.
9. ice cream cone
10. most of all

Set 27
1. Help me up.
2. if only I could
3. Plan a trip.
4. Tow the car.
5. Watch out!
6. bread and butter
7. Earn your keep.
8. Do it yourself.
9. cost of living
10. spoke too soon

Set 28
1. now and then
2. planet Earth
3. right or wrong
4. I mean it!
5. off duty
6. tough call to make
7. When do we leave?
8. Buy your ticket.
9. cream and sugar
10. dream of winning

Set 29
1. lost and found
2. Guess what happened.
3. Join hands.
4. nice to meet you
5. off and running
6. perfect timing
7. Rest a while.
8. Tie the knot.
9. Wash the car.
10. Chop the onion.

Set 30
1. bargains galore
2. cops and robbers
3. fair-weather friend
4. not right now
5. ran for mayor
6. pleasure trip
7. Good morning!
8. I don't know.
9. more than half
10. in and out

Set 31
1. I am hungry.
2. piece of cake
3. rough waters
4. treasure island
5. Where are you?
6. Bring it to me.
7. east of Elm Street
8. time to quit
9. far to travel
10. sharp as a tack

Set 32
1. Open the door.
2. Press your luck.
3. run-around
4. in big trouble
5. to each his own
6. What's on TV?
7. Yesterday's gone.
8. certain people
9. dawn's early light
10. each one of us

APPENDIX D. PRACTICE STIMULI, UNRESTRICTED PHONETIC CONTEXT

For use during
- Artificial larynx speech
- Combined methods of esophageal speech
- Tracheoesophageal speech

LEVEL I: TWO- TO FOUR-SYLLABLE PHRASES AND SENTENCES *(continued)*

Set 33
1. by the book
2. doesn't make sense
3. pretty good
4. Turn on the lights.
5. Where's my coat?
6. strong and healthy
7. meant to call
8. against the neck
9. Beat the system.
10. last to be served

Set 34
1. tall and handsome
2. around the block
3. Wait for the bus.
4. Maybe we can.
5. young as you feel
6. for an hour
7. by the way
8. caught a cold
9. Empty the trash.
10. spare a dime

Set 35
1. without much thought
2. off the hook
3. Saturday night
4. baked potato
5. Meet me at noon.
6. Finish your lunch.
7. ran out of salt
8. around the world
9. curbed his temper
10. stretch the truth

Set 36
1. Speak for yourself.
2. from the garden
3. made to order
4. your crystal ball
5. between two streets
6. collect back pay
7. Protect your hands.
8. ready to go
9. Laugh at yourself.
10. going, going, gone

Set 37
1. Cross the street.
2. Don't rock the boat.
3. Ring the bell.
4. twelve months
5. within my rights
6. Break the record.
7. Ask for more.
8. Swing your partner.
9. pick-up truck
10. Give it your best.

Set 38
1. friend or foe
2. out for a ride
3. wish you were here
4. Check the neck.
5. alone at last
6. Squeeze my hand.
7. now and then
8. red, white, and blue
9. Depend on me.
10. Reach for the stars.

Set 39
1. Set the table.
2. Welcome home!
3. as good as gold
4. Take my picture.
5. picnic basket
6. Obey the law.
7. my sister's son
8. Keep trying.
9. nosy neighbor
10. rush hour traffic

Set 40
1. dinner at six
2. sleeping soundly
3. two free tickets
4. Sample the cheese.
5. born in New York
6. Hang a picture.
7. of no interest
8. made a mistake
9. Keep it coming.
10. chill in the air

APPENDIX D. PRACTICE STIMULI, UNRESTRICTED PHONETIC CONTEXT

For use during   •   Artificial larynx speech
                 •   Combined methods of esophageal speech
                 •   Tracheoesophageal speech

LEVEL I: TWO- TO FOUR-SYLLABLE PHRASES AND SENTENCES *(continued)*

Set 41
1. always on time
2. midmorning tea
3. What do you want?
4. Sign the contract.
5. third from the right
6. Pick out a shirt.
7. tired of running
8. Strike a deal.
9. ghost of a chance
10. first at the scene

Set 42
1. sour cream and chives
2. church on Sunday
3. vase of flowers
4. Go north two miles.
5. buttered popcorn
6. Steal a kiss.
7. Patience pays off.
8. can't talk now
9. by the back door
10. taxi for two

Set 43
1. Stick with me.
2. Are my dues paid?
3. Suck a cough drop.
4. Good-bye for now.
5. Take up the fight.
6. Check up on Bob.
7. Pitch in and help.
8. matching bookends
9. vulgar language
10. because you asked

Set 44
1. Stop at nothing.
2. pet shop supplies
3. unless he asks
4. Defy the odds.
5. Forgive me.
6. Take advantage.
7. good company
8. Join the club.
9. Break the news.
10. woke to music

Set 45
1. heard a voice
2. Think about it.
3. south of my home
4. a day of rest
5. for Pete's sake
6. Cheer the team.
7. shirked his duty
8. made the best choice
9. We should wait.
10. Judge for yourself.

Set 46
1. gone fishing
2. what I wanted
3. Vote your conscience.
4. stock car races
5. Shop 'til you drop.
6. a stitch in time
7. out of control
8. postcard from Spain
9. cut the mustard
10. fifteen minutes

Set 47
1. Steer to the left.
2. Just sit tight.
3. Check out that car!
4. Pocket the cash.
5. deep and wide
6. guilty as charged
7. Compare prices.
8. forget to write
9. Bring a friend.
10. night on the town

Set 48
1. Pass out the cards.
2. Stop by later.
3. Tighten your belt.
4. Make four copies.
5. Keep out.
6. Don't count on it.
7. airplane tickets
8. Waste not, want not.
9. Yes, I want some.
10. in broad daylight

APPENDIX D. PRACTICE STIMULI, UNRESTRICTED PHONETIC CONTEXT

For use during
- Artificial larynx speech
- Combined methods of esophageal speech
- Tracheoesophageal speech

LEVEL II: FIVE- TO SEVEN-SYLLABLE PHRASES AND SENTENCES

Set 1
1. age before beauty
2. national treasure
3. We've gone too far to stop.
4. The battery is dead.
5. Thank you for your trouble.
6. Spring is my favorite season.
7. My relatives are here.
8. orange juice, rolls, and coffee
9. paper and pencil
10. Are you on vacation?

Set 2
1. Stand up for yourself.
2. What time is it?
3. The water is too hot.
4. May I try this on?
5. I'm glad you came today.
6. Bring the dessert tray please.
7. How long will we have to wait?
8. Do you want chicken or beef?
9. Talk to your doctor.
10. Pick out a pair of shoes.

Set 3
1. Anything is possible.
2. native Californian
3. room for improvement
4. Say it like you mean it.
5. That's all I have to say.
6. Which way should we take?
7. Don't leave me alone.
8. Parking is two dollars.
9. I forgot my homework.
10. Build your confidence.

Set 4
1. neighborly advice
2. This is my best friend.
3. Good things come to those who wait.
4. Learn something new every day.
5. Maybe I'll cash a check.
6. I'll take that as a yes.
7. Can you help me find it?
8. Where is the rest room?
9. See you tomorrow.
10. Is it in color?

Set 5
1. My vacation is in June.
2. This is a loaner.
3. We met last Thursday.
4. Keep your eyes on the road.
5. What are you doing?
6. Turn right at this corner.
7. Please mail this for me.
8. coffee with cream and sugar
9. You look nice in blue.
10. I'll see you next week.

Set 6
1. Thank your lucky stars.
2. rise to the occasion
3. What is your address?
4. My watch needs repair.
5. A table for two, please.
6. I have enough to share.
7. time off for good behavior
8. Draw a map for me.
9. away on business
10. Bring home the bacon.

Set 7
1. around the corner
2. That's the best I can do.
3. Whatever happens, don't quit.
4. I'm charging the battery.
5. Make mine a double.
6. Can you keep a secret?
7. building a nest egg
8. How long will it take to fix?
9. On Friday I'll call you.
10. Don't give it a thought.

Set 8
1. That's what friends are for.
2. Where are you going?
3. We think she'll be late.
4. Are we meeting next week?
5. home for the holidays
6. Set a good example.
7. whatever you say
8. My sister lives in Fresno.
9. I need to rent a car.
10. Practice makes perfect.

APPENDIX D. PRACTICE STIMULI, UNRESTRICTED PHONETIC CONTEXT

For use during
- Artificial larynx speech
- Combined methods of esophageal speech
- Tracheoesophageal speech

LEVEL II: FIVE- TO SEVEN-SYLLABLE PHRASES AND SENTENCES (*continued*)

Set 9
1. seven days a week
2. I can't find it anywhere.
3. Watch the water—don't slip.
4. Who knows where this will lead us?
5. Call me in the morning.
6. Be kind to yourself.
7. Don't talk with your mouth full.
8. Thanksgiving turkey
9. This is too easy.
10. May I have it "to go"?

Set 10
1. Who left the water on?
2. too late to stop him now
3. Heads I win, tails I lose.
4. Look at the bright side.
5. Don't quit—try harder.
6. The music is too loud.
7. It's time to eat dinner.
8. Bring a sweater.
9. Where did you find that?
10. Please clean my jacket.

Set 11
1. because of the weather
2. I'd like an answer today.
3. worth the time and effort
4. The light bulb is burned out.
5. When will you return?
6. Pass the salt and pepper.
7. Open your present.
8. You can't take it with you.
9. Let's go for a walk.
10. busy as a bee

Set 12
1. Next time I'll drive the car.
2. snug as a bug in a rug
3. Don't look now, but here comes Bill.
4. Our home has three bedrooms.
5. The car needs a tune-up.
6. no deposit, no return
7. slippery when wet
8. Beware of the dog.
9. down in the valley
10. Go the extra mile.

Set 13
1. Don't bother me right now.
2. Too bad you have a cold.
3. I can't believe my eyes!
4. The newspaper is downstairs.
5. Where's the nearest gas station?
6. Be there at eight o'clock.
7. Come in and stay awhile.
8. Sit down and rest your feet.
9. What a beautiful day.
10. How much do I owe you?

Set 14
1. That's just fine with me.
2. Let's play golf next Tuesday.
3. Carry a big stick.
4. How could we get lost?
5. It's too hot to sleep.
6. Did you hear a noise?
7. Wear your raincoat to class.
8. The show begins at nine.
9. She plays chess and checkers.
10. Fred will take two copies.

Set 15
1. I should be going.
2. Silence is golden.
3. Things are looking up.
4. How much is the car wash?
5. Wake up and smell the coffee.
6. Mail the letter to Boston.
7. Let's go out to dinner.
8. No one leaves 'til we find it.
9. Shake well before using.
10. calories per serving

Set 16
1. That's your opinion.
2. You can count on me.
3. sooner or later
4. I won't be here next week.
5. Where are the car keys?
6. The carpet needs vacuuming.
7. Drink plenty of water.
8. Read the instructions.
9. Call the fire department.
10. Make another set of keys.

APPENDIX D. PRACTICE STIMULI, UNRESTRICTED PHONETIC CONTEXT

For use during
- Artificial larynx speech
- Combined methods of esophageal speech
- Tracheoesophageal speech

LEVEL II: FIVE- TO SEVEN-SYLLABLE PHRASES AND SENTENCES (continued)

Set 17
1. Always tell the truth.
2. I'm only kidding.
3. The dog needs a walk.
4. Schedule my next appointment.
5. Put a light in the window.
6. Look up the number.
7. Should we hire an attorney?
8. Her plane has been delayed.
9. Leave a note on the windshield.
10. Open a charge account.

Set 18
1. Put it back in the oven.
2. caught in the middle
3. Don't eat between meals.
4. the name of the game
5. Have you had dinner?
6. Would you care to dance?
7. It's time to go home.
8. Take your medicine.
9. Steep the tea three minutes.
10. Make plenty of ice cubes.

Set 19
1. See me after class.
2. Could you do me a favor?
3. Think of me as your friend.
4. I don't understand.
5. Does this camera have film?
6. When will this be ready?
7. Remember to speak slowly.
8. Invest your money in stocks.
9. Stop to smell the flowers.
10. Paul is taller than Jim.

Set 20
1. better late than never
2. How much does it cost?
3. Press the button on the right.
4. Keep in touch with those you love.
5. one day at a time
6. I'll take twenty copies.
7. Thank you for being there.
8. Support your club members.
9. Go home for the holidays.
10. Check yourself in the mirror.

Set 21
1. not a cloud in the sky
2. I want my money back.
3. Someone is at the door.
4. Borrow it from your neighbor.
5. Turn off the oven.
6. on one condition
7. Make that dog stop barking!
8. Join an exercise club.
9. Is your passport up to date?
10. Paper towels will soak it up.

Set 22
1. Use your windshield wipers.
2. Enjoy yourself.
3. Did you warm up the car?
4. I'll pick you up at eight.
5. What's your telephone number?
6. Put a Band-Aid on it.
7. Grow your own vegetables.
8. It's freezing in here!
9. Be patient with yourself.
10. Always expect the best.

Set 23
1. as soon as possible
2. It always happens that way.
3. Put fruit in the basket.
4. I don't smoke anymore.
5. How much do I owe you?
6. That was a good movie.
7. Do I have a choice?
8. The trees are in bloom.
9. We parked three blocks away.
10. Turn your head to the left.

Set 24
1. Give it a lot of thought.
2. The news is at seven.
3. I wondered where you were.
4. Smile at least once a day.
5. Consider the source.
6. It's important to me.
7. Pardon me for asking.
8. Feel it in your throat.
9. Close the door behind you.
10. Which one is best for me?

APPENDIX D. PRACTICE STIMULI, UNRESTRICTED PHONETIC CONTEXT

For use during
- Artificial larynx speech
- Combined methods of esophageal speech
- Tracheoesophageal speech

LEVEL II: FIVE- TO SEVEN-SYLLABLE PHRASES AND SENTENCES (*continued*)

Set 25
1. It's like money in the bank.
2. more rain for tomorrow
3. They grew up together.
4. Step aside and let him pass.
5. Good to have met you.
6. Never say never.
7. Do you have spare pocket change?
8. Let some fresh air in.
9. Keep pace with the world.
10. We arrived at the same time.

Set 26
1. Ask me anything.
2. It is seven o'clock.
3. Discover yourself.
4. Make up for lost time.
5. Be kind to each other.
6. on the other hand
7. the road to recovery
8. Put things back where you found them.
9. Simplify your life.
10. Listen to me talk.

Set 27
1. It's only money.
2. open for business
3. Tomorrow will tell.
4. Do a good turn daily.
5. While there is life, there is hope.
6. She had a good cry.
7. Replace the batteries.
8. the strongest man alive
9. I need eight hours of sleep at night.
10. in relation to what?

Set 28
1. daily exercise
2. Let's have a cup of coffee.
3. person to person
4. I left my wallet at home.
5. My shoes are too tight.
6. a word to the wise
7. You asked me that before.
8. What did I tell you?
9. Five pennies make a nickel.
10. carrot cake for dessert

Set 29
1. only three days ago
2. I hear a car alarm.
3. Keep it to yourself.
4. Be quick to answer.
5. Quit while you're ahead.
6. State of the Union address
7. much ado about nothing
8. down to his last dollar
9. Go ahead and try.
10. How much do you weigh?

Set 30
1. Have you heard the news?
2. I'm afraid I will lose it.
3. When is your birthday?
4. mind over matter
5. double your money back
6. Get back on your feet.
7. shipping and handling
8. Don't buy what you don't need.
9. Two heads are better than one.
10. Beauty is but skin deep.

Set 31
1. Things aren't what they seem.
2. Pass the potatoes, please.
3. I don't mind at all.
4. Memories are made of this.
5. Knowledge is power.
6. Clean out the trunk of the car.
7. Look forward to spring.
8. the arm of the law
9. Do the best you can.
10. What do you mean by that?

Set 32
1. better safe than sorry
2. Try the yellow pages.
3. raining cats and dogs
4. Practice what you preach.
5. a cup of water
6. Sleep in on Saturday.
7. I'm in favor of it.
8. Help me wash the dishes.
9. No news is good news.
10. lemon in my tea

APPENDIX D. PRACTICE STIMULI, UNRESTRICTED PHONETIC CONTEXT

For use during
- Artificial larynx speech
- Combined methods of esophageal speech
- Tracheoesophageal speech

LEVEL II: FIVE- TO SEVEN-SYLLABLE PHRASES AND SENTENCES (continued)

Set 33
1. Give me one good reason.
2. Turn right at the next light.
3. No man is an island.
4. I have thought about it.
5. This jacket is too big.
6. We spent the day at the park.
7. Do what you want to do.
8. under lock and key
9. feather in my cap
10. Keep moving forward.

Set 34
1. Lend me a dollar.
2. under lock and key
3. vinegar and oil
4. ready for peace and quiet
5. Put it in the basement.
6. Did you bring your pictures?
7. feel like a million bucks
8. in the wink of an eye
9. Are those chairs for sale?
10. Believe it or not.

Set 35
1. Pick up the pieces.
2. Expect a miracle.
3. Another year has passed.
4. Do it every time.
5. middle of the night
6. Buy one, get one free.
7. Never lose control.
8. You puzzle me sometimes.
9. Things aren't what they seem.
10. He works for the newspaper.

Set 36
1. Follow the leader.
2. Look before you leap.
3. Walk around the block.
4. Don't try to explain.
5. There will be seven of us.
6. Go to the next page.
7. You can't teach him anything.
8. How can we agree to that?
9. Be ready at two-thirty.
10. I feel caught in the middle.

Set 37
1. Keep up the good work.
2. Practice makes perfect.
3. Is it safe to travel?
4. Close your mouth to swallow.
5. We're out of sugar.
6. did it on purpose
7. a sense of accomplishment
8. fifty-fifty chance
9. gets up with the chickens
10. Try and try again.

Set 38
1. All men are equal.
2. Put in a day's work.
3. Spend more time together.
4. I cross the bridge every day.
5. Exercise your rights.
6. Don't wait up for me.
7. a good sense of humor
8. Without sugar, please.
9. Both times I used slow speech.
10. You owe me five dollars.

Set 39
1. between you and me
2. Exit the back door.
3. Voice your opinion!
4. great day for a walk
5. Wait a little longer.
6. Don't make me laugh!
7. There are no short cuts.
8. I'm on top of the world.
9. Make room for me to sit.
10. The sign says "Do Not Enter."

Set 40
1. like music to my ears
2. reason for living
3. another time and place
4. May I be of help?
5. You look different today.
6. They're playing our song.
7. Better join now while you can.
8. What's the reason to go?
9. Could you explain it again?
10. Someone has to pay the bill.

APPENDIX D. PRACTICE STIMULI, UNRESTRICTED PHONETIC CONTEXT

For use during
- Artificial larynx speech
- Combined methods of esophageal speech
- Tracheoesophageal speech

LEVEL II: FIVE- TO SEVEN-SYLLABLE PHRASES AND SENTENCES (*continued*)

Set 41
1. all work and no play
2. Make up for lost time.
3. Bill it to insurance.
4. I don't know what will happen.
5. The best things in life are free.
6. Does the price include tax?
7. Wear something warm to the game.
8. Pleasant dreams, everyone.
9. Real men don't eat quiche.
10. He shot two under par.

Set 42
1. I'm almost finished.
2. May I have your attention?
3. We need another chair.
4. She spoke well of you.
5. There's a sale on aisle two.
6. vinegar and oil dressing
7. Trim a little off the sides.
8. ready to take his place
9. Blue is my color.
10. Stop me if you've heard this one.

Set 43
1. Good news travels fast.
2. What's wrong with this picture?
3. Come as soon as you can.
4. the first time I saw you
5. I'll need further directions.
6. Mention my name to her.
7. Return to sender.
8. after all is said and done
9. once in a lifetime
10. Let nothing stand in your way.

Set 44
1. I live around the corner.
2. We'll miss you while you're gone.
3. Plant a border of flowers.
4. much later than we thought
5. throughout the summer months
6. Think of a golden sunset.
7. Raise your hand to volunteer.
8. Keep the wind at your back.
9. Set a good example.
10. as many as you want

Set 45
1. Forget the whole thing.
2. mashed potatoes and gravy
3. Want to share a sandwich?
4. Some days you just can't win!
5. Time to take a break.
6. Let's get a head start.
7. I prefer the yellow one.
8. Have you flown before?
9. Is the post office open?
10. just because you don't know

Set 46
1. My credit card expired.
2. Will the rain stop you?
3. That was a long time ago.
4. You're too good to be true.
5. But you promised to help.
6. The book is due in two weeks.
7. I stood in a long line.
8. time for an oil change
9. requires more information
10. slept like a baby

Set 47
1. May I use the phone?
2. There's plenty of food.
3. It's in today's newspaper.
4. running for president
5. We were going to tell you.
6. Turn back the covers.
7. Pepper the salad.
8. neither rain, nor hail, nor sleet
9. American heroes
10. Close your eyes and relax.

Set 48
1. Will you be on time?
2. Raid the refrigerator.
3. Swim to the end of the pool.
4. power to make the difference
5. might be able to come
6. stars and stripes forever
7. Be true to yourself.
8. Take your vitamins.
9. your next appointment
10. clean as a whistle

APPENDIX D. PRACTICE STIMULI, UNRESTRICTED PHONETIC CONTEXT

For use during
- Artificial larynx speech
- Combined methods of esophageal speech
- Tracheoesophageal speech

LEVEL III: EIGHT-SYLLABLE OR MORE PHRASES AND SENTENCES

Set 1
1. A good start is an early morning walk.
2. He is on a low salt, fat-free diet.
3. Just the person I wanted to see!
4. One for the money and two for the show.
5. Take off your coat and have some tea.
6. You can go, or you can stay right here.
7. more than anything else in the world
8. Give credit where credit is due.
9. Take as many as you want.
10. I told you a hundred times.

Set 2
1. Do you have this book in paperback?
2. I couldn't have done it without you.
3. Take out the garbage and the recycling bin.
4. The car is low two quarts of oil.
5. Ask as many questions as you like.
6. May I have a glass of water?
7. For more information, call me.
8. between you, me, and the gate post
9. How do I get to the bus station?
10. We have two cats, a dog, and a bird.

Set 3
1. Bake at four hundred fifty for thirty minutes.
2. I'd like to open a savings account.
3. One today is worth two tomorrows.
4. just because you know the answer
5. My relatives are visiting.
6. Each person has to decide for himself.
7. Refrigerate after opening.
8. Schedule a shampoo and haircut.
9. Do you want chocolate or vanilla?
10. Take me to the nearest hospital.

Set 4
1. Freedom can survive only when it is shared.
2. How much do I owe you for the present?
3. Keep practicing until you get it right.
4. Take your time to do the job right.
5. You could call 9-1-1 or the fire department.
6. Pull over to the side of the road.
7. Bring me a hammer and screwdriver.
8. The bread is too stale to make a sandwich.
9. I want to make an appointment.
10. Sorry I'm late—the bus broke down.

APPENDIX D. PRACTICE STIMULI, UNRESTRICTED PHONETIC CONTEXT

For use during
- Artificial larynx speech
- Combined methods of esophageal speech
- Tracheoesophageal speech

LEVEL III: EIGHT-SYLLABLE OR MORE PHRASES AND SENTENCES (*continued*)

Set 5
1. Do you think you can remove this stain?
2. I'm nearly finished reading this book.
3. For whom are you going to vote?
4. My social security check is due.
5. Call the police to report a crime.
6. Look it up in the Yellow Pages.
7. It doesn't have a stamp on it.
8. The dog needs to go for a walk.
9. Remember to take your vitamins.
10. Some people say, "why?"; I say, "why not?"

Set 6
1. Add soap and bleach to the washing machine.
2. Our local park is a good place for a picnic.
3. Do you have these in black leather?
4. Income taxes are due April fifteenth.
5. Clap your hands to get attention.
6. Hold the flashlight in your left hand.
7. Thread the needle before you sew.
8. I have two tickets to see "Carmen."
9. Let's meet at the shopping center.
10. one less thing to worry about

Set 7
1. I'm nearly finished reading this book.
2. Let me help you put those things in the car.
3. Paris is beautiful this time of year.
4. Thank you for remembering my birthday.
5. Find ways to simplify your life.
6. Never do one thing when you can do two.
7. All things are difficult before they are easy.
8. Man is his own worst enemy.
9. Honesty is the best policy.
10. One today is worth two tomorrows.

Set 8
1. Thanks for helping me bring in the groceries.
2. You have a choice between red and yellow.
3. Before you go, I have something to tell you.
4. All people smile in the same language.
5. The washing machine is broken.
6. Try to set a good example.
7. I'll be back in a few minutes.
8. Divide it between the two of you.
9. Come to a full stop at the stop sign.
10. Choose a number between one and ten.

APPENDIX D. PRACTICE STIMULI, UNRESTRICTED PHONETIC CONTEXT

For use during
- Artificial larynx speech
- Combined methods of esophageal speech
- Tracheoesophageal speech

LEVEL III: EIGHT-SYLLABLE OR MORE PHRASES AND SENTENCES (continued)

Set 9
1. After dinner, let's go to the movies.
2. Store leftovers in plastic bags.
3. Is there a doctor in the house?
4. Don't tell anyone our secret.
5. Be quiet and listen to others.
6. That's the best one I've heard all day.
7. A hearing aid can make life exciting again.
8. Never open someone else's mail.
9. Radiation affected my teeth.
10. Could you check the air in my tires, please?

Set 10
1. Be a good neighbor and take in her mail.
2. I feel like a million dollars.
3. Pick up a loaf of bread and a gallon of milk.
4. That's the most beautiful sunset I've ever seen.
5. You must speak slowly to be understood.
6. No, you can't take that away from me.
7. Listen to the babbling of the brook.
8. Do the best you can; no one can fault you.
9. Take one tablet every two hours.
10. My car gets twenty miles to the gallon.

Set 11
1. Let me know if you don't understand me.
2. Do you want an apple or a pear?
3. The car needs gas and a quart of oil.
4. In case of emergency, break glass.
5. Let's take a stroll down by Lake Virginia.
6. roses, geraniums, and peonies
7. Spread newspaper and we'll cut the melon.
8. My insurance pays for my prescriptions.
9. beyond a reasonable doubt
10. I found a five-spot on the sidewalk.

Set 12
1. All people smile in the same language.
2. I'm sorry to hear you've been ill.
3. Stand on a chair to change the light bulb.
4. The bank is closed for the holiday.
5. Premium gas is two dollars per gallon.
6. Take the McArthur Boulevard exit.
7. You may borrow it for thirty days.
8. Do you want to follow me in your car?
9. Maybe I'm just fooling myself.
10. a slight chance of morning showers

APPENDIX D. PRACTICE STIMULI, UNRESTRICTED PHONETIC CONTEXT

For use during
- Artificial larynx speech
- Combined methods of esophageal speech
- Tracheoesophageal speech

LEVEL III: EIGHT-SYLLABLE OR MORE PHRASES AND SENTENCES *(continued)*

Set 13
1. I walked from one end of the mall to the other.
2. Point the way to the nearest service station.
3. The house rents for four hundred dollars.
4. You won't want to miss this special sale.
5. in celebration of your birthday
6. He was standing in the shadows.
7. Fortunately for Ted, he knew CPR.
8. Don't fix, I'll take you out to dinner.
9. Keep the cap on the medicine bottle.
10. Take the tour bus for a worry-free vacation.

Set 14
1. If at first you don't succeed, try, try again.
2. Does anyone know if the mail has come?
3. To tell the truth, it didn't occur to me.
4. Forgive and forget is a good rule.
5. There's so much I need to tell you.
6. He had left before I got there.
7. Sooner or later, Carl will notice it.
8. Leave a detailed message on my machine.
9. I am seeing a speech pathologist.
10. You should ask your doctor about that.

Set 15
1. Beat two eggs and add them to the batter.
2. None of the people I know chew tobacco.
3. I look forward to your visit.
4. How much would you charge to make the repairs?
5. Take two aspirin and call me in the morning.
6. You have been extremely helpful to me.
7. There's always room for improvement.
8. Don't take any wooden nickels.
9. fortieth wedding anniversary
10. In times like these, you learn who your friends are.

Set 16
1. Her car needs gas and a quart of oil.
2. I have keys to my car, house, and mailbox.
3. Put a stamp on it and mail it today.
4. Speak now or forever hold your peace.
5. The movie made us laugh loud and long.
6. Do you know who won the World Series?
7. It should be in the dictionary.
8. What's playing at the movie theater?
9. Turn left at the stoplight and go two blocks.
10. You've given me a reason for living.

APPENDIX D. PRACTICE STIMULI, UNRESTRICTED PHONETIC CONTEXT

For use during • **Artificial larynx speech**
 • **Combined methods of esophageal speech**
 • **Tracheoesophageal speech**

LEVEL III: EIGHT-SYLLABLE OR MORE PHRASES AND SENTENCES *(continued)*

Set 17
1. I find myself asking the same question.
2. Let's be perfectly clear on the matter.
3. Do you have time to go over the list?
4. She went to the supermarket.
5. The crickets are very noisy tonight.
6. How many people will be able to go?
7. Give me your address and I'll send it to you.
8. Excuse me for interrupting.
9. Buy some paper tissue and toothpaste.
10. You should know he is a neck breather.

Set 18
1. All the stores are closed for the holiday.
2. Who would you nominate for president?
3. Take advantage of this service.
4. Sometimes it's a struggle to make ends meet.
5. I bought a money belt for the trip.
6. Catch the six o'clock weather forecast.
7. The leaves are their prettiest in the fall.
8. holding a bouquet of flowers
9. Don't sit under the apple tree.
10. Brief practice sessions throughout the day are best.

Set 19
1. If I'm not there by three, start without me.
2. Put butter and gravy on my mashed potatoes.
3. The next bus will take you to Union Square.
4. Fill out a credit application.
5. Did you misunderstand what I said?
6. Come to work early and stay late.
7. Time is the stuff life is made of.
8. I don't know when I've been happier.
9. What is the balance in my checking account?
10. The newsletter will be mailed the first of May.

Set 20
1. Honesty is the best policy.
2. You shouldn't feed the dog table scraps.
3. Sooner or later you have to go home.
4. I knitted two caps in an afternoon.
5. Change the rules if you're tired of the game.
6. There are times when you need to be alone.
7. The solution is inside of you.
8. Is the snapper fresh or frozen?
9. Where do we keep the first-aid kit?
10. A motel is better than a campground.

APPENDIX D. PRACTICE STIMULI, UNRESTRICTED PHONETIC CONTEXT
For use during   •   Artificial larynx speech
                •   Combined methods of esophageal speech
                •   Tracheoesophageal speech

LEVEL III: EIGHT-SYLLABLE OR MORE PHRASES AND SENTENCES *(continued)*

Set 21
1. Do you want your fish baked or fried?
2. I have an appointment for three o'clock.
3. The sports section has the details.
4. Our apartment is on the third floor.
5. Is the elevator working?
6. Ask for a chocolate ice cream cone.
7. Jewelry should be kept in a safe place.
8. raindrops falling against the window pane
9. Weatherman says a tornado is coming.
10. It took me five hours to rake the leaves.

Set 22
1. Give me your address and phone number.
2. Let's take a trip south of the border.
3. Radio is more interesting than television.
4. I lost my ring last Saturday.
5. The basement is the coldest place in my house.
6. An owl softly hooted in the night.
7. Billboards advertising smoking should be banned.
8. hundreds of books on the bookshelf
9. Put clothes in the closet and chest of drawers.
10. Is it as deep as the Grand Canyon?

Set 23
1. If you're cold, put on a sweater.
2. No one knows what he can do until he does it.
3. The store is closed on Saturday.
4. Where did I put my keys and my wallet?
5. She ordered a toasted cheese and ham sandwich.
6. My stomach has been acting up.
7. a lucky shamrock in my pocket
8. I never know when she will be home.
9. fourteen-carat gold necklace and bracelet
10. He followed her into the dressing room.

Set 24
1. An opinion is one man's point of view.
2. He kept a notebook of all his expenses.
3. My gray wool suit is in the cleaners.
4. Set the table with a fork, knife, and spoon.
5. I never thought of it that way before.
6. You're comparing apples with oranges.
7. Do you want green beans, spinach, or broccoli?
8. These are a few of my favorite things.
9. It comes in red, white, blue, and green.
10. the spicier the sauce, the better

APPENDIX D. PRACTICE STIMULI, UNRESTRICTED PHONETIC CONTEXT

For use during
- Artificial larynx speech
- Combined methods of esophageal speech
- Tracheoesophageal speech

LEVEL III: EIGHT-SYLLABLE OR MORE PHRASES AND SENTENCES (continued)

Set 25
1. Friends and family always come first.
2. My sister called from St. Petersburg.
3. The trees in the park are full of blossoms.
4. Keep a box of matches handy.
5. Anybody for a bike ride?
6. Write a postcard to your friends back home.
7. It has an automatic transmission.
8. Lasagna is not what I ordered.
9. Give me the directions one more time.
10. I'd like a roll of color print film.

Set 26
1. I need cream and sugar for my coffee.
2. Refrigerate after opening.
3. When you can't sleep, try reading a good book.
4. The local department store should carry it.
5. a surprise party with cake and ice cream
6. Live like you expect a miracle.
7. I feel responsible for my actions.
8. Yesterday my sister returned to work.
9. Traffic was moving at a snail's pace.
10. Figure it out using the calculator.

Set 27
1. Does this bus go to the museum?
2. Silence may be golden, but I want to talk.
3. The upcoming election should be interesting.
4. As a consumer, I read the labels.
5. Try not to hold your breath when you speak.
6. Remember daylight savings time.
7. I should be home by seven o'clock.
8. Have you ever gambled at Reno?
9. Which is your favorite national holiday?
10. Change into a sweat suit to go for a walk.

Set 28
1. But officer, I was only going fifty-five!
2. If you're cold, put on a sweater.
3. He plays the piano quite well.
4. Meet me at the entrance to the park.
5. These stoma covers are quite stylish.
6. I traded it in at eighty thousand miles.
7. Your opinion is just that—your opinion.
8. Everyone deserves a fair trial.
9. information stored on the computer
10. Are you going to vote this election?

APPENDIX D. PRACTICE STIMULI, UNRESTRICTED PHONETIC CONTEXT

For use during
- Artificial larynx speech
- Combined methods of esophageal speech
- Tracheoesophageal speech

LEVEL III: EIGHT-SYLLABLE OR MORE PHRASES AND SENTENCES *(continued)*

Set 29
1. Having a pet is a big responsibility.
2. Lock your car if you leave it in the parking lot.
3. The waitress served us hot coffee and rolls.
4. at the Vietnam Memorial
5. I left my glasses in the car.
6. We protected our eyes during the eclipse.
7. This is an artificial larynx.
8. Don't talk to me during the Super Bowl.
9. Free nothing! They expected a donation.
10. Only a magician could make that happen.

Set 30
1. It is better to give than to receive.
2. Some movies make us laugh loud and long.
3. The zoo had a penguin, a kangaroo, and a lion.
4. When will my glasses be ready?
5. Help me with this crossword puzzle.
6. I leave the day after tomorrow.
7. recycling paper, plastic, and glass
8. You've got my interest—what do you want?
9. Defrost the roast in the microwave.
10. The Red Cross is there in a disaster.

Set 31
1. Ask directions to the nearest motel.
2. Remember, good speech takes practice.
3. There are only so many hours in a day.
4. Stay out of trouble; follow the rules.
5. Is there anything good on TV tonight?
6. Oops! I almost backed into you!
7. I wish you well in your venture.
8. Be careful what you ask for; you might get it!
9. Have you read your horoscope today?
10. We are the grandparents of five children.

Set 32
1. It will be partly cloudy tomorrow.
2. My million dollars didn't come in the mail.
3. She made the roast and I made the salad.
4. Today is the first day of the rest of your life.
5. I was just about to call you!
6. How many acres is the farm?
7. We're part of the twenty-first century.
8. There are certain guidelines we must follow.
9. Carolers sang outside our window.
10. Does he play professional sports?

APPENDIX D. PRACTICE STIMULI, UNRESTRICTED PHONETIC CONTEXT

For use during
- Artificial larynx speech
- Combined methods of esophageal speech
- Tracheoesophageal speech

LEVEL III: EIGHT-SYLLABLE OR MORE PHRASES AND SENTENCES *(continued)*

Set 33
1. Can you keep a secret if I tell you?
2. We're probably too late for the first show.
3. I will help you on one condition.
4. Jackson's picture is on the twenty.
5. May I make a long distance call?
6. That was no knockout; he tripped!
7. Have you eaten in the train's dining car?
8. Submit your resume to our main office.
9. Void where prohibited by law.
10. I'd like my steak cooked medium-rare.

Set 34
1. There has to be a good explanation.
2. He's a veteran of World War II.
3. I'm writing a book about my life.
4. children building sand castles by the sea
5. When you slammed the door, the cake fell.
6. This pot roast will make good hash tomorrow.
7. Someone is signaling for your attention.
8. Mexico is south of the border.
9. You'll find the blankets in the cedar chest.
10. Do you have change for a dollar?

Set 35
1. Don't bite off more than you can chew.
2. It's time to get ready for speech class.
3. She found the newspaper in the bushes.
4. Why don't you start all over again?
5. Carpet the upstairs bedroom and bath.
6. The ringing in my ears went away.
7. Egg yolks, cheese, and lemons are yellow.
8. Join hands and form a semicircle.
9. tombstones from the seventeen hundreds
10. They don't make movies like they used to.

Set 36
1. There's a pot of gold at the end of the rainbow.
2. I pledge allegiance to the flag.
3. A caterpillar will become a butterfly.
4. It made the hair stand up on my neck.
5. June, July, and August are summer months.
6. If life gives you a lemon, make lemonade.
7. from Atlantic to Pacific
8. My umbrella is too wet to fold.
9. Offer to pay for everybody's lunch.
10. Where could we go for dinner that's cheap?

APPENDIX D. PRACTICE STIMULI, UNRESTRICTED PHONETIC CONTEXT

For use during
- Artificial larynx speech
- Combined methods of esophageal speech
- Tracheoesophageal speech

LEVEL III: EIGHT-SYLLABLE OR MORE PHRASES AND SENTENCES *(continued)*

Set 37
1. Carry an umbrella in case it rains.
2. It's time to get ready for speech class.
3. We're having company for dinner tonight.
4. The museum is across the street.
5. Leave me a note about where you're going.
6. Who ever heard of a flying pig?
7. May I beg, steal, or borrow your pen?
8. I didn't mean to hurt your feelings.
9. Problems arise when people don't call.
10. Do you smell something cooking on the stove?

Set 38
1. Green is the color of frogs, grass, and money.
2. My favorite month of the year is September.
3. They guarantee the lowest prices.
4. Watch out for pedestrians in the crosswalk.
5. Do you know how to use a computer?
6. Fill out the card and return it to me.
7. A cruise ship is the only way to go.
8. Tune the radio to ninety-two point five.
9. Several messages have been sent to them.
10. I breathe through an opening in my neck.

Set 39
1. A warm bath before bed makes me sleepy.
2. Check your calendar to see if you are free.
3. My neighbor met me at the back fence.
4. Loan me your stapler and scotch tape.
5. The pilot says we're at thirty thousand feet.
6. Do you have paper and pen handy?
7. Painting the house is our next big project.
8. Experiment with several devices.
9. The speaker held us hostage with his words.
10. Winter brought snow to the mountains.

Set 40
1. I need to gas and wash the car.
2. She called at seven o'clock this morning.
3. This house rents for four hundred dollars.
4. We could hear the sirens for ten minutes.
5. Enough soap and water will make this place shine.
6. milk and cheese fresh from the dairy
7. Here's a map with the directions.
8. An insect is on your collar.
9. Turn up the volume—I can't hear.
10. The landlord slipped a note under my door.

APPENDIX D. PRACTICE STIMULI, UNRESTRICTED PHONETIC CONTEXT

For use during
- Artificial larynx speech
- Combined methods of esophageal speech
- Tracheoesophageal speech

LEVEL III: EIGHT-SYLLABLE OR MORE PHRASES AND SENTENCES *(continued)*

Set 41
1. My doorbell rang in the middle of the night.
2. We only hear what we want to hear.
3. How many goals has the hockey team scored?
4. Wrinkles are memories of lots of smiles.
5. The sound of the chimes floated in the night air.
6. a cup of coffee and the morning paper
7. Is there a telephone in this building?
8. Can you see the clock from where you're sitting?
9. Turn on the electric blanket.
10. They look enough alike to be twins.

Set 42
1. This is the way I want you to do it.
2. Are there any skeletons in your closet?
3. Look at your lips in the mirror.
4. Clean the ashes from the fireplace.
5. My wife painted this vase many years ago.
6. When you think of the answer, call me.
7. Did you forget the combination?
8. souvenir of our vacation together
9. The grandfather clock struck twelve times at midnight.
10. He recorded the words in his speech journal.

Set 43
1. Close your eyes, take a breath, and relax.
2. Have you tried an amplifier?
3. maximum hospital stay of ten days
4. Listen to the roar of the ocean.
5. not sharp enough to cut warm butter
6. We have reservations for May 18.
7. Permit me to introduce myself.
8. nothing like lemonade in the summertime
9. Do you have any identification?
10. She puts the icing on the cake.

Set 44
1. Dunking doughnuts in milk is a treat.
2. Seasons come and go, but I like fall best.
3. We had ham, eggs, and toast for breakfast.
4. Have you ever played a practical joke?
5. jazz festival in Monterey
6. balloons, confetti, and streamers
7. Leave time for questions and answers.
8. covered in ashes from head to toe
9. Turn off the lights when you leave the room.
10. I'm sorry, you have the wrong number.

APPENDIX D. PRACTICE STIMULI, UNRESTRICTED PHONETIC CONTEXT

For use during
- Artificial larynx speech
- Combined methods of esophageal speech
- Tracheoesophageal speech

LEVEL III: EIGHT-SYLLABLE OR MORE PHRASES AND SENTENCES *(continued)*

Set 45
1. Hank flew to Paris, Frankfurt, and London.
2. Those who learn nothing have nothing to forget.
3. stood at the altar to get married
4. Never accept a ride from someone you do not know.
5. I owe you an apology.
6. going to attend a family reunion
7. We made five hundred dollars with our fund-raiser.
8. Excuse me, but I was sitting there.
9. Send these flowers to 33 Elm Street.
10. Thank you for your hospitality.

Set 46
1. Sarah called at seven o'clock this morning.
2. Valentine's Day is February 14.
3. Bring refreshments to the next meeting.
4. I haven't done that since I was a kid.
5. Lemon juice will remove a stain.
6. Update your mailing list yearly.
7. Has anybody seen Rudy today?
8. a variety of sizes and colors
9. passed the test with flying colors
10. We have pot roast, baked chicken, or shrimp.

Set 47
1. I see my doctor next Tuesday.
2. Man is his own worst enemy.
3. To open it, remove the label first.
4. a hammock under an old shade tree
5. Behave yourself while I am gone.
6. Scramble some eggs and toast some bread.
7. Roberto opened up his own business.
8. Install a new set of spark plugs.
9. The weather seems to be worsening.
10. Love awakens the best in us.

Set 48
1. Use the stairs in case of an emergency.
2. Would you rather play chess or checkers?
3. Count your blessings each day of your life.
4. Fourteen people came to the meeting.
5. Happiness comes to those who seek it.
6. listening to rhythm and blues
7. Please sign this get-well card for Mary.
8. The newspaper is late again this morning.
9. Use humor in your presentation.
10. You can catch a ride with me to class.

APPENDIX D. PRACTICE STIMULI, UNRESTRICTED PHONETIC CONTEXT

LEVEL IV: ORAL READING OF PARAGRAPHS

Note: There are 10 sentences in each paragraph. The first letter of each sentence appears in BOLD to assist the clinician in scoring.

Paragraph 1: Turn on Your Headlights for Safety

Headlights have been a standard feature on automobiles for many years. The accepted rules for use of headlights include turning your lights on between the hours of dusk and dawn. Special weather conditions such as fog and rain may also require use of the vehicle's headlights. Generally, the use of high beams is reserved for night driving on dark roads when there are no other cars around. Recently, you may have noticed more cars than usual with their headlights on during the daytime. The reason is that, as of 1995, General Motors has made daytime headlights a standard feature on several of their new models. These "running lights" do not have as much glare as regular headlights and are designed to come on automatically when the car is started. The idea is to alert oncoming drivers of the car's presence. Running lights have already been in use in Canada and Scandinavian countries for a number of years. Only time will tell whether the use of running lights will reduce traffic accidents in the daylight hours. (175 words)

Paragraph 2: When Is the Best Time to Exercise?

Every morning without fail, your neighbor across the street rises at six, dons a bright yellow sweat suit and heads out for her five-mile walk. Al, your best friend, always stops by for a chat as he walks his golden retriever in the late afternoon. So who is getting the most benefit from their exercise? You've probably read or heard that an early morning workout is the best time to exercise. Other sources insist that afternoon exercise can offer a much-needed energy "pickup." The answer to when is the best time to exercise is quite simple. The best time to work out is the time that is most convenient for you. If you choose a time that you will be most likely to take that walk, you will be more likely to stick with your routine. And remember, vigorous exercise after a heavy meal is probably not a good idea. During digestion, your digestive system needs extra blood, leaving less for your heart and muscles. (165 words)

Paragraph 3: When Autumn Leaves

Every fall a fantastic display of color splashes across the New England countryside. Hillsides and forests turn into a rainbow of brilliant yellows, fire-engine reds, burning golds, and velvety browns. People travel from all over the country—by car, bus, train, and plane—to share this wonderful sight. Nature hikes are the perfect way to capture the color by gathering specimens, taking photographs, or making journal observations. The New England states receive their visitors with open arms, often putting on parades, festivals, and concerts. The celebration spills over into restaurant dining which includes New England clam chowder and Maine red lobster. Tourists armed with cameras are rewarded with picture-postcard views of steepled churches and farmhouses nestled in lush valleys. Or, if they venture to the Atlantic coast, they will find seagulls, harbor seals, and an array of fishing boats. A trip to see the golden autumn splendor will not soon be forgotten. Make your plans to experience New England next October or November. (163 words)

APPENDIX D. PRACTICE STIMULI, UNRESTRICTED PHONETIC CONTEXT

LEVEL IV: ORAL READING OF PARAGRAPHS *(continued)*

Paragraph 4: *Time to Fly the Flag*

Who has not experienced the thrill of seeing the American flag pass by during a parade? The design of our flag is fairly simple. Thirteen horizontal red-and-white stripes border fifty white stars on a deep blue background. Did you know there are rules of etiquette regarding displaying the American flag? Most everyone agrees that the flag may be flown during the hours from sunrise to sunset. The flag should not be allowed to hang and become wet in rain, sleet, or snow. The flag should be suspended from a pole with the Union section of the flag nearest the top of the staff. If the flag is to be displayed on a wall, it should hang flat with the Union section in the upper left corner. You may choose to fly your flag every day or only on special occasions, such as Lincoln's and Washington's birthdays, Memorial Day, Flag Day, Veterans' Day, and the Fourth of July. When a flag shows wear or is damaged, it should be removed from display and privately burned. (174 words)

Paragraph 5: *And Your Name Is . . .?*

Do you wish you could remember the name of that nice young man you just met? There are several memory tricks that may help you recall his name the next time you need it. For example, let's say the name of the gentlemen you just met is Eugene Hauck. When you are first introduced, look Eugene in the eyes as you shake hands with him. Make a point of using his name several times in the first few minutes of the conversation. Use phrases like "Nice to meet you, Eugene Hauck" or "Where do you work, Eugene?" Use the "link" method: Pair something familiar to you with something unfamiliar (his name). In this case, "Hauck" (unfamiliar) is pronounced the same as "hawk" (familiar). Visualize Eugene, standing there in his blue "jeans" (Gene) with a hawk (Hauck) on his arm. The next time you meet Eugene, your visual memory trick may help you extend your hand, smile, and say "Nice to see you again, Eugene Hauck." (165 words)

Paragraph 6: *I Hear What You're Saying*

As we get older, our ears tend to lose their sensitivity to sound, whether it be music or the spoken word. We blame the loss on heredity—hearing loss may be due to aging just as thinning hair or the need for reading glasses. However, other types of hearing loss may result from "ear abuse"—the needless exposure of our ears to excessive noise. Many individuals fail to wear ear protection while discharging firearms or operating loud machinery. The frequent use of headphones with the volume turned up may cause damage. When you have difficulty hearing the music, don't go for the volume control. Adjust the bass-treble control of your stereo to match your hearing needs. To compensate for loss of sensitivity for the higher frequencies, turn up the treble tone control on your stereo. This simple technique will improve your listening enjoyment of your CDs, records, and tapes. On occasion, you may want to turn up the volume to hear the full frequency range of your favorite opera—but remember to be kind to your ears. (177 words)

APPENDIX D. PRACTICE STIMULI, UNRESTRICTED PHONETIC CONTEXT

LEVEL IV: ORAL READING OF PARAGRAPHS *(continued)*

Paragraph 7: *Tired of Living a Life of Grime?*

Are you tired of cleaning the bathroom sink, toilet, and shower only to discover fresh mold and mildew in a few days? The moisture-rich environment of the bathroom is a mold and mildew heaven. A few simple tips will help you get the upper hand on this grimy situation. Arm yourself with rubber gloves and ammonia or bleach solution (NEVER the two together!) and prepare to scrub vigorously. A cup of bleach to five gallons of water, a scouring pad, and a little elbow grease should do the trick. For the mirror and glass shower doors, try mixing water and vinegar plus a little alcohol and ammonia. The alcohol speeds the drying process and the vinegar eliminates smearing. When you're finished scrubbing, lemon oil applied to the inside of the dried shower door will prevent soap scum from sticking to it. Toss plastic shower curtains into the washing machine with a load of towels and hot, soapy water. For the finishing touch, pour white vinegar into the toilet bowl and allow it to sit overnight. (175 words)

Paragraph 8: *How Dry I Am*

Removal of your larynx has left you with an opening in the front of your neck called a stoma. Breathing now occurs at the level of the stoma, and the air is no longer warmed, moisturized, or filtered before entering the trachea and lungs. This situation may result in crusting around the stoma, mucus buildup inside the stoma, and increased coughing. You may prevent these problems by finding ways to increase humidification. The simplest method is to wear a stoma cover, which acts as a filter for the incoming air. Some of the exiting air is trapped under the stoma cover, providing warm moist air at the entrance to the stoma. There are several commercial humidifiers that provide filtering, moisturizing, and warming. Using a room humidifier during sleep may be helpful. Or you may want to make use of a boiling teakettle or the steam from the bathroom sink. No matter which method you use, it is important to compensate for the dry air going into your stoma. (167 words)

Paragraph 9: *It All Tastes the Same to Me*

Taste, complemented by the sense of smell, is an important aspect of eating pleasure and involves the sensations of sweet, salty, sour, and bitter. Chemotherapy, radiation therapy, or the surgery may alter a laryngectomee's sense of taste and smell. The result may be a bitter or metallic taste to foods, especially proteins such as meat. Good nutrition is vital to individuals who have had cancer, so it is important to find ways to compensate for the problem. Choose and prepare foods that are your traditional favorites. If beef has an odd taste or smells peculiar to you, try other meats, such as chicken or pork, fish, eggs, or dairy products. Before cooking, marinate meat in apple, orange, or pineapple juice, sweet wine, salad dressing, or sweet-and-sour sauce. A variety of herbal seasonings—basil, oregano, or rosemary—may spark up the dish. Many laryngectomees report the ability to taste the tartness of oranges or lemons. Vegetables such as peas, squash, green beans, or spinach may be improved by adding bacon, ham, or onion. (172 words)

APPENDIX D. PRACTICE STIMULI, UNRESTRICTED PHONETIC CONTEXT

LEVEL IV: ORAL READING OF PARAGRAPHS (*continued*)

Paragraph 10: *You Auto Know Better*

A number of car oddities as well as classics were produced in the 1950s and '60s. The pink and white Dodge Custom Royal Lancer LaFemme sported huge tail fins and was equipped with a cosmetic kit and matching umbrella. For $2,068 you could buy a fully loaded Studebaker with a bizarre design: its front looked like its back. Edsel, the ugly duckling of cars, with its push-button transmission and electric windows, arrived in the late 1950s. Manufacture of the popular De Soto Adventurer was discontinued in 1961. In 1965, Ralph Nader condemned the Chevrolet Corvair, saying it could flip over in a sharp turn. Meanwhile, the Ford Mustang made its debut and became one of the most beloved cars of the decade. Walt Disney made a movie called The Love Bug based on the adventures of Herbie, a Volkswagen beetle. High school and college students put roll bars and oversized tires on their Volkswagens to create dune buggies. And no car was considered complete without the first car stereo, the 8-track tape player. (173 words)

Paragraph 11: *Update That First-Aid Kit*

All of us want to be prepared for emergencies when someone becomes ill or suffers a minor injury. Having a first-aid kit that contains appropriate and updated materials is a good start. In your first-aid kit, you should have hydrogen peroxide for cleaning and disinfecting wounds. Do not use alcohol because it may dry and irritate the cut. Cotton balls or swabs as well as sterile gauze pads are useful for applying hydrogen peroxide. After cleaning the wound, dry it and lightly apply an antibiotic cream to promote healing. A supply of various-sized adhesive bandages, large gauze pads, and surgical tape is recommended. Tweezers, a small pocket knife, and a pair of blunt scissors may come in handy. You will want to include a pen light and a small hand mirror in your kit. It is a good idea to have three first-aid kits: one in your car, one at work, and one in your home. (157 words)

Paragraph 12: *Mean What You Say*

Have you ever really listened to the expressions we have in the English language? Our daily conversations contain many idioms, or speech forms that are peculiar to our language. Idioms, interpreted literally, make no sense at all. You have to know English very well to get the "hidden meaning." People who do not speak English as their first language often find our expressions confusing. For example, "eat your heart out" may be our response when we think others are envious of our good fortune. When someone has lost his or her job and feels desperate, they moan "I'm at the end of my rope." A good friend who "knows the ropes" may be able to "pull some strings" and help them "make ends meet." The person who cannot keep a secret is guilty of "spilling the beans." And there are those who waste our time "beating around the bush" while others are able to "hit the nail on the head." So, unless you "get my drift," you'll be "going around in circles" trying to figure out what was just said. (180 words)

APPENDIX D. PRACTICE STIMULI, UNRESTRICTED PHONETIC CONTEXT

LEVEL IV: ORAL READING OF PARAGRAPHS *(continued)*

Paragraph 13: Childhood Memories

When I was a youngster, my parents and I spent our summer vacations on my grandmother's farm. Each June, we loaded our suitcases into the car and headed north to Tennessee. During the long hours on the road, I entertained myself reading comic books saved just for this journey. At grandma's house, I eagerly joined my cousin for an adventuresome two weeks of farm living. Early in the morning, before the sun had risen, we quickly dressed and headed for the barn. The strong odors of hay, manure, and warm milk surrounded us as we watched my uncle milk the cows. After breakfast, we headed for the pond and took turns skimming rocks or dabbling our fishing poles in the water. Then there was the picking of berries—we braved the thorns and suffered a few bee stings to taste the tender blackberries. When we collected enough berries in a pail, grandma baked them into a delicious pie. Grandma passed away years ago and the farm was sold, but my memories of those wonderful days will always be with me. (180 words)

Paragraph 14: Where's My Wallet?

You wait in a long line to pay for your purchase at a local department store. The clerk rings up the sale and asks for $10.92. As you reach for your wallet, you discover, to your horror, that it is missing. After much searching, you face the fact that your wallet has been stolen. The first thing you should do is cancel your credit cards, department store charge cards, and your automated teller machine card. Be sure to have your account numbers available when you make your calls to the bank, department stores, and credit card companies. If your checkbook was in your wallet, you should cancel your checking account and open a new one. Notify the police of your loss; a police report is frequently required by the insurance company and the credit card companies in the event that someone does try to use your cards. Carefully check your monthly statements for any goods or services that you did not purchase. Knowing what to do when you lose your wallet can save you unwanted bills and frustration. (178 words)

Paragraph 15: Laughter is Good Medicine

Feeling blue, down in the dumps, out in the cold, or all alone in the world? What you need is a good dose of humor, laughter, and funny business. Change your attitude, and put yourself in the company of others who see the funny side of life. Laughter fights the effects of daily stress by pumping up the immune system, and it causes relaxation by releasing muscular tension. People are thirty times more likely to laugh in the company of others than when they are alone. So get up off your duff and start dialing—invite friends over for dinner, to play a game of cards, or to reminisce about old times. Share humor with others: retell the best jokes or humorous stories, learn the art of delivering a carefully timed punch line. Wake up smiling to lively music on your clock radio or tune in to a cartoon show on television while you sip your morning tea. The happier you are, the healthier you are. Who knows, a good sense of humor may be the key to survival, better than any "medicine." (184 words)

APPENDIX D. PRACTICE STIMULI, UNRESTRICTED PHONETIC CONTEXT

LEVEL IV: ORAL READING OF PARAGRAPHS *(continued)*

Paragraph 16: *Did You Get Your Shot Yet?*

Each fall as the flu season approaches, Americans are faced with the dilemma of whether to get a flu shot. No one looks forward to the headache, aching muscles, sore throat, fever, and nausea common to most flu viruses. These symptoms of the flu last approximately a week. Fifty million Americans contract the flu annually, resulting in millions of lost work hours. Though the flu vaccine is widely available, very few people take advantage of this protective step. The flu vaccine is a must for people over the age of 65 or those who have heart disease, respiratory conditions, or diabetes. Likewise, individuals who have immune disorders and health care workers should be vaccinated. There are many strains of the flu virus requiring revaccination each year to protect against the current flu virus. To date, the flu vaccine is available only by injection and can be obtained from your physician or public health agency. The cost may be as little as $10, a small price to pay for immunity from the flu. (172 words)

Paragraph 17: *Don't Look Now But . . .*

Next time you are at the grocery store, take a good look around you. The floor plan has been carefully designed to slow down the shopper and encourage impulse buying. From the moment you enter the supermarket, you are being "set up" to buy, buy, buy. For example, seasonal bargains such as Halloween candy or picnic supplies are located at the store's entry. The bakery and deli are usually located near the entrance to entice you with the smell of fresh-baked bread. Also close to the front is the produce section, a colorful display of fruits and vegetables arranged to attract your attention. Related items are conveniently placed together—e.g., salad dressing and croutons are next to the salad vegetables. Notice the milk is shelved at the rear of the store. If you "just came in to buy milk," walking to the back of the store exposes you to many temptations. In the checkout line, an array of candies, gum, batteries, and magazines invite you to make one last impulse buy. (171 words)

Paragraph 18: *Protect Those Peepers*

Most of us know we should wear sunscreen to protect our skin from the harmful rays of the sun. But are you equally aware of the potential damage sunlight can do to your eyes? Exposure to intense sunlight reflecting off snow or water can cause sunburn of the cornea, the clear front surface of the eye. Although the damage is not permanent, the condition is painful. Long-term exposure to ultraviolet (UV) light can cause more serious damage: macular degeneration, a leading cause of blindness. People who spend long hours outdoors unprotected from the sun are three times more likely to develop cataracts than those who have less exposure. There are several things you can do to protect your eyes on bright sunny days. Wear a large-brimmed hat and UV-blocking sunglasses. Sunglasses do not have to be expensive to provide adequate protection; virtually all sunglasses provide good UV blocking. If your eyes are very sensitive to light, you may want to buy sunglasses that provide 99% protection from UV rays. (169 words)

APPENDIX D. PRACTICE STIMULI, UNRESTRICTED PHONETIC CONTEXT

LEVEL V: STRUCTURED CONVERSATION (Respond in two to three sentences.)

Set 1

1. Describe how to change the batteries in the artificial larynx.
2. Think of four tourist spots to visit with out-of-town guests in a weekend.
3. Would it be a good idea to be able to "see" the future?
4. If you could have dinner with a famous person, what would you talk about?
5. What television show do you enjoy and why?
6. How do you use a mail order catalog?
7. True or false: Large doses of vitamin C are worthless against the common cold.
8. How would winning a $1 million lottery change your life?
9. What is the difference between a letter and a postcard?
10. "A woman's place is in the home." Is this a valid statement today?

Set 2

1. What city in the world would you like to visit and why?
2. Off you go to a desert island for one year. Choose one person to take with you.
3. What do you consider the necessary ingredients to a long and happy life?
4. Describe how you would change the oil in your car.
5. Explain the saying "Like father, like son."
6. Barring difficulties with finances, schooling, and circumstances—what career would you like to have had?
7. Was putting a man on the moon a waste of taxpayer's money?
8. Can you think of two uses for a belt besides holding your pants up?
9. What would you do if your menu was written in French?
10. What could it mean if someone frequently looked at their watch while you were talking?

Set 3

1. Do you think socialized medicine is the answer to caring for the geriatric population in the United States?
2. What are two things you'd like to know before loaning someone money?
3. What is your favorite pastime?
4. What is the most unusual pet you've ever had?
5. Do you consider yourself lucky? Why or why not?
6. How do you return an item to the store for a refund?
7. Define "family."
8. What three plants would you like to have in your garden?
9. Name a movie you especially enjoyed and tell why.
10. Do you dream in color? How do you know?

Set 4

1. What was your favorite job during your life?
2. Is communication an important part of your life? Why or why not?
3. Who was the most interesting person you ever met?
4. Describe the best car you ever owned.
5. What are the benefits of a smoke detector?
6. You've won $1,000. What will you do with it?
7. How do you feel about spiders and snakes?
8. If you received an obscene phone call, what would you do?
9. Tell two ways you could apologize to someone.
10. What are important qualities for a physician to have?

APPENDIX D. PRACTICE STIMULI, UNRESTRICTED PHONETIC CONTEXT

LEVEL V: STRUCTURED CONVERSATION *(continued)*

Set 5
1. Explain the saying "You can't teach an old dog new tricks."
2. How would you obtain a copy of your birth certificate?
3. Why might you need to rent a car?
4. Talk about your favorite kinds of music.
5. What would you do if you ran out of gas?
6. How do you feel about being on time?
7. Tell me three things you do on a weekly basis.
8. Which is better, contact lenses or glasses?
9. If you could save one thing from a fire in your home, what would it be?
10. What was the most meaningful present you've received?

Set 6
1. Explain the saying "Kill two birds with one stone."
2. What have you done to secure your home?
3. How is a discussion better than an argument?
4. What could someone do to improve his or her credit rating?
5. Do you prefer paper or plastic for your groceries? Why?
6. What are you afraid of?
7. Provide three uses for rubbing alcohol.
8. Describe how to wrap a present.
9. What new skill would you like to learn and why?
10. Talk about the most beautiful city you've visited.

Set 7
1. Would you rather take a leisurely vacation or a touring vacation? Why?
2. Explain the saying "The best things in life are free."
3. Tell me two things you could do for a headache.
4. Describe how to sew a button on a shirt or blouse.
5. What are the ingredients in French toast?
6. What are three things you do on a daily basis?
7. Tell about a time when you felt embarrassed.
8. What are the qualities that make your best friend so special to your life?
9. Where were you born and how many brothers and sisters did you have?
10. Why do people clip coupons?

Set 8
1. Name two things that cost less today than they did five years ago.
2. How would you go about finding a reputable carpet cleaning service?
3. Relate a good deed you performed in the last month.
4. What's so important about washing your hands?
5. After you leave here, what are you going to do today?
6. Do you think the draft should be reinstated? Why or why not?
7. What part of the newspaper do you most enjoy reading?
8. What is the scariest movie you ever watched?
9. Describe how to withdraw money from an automated teller machine.
10. How do other people react to your use of alaryngeal speech?

APPENDIX D. PRACTICE STIMULI, UNRESTRICTED PHONETIC CONTEXT

LEVEL V: STRUCTURED CONVERSATION (continued)

Set 9
1. Describe how you keep your stoma clean.
2. What items do you recycle?
3. How good a driver are you? How do you know?
4. Confess: What "fad" did you participate in?
5. Name several foods you like to eat cold.
6. Would you rather visit a zoo or an art museum? Why?
7. What items would you expect to find in a lady's purse?
8. Have you ever had a reaction to a prescription medicine?
9. What makes you laugh?
10. How did you celebrate your last birthday?

Set 10
1. Explain the saying "Don't rain on my parade."
2. What would you do if you received the wrong order in a restaurant?
3. How do you open a charge account?
4. What were you doing the day President Kennedy was shot?
5. In what ways do you exercise?
6. Why do we have time zones in the United States?
7. How can you tell the difference between a real and a fake diamond?
8. Should sports stars be paid millions of dollars?
9. What qualities make for a good listener?
10. Where did you grow up and when did you leave home?

Set 11
1. What is the happiest month of the year for you? Why?
2. When might "honesty" not be the best policy?
3. Describe how to make a BLT sandwich.
4. Have you ever been on TV news or in the newspaper?
5. Who is "Uncle Sam?"
6. What do you know about lightning?
7. Think of several items usually stored in a safe-deposit box.
8. What things contribute to a good night's sleep?
9. Do you think a four-day work week is a good idea?
10. What are some ways to entertain a child?

Set 12
1. Tell two ways to let someone know you love him or her.
2. What are the advantages to living in an apartment?
3. Would you describe yourself as having a type A or type B personality?
4. How can you find out what the weather is going to be like this weekend?
5. Which states border California?
6. What is the purpose of "taking a vacation"?
7. What is hard for you to remember?
8. Predict the items you would find in a car trunk.
9. Finish the sentence: "Something you may not know about me is _____."
10. What did you eat for your last meal?

APPENDIX D. PRACTICE STIMULI, UNRESTRICTED PHONETIC CONTEXT

LEVEL V: STRUCTURED CONVERSATION *(continued)*

Set 13
1. Describe how you would make reservations at a local restaurant for dinner.
2. How do you respond to rudeness?
3. Which do you prefer—radio or television? Why?
4. Name two activities you could do on a rainy day.
5. Comment on the price of gasoline.
6. What do you wish other people knew about smoking?
7. Who is the most "famous" person you've met?
8. Where is the nearest drugstore to your home?
9. Do you believe in ESP? Why or why not?
10. Provide the steps involved in balancing your checkbook.

Set 14
1. Explain the saying, "The grass is always greener on the other side of the fence."
2. What are two ways you could return a favor.
3. Which would you prefer to own, a sports car or a four-wheel drive vehicle?
4. Tell how to make a pot of coffee (or tea).
5. What does New York City have to offer?
6. Do you remember who you voted for in your first election?
7. In what ways can a guest show his or her appreciation?
8. Name some things that contribute to air pollution.
9. Compose a short ad for a "roommate."
10. What would you consider a good financial investment?

Set 15
1. What is the best first aid for a minor burn?
2. How do you want people/history to remember you?
3. Explain the difference between a solid line and a broken line on the highway.
4. Give a safety tip for cooking outdoors on the barbecue grill.
5. What is the purpose of the Statue of Liberty?
6. True or false: Silence is golden.
7. Would you be willing to be a "guinea pig" for an experimental drug to cure cancer?
8. Are there any topics you can think of that are not listed in the Yellow Pages?
9. Go through the steps for making up the bed.
10. Relate three things that are wrong with our federal government.

Set 16
1. Describe how you would shop for a new car.
2. Which is better, a shower or a bath? Why?
3. What do other people do that irritates you?
4. What is the difference between a governor and a mayor?
5. Is it better to remember yesterday or look ahead to tomorrow?
6. Walk me through the steps to make spaghetti.
7. Are cigars safer to smoke than cigarettes?
8. What does the phrase "baseball, motherhood, and apple pie" mean to you?
9. Which holiday of the year do you enjoy most? Why?
10. You've been asked to write a column for the newspaper. What's the topic?

APPENDIX D. PRACTICE STIMULI, UNRESTRICTED PHONETIC CONTEXT

LEVEL V: STRUCTURED CONVERSATION (*continued*)

Set 17
1. What should you know about a used car before you buy it?
2. Do you think passive smoking is a serious health hazard?
3. What is the purpose of the "World Series"?
4. What is your definition of a relaxing evening at home?
5. Describe the "black sheep" in your family.
6. Close your eyes and describe what you are wearing.
7. Have you ever had something stolen from you?
8. If you had the power to read other people's minds, would you?
9. Why might someone become a vegetarian?
10. Would you describe yourself as a "talker" or a "listener"?

Set 18
1. Who has been your friend for the most years?
2. Which do you think is more effective, an electric or a manual toothbrush?
3. What's the matter with kids today?
4. What magazines do you enjoy reading?
5. Finish the statement: "I wish someone would invite me to _____."
6. Decide what you would do if you found a briefcase containing $500,000.
7. What steps do you have to take to make an international phone call?
8. If you could have a brief conversation with the President of the United States, what would you say to him?
9. Describe your wife (husband, son, daughter) to me.
10. Explain the saying, "Too many cooks spoil the broth."

Set 19
1. Make a suggestion for cheering up a friend.
2. Where do francs, pesos, pounds, and lira come from?
3. Describe your living room.
4. How would you react if someone pushed you from behind as you boarded a bus?
5. Explain the steps in starting a car.
6. What are you an "expert" about?
7. You've won a free dinner for two at a fine restaurant. What would you like to eat?
8. How did you get your nickname?
9. What do you keep putting off until tomorrow?
10. Do you watch soap operas? Which is your favorite?

Set 20
1. What are some ways to treat indigestion?
2. Tell about a time in your life when you felt proud.
3. How would you challenge a bill for services you did not receive?
4. Give brief instructions for how to play your favorite game.
5. What can you do about your mail while you're away on vacation?
6. What are the worst weather conditions you've experienced?
7. Describe the flowers you were sent.
8. Make a suggestion for getting an ink stain out of your favorite garment.
9. Do you have a collection of anything?
10. What do you wish young people knew about drinking?

APPENDIX D. PRACTICE STIMULI, UNRESTRICTED PHONETIC CONTEXT

LEVEL V: STRUCTURED CONVERSATION *(continued)*

Set 21
1. How would you plan a surprise birthday party for your spouse or best friend?
2. What would you change about the way the six o'clock news is presented?
3. List the supplies you need to plant a vegetable garden.
4. What is the largest public event you've attended?
5. Have you ever been fishing? Did you catch anything?
6. Give directions to the nearest fire station.
7. If you've ever worn a lapel button, what did it say?
8. How can you ensure you will pass through the airport security easily?
9. Describe how you would shop for a new home or apartment.
10. You and your friend spot a fifty dollar bill on the sidewalk. How do you resolve who gets it?

Set 22
1. What is the nicest compliment you've ever received?
2. Describe an amazing animal trick you've seen.
3. Can you think of two uses for a shoestring besides tying your shoes?
4. How would you organize your pictures to put them in a photo album?
5. Tell why you quit a job.
6. How many states have you visited?
7. Suggest several of your favorite appetizers to begin the meal.
8. What discontinued product do you wish they'd bring back?
9. Who is the smartest person you've known?
10. What is the difference between a rumor and fact?

Set 23
1. Would you rather live in a big city or a small town? Why?
2. Finish the sentence: The best year of my life was ____. Why?
3. What are some tips for making a good fire in the fireplace?
4. Without giving its name, describe an animal.
5. If you could change one thing about your car, what would it be? Why?
6. Name three ways to keep dust and foreign objects out of the stoma.
7. How much does it cost to take speech therapy lessons?
8. Which vegetable do you hate?
9. Report the most unusual vanity license plate you've seen.
10. What would you do if you borrowed your friend's watch and broke it?

Set 24
1. Do you remember your first traffic ticket?
2. Who has it worse—short people or tall people?
3. If you could make a song request, what would be the song?
4. What are some things people do to bring them good luck?
5. What is proper etiquette when you dial the wrong number?
6. How do you keep your glasses clean?
7. What is the most unusual food you've eaten?
8. Did you ever enter a contest? What kind and did you win?
9. What's wrong with "whining"?
10. What would you do if someone began telling you a joke you already knew?

APPENDIX D. PRACTICE STIMULI, UNRESTRICTED PHONETIC CONTEXT

LEVEL V: STRUCTURED CONVERSATION (*continued*)

Set 25
1. Explain the saying "Don't count your chickens before they hatch."
2. What activity do you wish you were brave enough to do?
3. Describe your neighbor who lives across the street (or hall) from you.
4. Have you ever lied about your age?
5. What is the purpose of the "Great American Smoke-Out"?
6. If you needed a policeman, how would you contact him or her?
7. Name five things we would find in your refrigerator.
8. What do other motorists do that annoys you?
9. For fun, what animal would you be and why?
10. What were your friends doing that your parents wouldn't give you permission to do?

Set 26
1. Confess: Did you ever sneak into a movie as a kid?
2. Off you go to a desert island for one year. Choose two books to take with you.
3. Describe how you would check the air pressure in your car's tires.
4. Explain how you keep water out of the stoma during bathing.
5. What is your favorite candy?
6. Have you ever lost anything expensive?
7. Tell about help you received from a perfect stranger.
8. Name three things that are positive about our local government.
9. What would you do if the clerk accidentally gave you too much change?
10. Explain how to make toast.

Set 27
1. Would you rather have a "free" chauffeur or a chef for a month?
2. Where do your closest relatives live?
3. Share two of your strengths.
4. Share two of your weaknesses.
5. Which of the tastes do you prefer: sweet, sour, bitter, or salty?
6. What are some ways to cover windows to maintain our privacy?
7. If you could change one incident in your past, what would it be?
8. How can you prepare for a natural disaster?
9. Describe how you would shop for a new television.
10. What would you do if you realized you were driving the wrong way down a one-way street?

Set 28
1. What are the benefits of owning your own home?
2. In what ways are you generous?
3. Without giving its name, describe a fruit.
4. Why is it important for you to wear some type of medical identification?
5. What foreign language would you like to learn? Why?
6. Think of several ways to protect yourself from phone scams.
7. What do you enjoy most about the summer months?
8. If you had a power outage, how would you save the food in your refrigerator?
9. What does it mean to have a "contagious" disease? Give an example.
10. If someone hangs up on you while you're using alaryngeal speech, how does that make you feel?

APPENDIX D. PRACTICE STIMULI, UNRESTRICTED PHONETIC CONTEXT

LEVEL V: STRUCTURED CONVERSATION *(continued)*

Set 29

1. True or false: Absence makes the heart grow fonder.
2. What is your favorite piece of furniture in your house?
3. If you could be invisible for a day, where would you go?
4. Talk about a time when you were homesick.
5. Do you believe wearing seat belts saves lives?
6. What is the most money you've found on the street?
7. Have you ever done something on a dare?
8. What movie did you see that you wish you hadn't?
9. What are some products made from milk?
10. Who was the recipient of your first crush?

Set 30

1. Do you believe in astrology? Do you know your "sign"?
2. What radio show do you enjoy and why?
3. How can friends and family be supportive to the laryngectomee?
4. Name something money cannot buy.
5. What is the significance of having a fever?
6. Is there a time when taking the bus would be easier than driving a car?
7. No one is looking—what is your favorite "junk food"?
8. Talk about the ugliest city you've visited.
9. What should you do if your credit cards are stolen?
10. Talk about first aid for a minor cut on your finger.

Set 31

1. Describe how you would get from your house to our clinic (my office).
2. Do you prefer to eat in or dine out?
3. What is it about your favorite holiday song?
4. How can you protect yourself and your belongings in a hotel?
5. Suggest a couple of ways to get your friend out of a bad mood.
6. Tell me how to get to your house from the nearest bus stop.
7. Think of some uses for baking soda.
8. Which cartoon character still makes you laugh?
9. Whose pictures do you carry in your wallet?
10. Would you rather take the bus or the train on a cross-country trip?

Set 32

1. Name several foods that can be eaten raw.
2. How can you take advantage of flying by getting cheaper airline tickets?
3. What are some secrets to a lasting marriage?
4. Why do football referees throw yellow hankies?
5. Have you ever shrunk anything in the washer or dryer?
6. Would you rather attend the opera or a jazz concert?
7. How can you tell a person is from the South?
8. Would you say anything to a person who illegally parked in a handicapped parking space?
9. If you've misplaced your keys, what steps do you take to find them?
10. Do you believe you make things happen or that things happen to you?

APPENDIX D. PRACTICE STIMULI, UNRESTRICTED PHONETIC CONTEXT

LEVEL V: STRUCTURED CONVERSATION (continued)

Set 33
1. Which period would you choose to live—past, present, or future—and why?
2. What three ingredients make for a stirring parade?
3. Would you report a shoplifter to the store management?
4. Think of some ways to stay cool during the summer.
5. In your opinion, who has been the best President during your lifetime?
6. Name something you do that should be done slowly and carefully.
7. Who is your favorite author? What is your favorite novel?
8. Which do you think has more calories, a baked potato or French fries? Why?
9. What can you do to protect your skin from the sun?
10. What are some things you can do if another car is following you too close?

Set 34
1. Explain the saying "Do unto others as you would have them do unto you."
2. How do you select what to wear for the day?
3. How would you respond to a stranger's question, "What happened to you"?
4. Do you agree with mandatory retirement at age 65 years? Why or why not?
5. Make a list of items to have in your pantry for an emergency.
6. If you accidentally dented the unoccupied car next to you, what would you do?
7. Without giving its name, describe a vegetable.
8. If you were invited to the White House for dinner, would you go?
9. How did you get your name?
10. Compose a thank you note to your nephew for a key chain he sent you.

Set 35
1. How can you tell whether a melon is ripe?
2. You and another driver spot an available parking space at the same time. How do you resolve who gets the space?
3. Have you ever written anything on a rest room wall?
4. Off you go to a desert island for one year. Choose three foods to take with you.
5. What are the benefits of a college education?
6. How many "lives" is a cat supposed to have? Why?
7. What's your favorite excuse for being late?
8. What do you wish someone would invent?
9. Relate a dream that seemed very real to you.
10. If you came home and your front door was ajar, what would you do?

Set 36
1. Close your eyes and describe this room.
2. What do your keys unlock?
3. Who was Franklin Delano Roosevelt?
4. Have you ever gotten into trouble for standing up for your beliefs?
5. Name some items associated with Halloween.
6. When you go out to lunch with three of your friends, should the check be split evenly four ways?
7. What is the purpose of the "Rose Bowl"?
8. Do you remember whose pictures are on the five, ten, and twenty dollar bills?
9. If you drove 50 miles north of our city, where would you be?
10. When is your next doctor's appointment?

APPENDIX D. PRACTICE STIMULI, UNRESTRICTED PHONETIC CONTEXT

LEVEL V: STRUCTURED CONVERSATION *(continued)*

Set 37
1. What is your policy about tipping in a restaurant?
2. How might you brighten the day for a shut-in?
3. What is the purpose of physical therapy?
4. Do you know a popular tourist attraction in England?
5. What are ways you can get an urgent message to someone?
6. Where is the rest room in this building?
7. What does it mean to "get up on the wrong side of the bed"?
8. What is the proper procedure for burning leaves?
9. Why is "freedom of speech" so important to Americans?
10. Explain why a certain team is your favorite sports team.

Set 38
1. Have you ever won a prize? What did you do to win it?
2. What could you do with those leftover vegetables in the refrigerator?
3. How did you earn your first paycheck?
4. After leaving class, you realize you accidentally picked up the wrong jacket. What do you do?
5. Describe how you would groom your dog or cat.
6. Who is your hero?
7. Would you honor the picket line at your local grocery store?
8. If you forget someone's name, how might you "cover up"?
9. Describe how we benefit from the taxes we pay.
10. What was the last television program you watched?

Set 39
1. What are your options if you're stuck in an elevator?
2. Five years from now, what will you be doing?
3. Finish the sentence: "My idea of a relaxing activity would be _____."
4. How might you solve the problem of loose dentures?
5. Compose a brief ad for a housekeeper.
6. Do you know anyone who has had a baby in the last year?
7. Which states border Tennessee?
8. Predict how much it would cost to own a dog for a year.
9. You're dining at a friend's home and find a dead fly in your salad. What do you do?
10. What is Mardi Gras?

Set 40
1. What do you know about your family tree?
2. Summarize the top news story of the day.
3. Before you'd see a dentist, what would you like to know about him or her?
4. How would you look up a word in the dictionary that you didn't know how to spell?
5. What are some symptoms that let you know you are ill?
6. Give us the recipe for your favorite dessert.
7. What items would you expect to find in a man's wallet?
8. Do you prefer to use an umbrella or a raincoat when it's raining?
9. Tell what you know about earthquakes.
10. Share your personal motto you live by.

APPENDIX D. PRACTICE STIMULI, UNRESTRICTED PHONETIC CONTEXT

LEVEL V: STRUCTURED CONVERSATION *(continued)*

Set 41

1. Report a stressor in your life and what you're doing to lessen its effect.
2. How can you tell whether or not someone is telling the truth?
3. If you didn't have a driver's license, how else might you identify yourself?
4. In the history of the United States, who do you think has been the best president?
5. What does Reno, Nevada have to offer?
6. In what ways did you become more like your mother or father as you grew up?
7. Architecturally speaking, what is the most dramatic building in your city?
8. Give us at least two good home remedies for a cold.
9. Do you believe in "flying saucers"? Why or why not?
10. What is your favorite flavor of ice cream? Your favorite toppings?

Set 42

1. What are the lyrics to one of your favorite songs?
2. Explain how the artificial larynx (or esophageal speech or tracheoesophageal prosthesis) "works."
3. If you were invited to two parties, how would you decide which one to attend?
4. Tell us about your first car.
5. When you're too tired to cook, what are your options?
6. What is something special you have that you can offer to others?
7. Leave a message on my voice mail that you are unable to make it to therapy.
8. You're in the grocery checkout—you've forgotten your checkbook. What do you do?
9. Where is the television located in your home?
10. Describe an unexpected present that you received.

Set 43

1. How would you get rid of a guest who has overstayed his or her welcome?
2. Who was Abraham Lincoln?
3. Name a good cause that you would be willing to picket for.
4. Would you report the person taking bottles and cans from your recycling bin?
5. Is there a television commercial that you think is pretty effective?
6. When was the last time you attended a wedding?
7. Think of several items usually stored in your attic.
8. Describe the countryside in New England during the late fall.
9. Explain the saying: "People who live in glass houses shouldn't throw stones."
10. Explain how you would make your favorite casserole (or another dish).

Set 44

1. Describe yourself to someone who has never seen you.
2. If you wanted to know more about arthritis, how could you get more information?
3. Who were the original forty-niners? Who are the current forty-niners?
4. What is something your mother or father taught you that you have never forgotten?
5. If you had the power to make a new law, what would that law be?
6. What would the title of a book about your life be?
7. In what ways can a host make sure his or her guests are comfortable?
8. What is celebrated on St. Patrick's Day?
9. What two things would you want to know before you went on a special diet?
10. On what occasion would you use candles?

APPENDIX D. PRACTICE STIMULI, UNRESTRICTED PHONETIC CONTEXT

LEVEL V: STRUCTURED CONVERSATION *(continued)*

Set 45

1. If you had the ability to read other people's minds, how would you use it?
2. What, if anything, is wrong with the movies of today?
3. What is your idea of a perfect evening?
4. Predict your life five years from now.
5. Think of an invention that has had a positive influence on your life.
6. Express your views about illegal immigrants.
7. What can you do for a toothache until you see the dentist?
8. Share an important decision you've made recently.
9. What errands do you need to do before the week is over?
10. How much longer do you think Social Security will be in effect?

Set 46

1. Describe the inside of your medicine cabinet.
2. Have you ever "gotten away" with something?
3. Would you consider getting a puppy? Why or why not?
4. What are some ways to reduce dry mouth after radiation?
5. Where is the most unusual place you've fallen asleep?
6. Finish the sentence: "I really should _____."
7. What kind of weather do you prefer? Why?
8. It's two o'clock AM and the faucet is drip-drip-dripping. What would you do?
9. What does it take to renew your driver's license?
10. True or false about yourself: I like being alone.

Set 47

1. Describe how you would take care of a special potted plant.
2. What is a "skeleton" key?
3. Recall a time when you saved for something you really wanted.
4. On what occasion would you use candles?
5. What would you do if you had trouble hearing others talk?
6. What is meant by the saying "two heads are better than one"?
7. Would you rather work a crossword puzzle or play cards?
8. Have you ever been wrongly accused of something?
9. What kind of artwork would you like to hang in your living room?
10. If you could have one wish, what would that wish be? Why?

Set 48

1. Complete the sentence: "One thing I like about myself is _____."
2. Give two suggestions for increasing the humidity in your home.
3. Why is September a special month for you?
4. What are two things you'd like to know before buying medical insurance?
5. Tell a personal sacrifice you have made in your life.
6. Who would you like to invite to Thanksgiving dinner?
7. Name at least three community servants.
8. What are some items that come in pairs?
9. What does it mean to be wealthy?
10. Think of some ways to stay warm in the winter.

APPENDIX D. PRACTICE STIMULI, UNRESTRICTED PHONETIC CONTEXT

LEVEL VI: SPONTANEOUS AND EXTENDED CONVERSATION

1. Discuss a recently read book or journal article.
2. What year of your life would you like to repeat? Why?
3. Describe the most exotic vacation you've ever taken.
4. Debate political issues surrounding an upcoming election.
5. Tell about your first car: make and model, cost, performance, "fun" value.
6. Describe the teacher who had the most influence on you during your school years.
7. Go through your wallet or purse and talk about some of the items.
8. Teach stoma hygiene care to a new laryngectomee in the group.
9. Make a phone call to a local airline to inquire about rates to a certain city.
10. Recommend a good pet and tell about the care and feeding involved.
11. What has been your greatest challenge in life? Explain.
12. If you could make a new law, what would that law be? How would you enforce it?
13. Describe the most unusual job you've had.
14. In how many cities (countries) have you lived during your life?
15. How do you feel about loaning friends money?
16. Tell a humorous story about your grandchild (or spouse, child, friend, pet).
17. What is the most unusual prize you've won?
18. With whom have you enjoyed the longest friendship? What is the secret of your friendship?
19. Tell the story line of the best movie you've seen.
20. Describe your morning routine (i.e., from wake up until noon).
21. Make a phone call to the local library and ask information about a certain topic or book.
22. What is the most interesting autobiography (or biography) you've read?
23. Share memories of a wedding you attended.
24. Tell about when your first child was born.
25. What is the most important decision you've made in your life?
26. Role play an interaction at the bank (e.g., cashing an out-of-state check).
27. Tell about the best live play you've seen.
28. Discuss the advantages and disadvantages of credit cards.
29. Describe your last visit to your doctor.
30. Give your opinion about gun control.
31. Read and discuss a newspaper article or current event topic.
32. What ideas do you have for solving the homeless problem?
33. In the upcoming election, how are you going to vote about proposition _____?
34. Call a store and ask hours of operation or if they have a specific product.
35. If you've served in the military, share an experience you had.
36. Share memories of a special holiday.
37. Would you prefer to live in a warm climate year round or have seasons? Why?
38. Discuss the role of "good manners" in society. Give examples.
39. Role play an interaction at the store (e.g., returning damaged goods).
40. Share memories of a special event in your life.
41. Call a travel agency and inquire about a vacation package to a certain city.
42. Talk about having a brother or sister (if you do!).
43. Read a question from the advice column in the newspaper. Provide your solution before reading the published answer.
44. What do you consider the secret to a long and happy life? Why?
45. Do you prefer living in the city or the country? What are benefits/drawbacks of each?
46. Go through the steps you would take to find and purchase a used car.
47. What are the pros and cons of being married?

APPENDIX D. PRACTICE STIMULI, UNRESTRICTED PHONETIC CONTEXT

LEVEL VI: SPONTANEOUS AND EXTENDED CONVERSATION *(continued)*

48. How might a person earn extra money?
49. In what order do you read the daily newspaper?
50. Role play calling the doctor's office to make an appointment.
51. Relate the worst night you ever spent in a hotel (or motel).
52. Express your ideas for decreasing vandalism—for example, public transportation and buildings.
53. If you were the President of the United States, what would be your goals for the country?
54. Tell what you know about diabetes (or high blood pressure, asthma, emphysema).
55. Has your car ever run out of gas? How did you resolve the problem?
56. Have you ever been on a diet? What kind? How successful were you?
57. What do you consider the most important lesson you've learned in life?
58. How would your life change if you won the lottery? How would you deal with people asking you to donate to their cause? With the fame and loss of privacy?
59. Describe your dream house, including room arrangements, special features, colors, furniture. Don't forget the yard!
60. Verbally pack your suitcase for a two week vacation to Florida (Hawaii, etc.).
61. Role play ordering in a restaurant (clinician supplies menu).
62. Discuss the precautions you take to keep yourself healthy.
63. What role does music play in your life? What is your favorite type of music? instrument? Who is your favorite singer? How does music make you feel?
64. If you were to visit a new laryngectomee, what are some things you would want to tell him or her in that first conversation?
65. You and three friends have won an all expenses paid weekend in San Francisco. What sights will you see? Where will you eat?
66. Summarize this past year of your life.
67. Tell us about something you haven't done since you were a kid.
68. In a dream, you're hosting an all-star dinner. You may invite 10 famous people (living or dead) to dinner. Who are they and why did you select each person?
69. Tell about a time you received a traffic ticket (or talked yourself out of one!).
70. What question have you been wishing I would ask you? Ask it and answer it.

Consonant Contrast Drills

APPENDIX E. CONSONANT CONTRAST DRILLS

INITIAL POSITION IN WORDS

Initial /p/ vs. /b/ contrasts
Set 1
1.	pearl	burl
2.	ped	bed
3.	pub	bub
4.	pull	bull
5.	pert	Bert
6.	pony	bony
7.	pot	bought
8.	pin	bin
9.	poop	boop
10.	peach	beach

Set 2
1.	peas	bees
2.	pig	big
3.	pond	bond
4.	pun	bun
5.	pout	bout
6.	Powell	bowel
7.	pang	bang
8.	purr	burr
9.	peep	beep
10.	pudge	budge

Initial /p/ vs. /m/ contrasts
Set 1
1.	pith	myth
2.	pope	mope
3.	pock	mock
4.	pick	Mick
5.	pod	mod
6.	purge	merge
7.	pine	mine
8.	pooch	mooch
9.	pitch	Mitch
10.	pace	mace

Initial /p/ vs. /b/ vs. /m/ contrasts
Set 1
1.	pad	bad	mad
2.	pop	bop	mop
3.	putt	butt	mutt
4.	pack	back	Mack
5.	Pete	beat	meet
6.	pale	bale	male
7.	pug	bug	mug
8.	pole	bowl	mole
9.	pore	bore	more
10.	pan	ban	man

Set 2
1.	pus	bus	muss
2.	peek	beak	meek
3.	pit	bit	mitt
4.	path	bath	math
5.	peg	beg	Meg
6.	puck	buck	muck
7.	pain	bane	main
8.	pass	bass	mass
9.	pile	bile	mile
10.	pen	been	men

Set 3
1.	paid	bade	made
2.	puff	buff	muff
3.	pier	beer	mere
4.	pet	bet	met
5.	ping	bing	ming
6.	pound	bound	mound
7.	pat	bat	mat
8.	pike	bike	mike
9.	patch	batch	match
10.	pill	bill	mill

APPENDIX E. CONSONANT CONTRAST DRILLS

INITIAL POSITION IN WORDS (continued)

Initial /t/ vs. /d/ contrasts

Set 1

1.	ten	den
2.	tad	dad
3.	tuck	duck
4.	time	dime
5.	towel	dowel
6.	tug	dug
7.	tome	dome
8.	tall	doll
9.	Tim	dim
10.	type	dike

Set 2

1.	tire	dire
2.	town	down
3.	tummy	dummy
4.	team	deem
5.	tin	din
6.	tomb	doom
7.	tongue	dung
8.	tore	door
9.	tune	dune
10.	ten	den

Initial /t/ vs. /n/ contrasts

Set 1

1.	tape	nape
2.	tat	gnat
3.	toad	node
4.	tease	knees
5.	tier	near
6.	tight	night
7.	toys	noise
8.	tap	nap
9.	tone	known
10.	Todd	nod

Set 2

1.	tag	nag
2.	taught	naught
3.	took	nook
4.	tile	Nile
5.	tail	nail
6.	ton	none
7.	toes	nose
8.	tot	not
9.	teal	kneel
10.	tech	neck

Initial /t/ vs. /d/ vs. /n/ contrasts

Set 1

1.	Tate	date	Nate
2.	tame	dame	name
3.	Ted	dead	Ned
4.	tear	dear	near
5.	tam	dam	Nam
6.	tub	dub	numb
7.	taupe	dope	nope
8.	toes	does	nose
9.	tot	dot	not
10.	teed	deed	need

Set 2

1.	til	dill	nil
2.	tale	dale	nail
3.	tech	deck	neck
4.	tell	dell	Nell
5.	tab	dab	nab
6.	tan	Dan	Nan
7.	ton	done	none
8.	tote	dote	note
9.	toll	dole	knoll
10.	tog	dog	nog

Initial /k/ vs. /g/ contrasts

Set 1

1.	cape	gape
2.	cuss	Gus
3.	coat	goat
4.	cot	got
5.	cause	gauze
6.	Kyle	guile
7.	con	gone
8.	core	gore
9.	curd	gird
10.	Kate	gate

Set 2

1.	cave	gave
2.	cap	gap
3.	cull	gull
4.	come	gum
5.	card	guard
6.	could	good
7.	curl	girl
8.	cash	gash
9.	cool	ghoul
10.	came	game

APPENDIX E. CONSONANT CONTRAST DRILLS

INITIAL POSITION IN WORDS (continued)

Initial /s/ vs. /z/ contrasts
Set 1

1.	seek	Zeke
2.	sane	Zane
3.	sue	zoo
4.	send	Zen
5.	saps	zaps
6.	sack	Zack
7.	sag	zag
8.	sone	zone
9.	seal	zeal
10.	sip	zip

Set 2

1.	sues	zoos
2.	sit	zit
3.	Seus	Zeus
4.	see	zee
5.	sink	zinc
6.	sing	zing
7.	sipper	zipper
8.	saps	zaps
9.	sags	zags
10.	sap	zap

Initial /f/ vs. /v/ contrasts
Set 1

1.	face	vase
2.	fail	vail
3.	fest	vest
4.	fetch	vetch
5.	fend	vend
6.	ferry	very
7.	fat	vat
8.	file	vile
9.	fine	vine
10.	fern	Vern

Initial /f/ vs. /v/ contrasts
Set 2

1.	foul	vowel
2.	fast	vast
3.	fan	van
4.	feel	veal
5.	few	view
6.	fear	veer
7.	fault	vault
8.	final	vinyl
9.	feign	vain
10.	focal	vocal

Initial /tʃ/ vs. /dʒ/ contrasts
Set 1

1.	chokes	jokes
2.	Chan	Jan
3.	chunk	junk
4.	chalk	jock
5.	chew	Jew
6.	cheer	jeer
7.	choker	joker
8.	char	jar
9.	chest	jest
10.	chitter	jitter

Set 2

1.	chaw	jaw
2.	cheap	jeep
3.	chess	Jess
4.	Chet	jet
5.	chigger	jigger
6.	chinks	jinks
7.	choke	joke
8.	chug	jug
9.	chump	jump
10.	chews	Jews

APPENDIX E. CONSONANT CONTRAST DRILLS

FINAL POSITION IN WORDS

Final /p/ vs. /b/ contrasts
Set 1

1.	cop	cob
2.	cup	cub
3.	lap	lab
4.	rip	rib
5.	sop	sob
6.	gop	gob
7.	lop	lob
8.	pup	pub
9.	slap	slab
10.	rip	rib

Final /p/ vs. /m/ contrasts
Set 1

1.	whip	whim
2.	top	Tom
3.	cape	came
4.	nape	name
5.	type	time
6.	dip	dim
7.	dope	dome
8.	clap	clam
9.	steep	steam
10.	ripe	rhyme

Final /p/ vs. /b/ vs. /m/ contrasts
Set 1

1.	rip	rib	rim
2.	tap	tab	tam
3.	cup	cub	come
4.	cap	cab	cam
5.	gape	Gabe	game
6.	rope	robe	roam
7.	mop	mob	mom
8.	slap	slab	slam
9.	sup	sub	some
10.	lap	lab	lamb

Final /t/ vs. /d/ contrasts
Set 1

1.	vent	vend
2.	brought	broad
3.	fret	Fred
4.	hat	had
5.	mate	made
6.	threat	thread
7.	wrought	rod
8.	neat	need
9.	right	ride
10.	bet	bed

Final /t/ vs. /n/ contrasts
Set 1

1.	that	than
2.	suit	soon
3.	wit	win
4.	gout	gown
5.	gut	gun
6.	sate	sane
7.	fight	fine
8.	fought	fawn
9.	fit	fin
10.	might	mine

Final /t/ vs. /d/ vs. /n/ contrasts
Set 1

1.	trait	trade	train
2.	rat	rad	ran
3.	beat	bead	bean
4.	Bart	bard	barn
5.	rate	raid	rain
6.	debt	dead	den
7.	wrote	road	roan
8.	mat	mad	man
9.	cot	cod	con
10.	great	grade	grain

APPENDIX E. CONSONANT CONTRAST DRILLS

FINAL POSITION IN WORDS (continued)

Final /t/ vs. /d/ vs. /n/ contrasts
Set 2

1.	greet	greed	green
2.	cat	cad	can
3.	fat	fad	fan
4.	sight	side	sign
5.	mate	made	main
6.	coat	code	cone
7.	fate	fade	feign
8.	light	lied	line
9.	it	id	in
10.	brought	broad	brawn

Final /k/ vs. /g/ contrasts
Set 1

1.	cock	cog
2.	wick	wig
3.	lack	lag
4.	tack	tag
5.	luck	lug
6.	brick	brig
7.	buck	bug
8.	hawk	hog
9.	peck	peg
10.	snack	snag

Set 2

1.	rack	rag
2.	chuck	chug
3.	Dick	dig
4.	flack	flag
5.	frock	frog
6.	pick	pig
7.	stack	stag
8.	back	bag
9.	clock	clog
10.	leak	league

Final /s/ vs. /z/ contrasts
Set 1

1.	lace	laze
2.	fuss	fuzz
3.	lease	Lee's
4.	loose	lose
5.	ice	eyes
6.	piece	peas
7.	hearse	hers
8.	grace	graze
9.	fleece	fleas
10.	race	raise

Set 2

1.	spice	spies
2.	bus	buzz
3.	cross	craws
4.	rice	rise
5.	niece	knees
6.	dose	doze
7.	face	faze
8.	cease	seize
9.	price	prize
10.	purse	purrs

Final /f/ vs. /v/ contrasts
Set 1

1.	surf	serve
2.	shelf	shelve
3.	safe	save
4.	leaf	leave
5.	thief	thieve
6.	half	have
7.	grief	grieve
8.	waif	waive
9.	fife	five
10.	calf	calve

APPENDIX E. CONSONANT CONTRAST DRILLS

FINAL POSITION IN WORDS (continued)

Final /θ/ vs. /ð/ contrasts
Set 1

1.	sheath	sheathe
2.	sooth	soothe
3.	mouth [noun]	mouth [verb]
4.	teeth	teethe
5.	loath	loathe
6.	wreath	wreathe
7.	teeth	teethe
8.	sheath	sheathe
9.	sooth	soothe
10.	mouth [noun]	mouth [verb]

Final /tʃ/ vs. /dʒ/ contrasts
Set 1

1.	bench	binge
2.	Mitch	Midge
3.	etch	edge
4.	March	Marge
5.	search	surge
6.	cinch	singe
7.	lunch	lunge
8.	batch	badge
9.	perch	purge
10.	rich	ridge

Practice Stimuli, Restricted Phonetic Context

APPENDIX F. PRACTICE STIMULI, RESTRICTED PHONETIC CONTEXT
For use during injection method for obstruents in esophageal speech.

LEVEL I: ONE-SYLLABLE WORDS BEGINNING WITH UNVOICED (UV) OBSTRUENTS PLUS MID AND LOW VOWELS

- Unvoiced obstruents /p/, /t/, /k/, /f/, /s/, /ʃ/, /θ/, /tʃ/, /sp/, /st/, /sk/, and /h/ as a "modified" /k/
- Mid and low vowels /a/, /o/, /ɔ/, /ʌ/, /æ/, /e/, and /ɛ/

/p/ words Set 1	/t/ words Set 1	/k/ words Set 1	/f/ words Set 1	/s/ words Set 1
1. pop	1. top	1. cop	1. fall	1. sarge
2. poach	2. taupe	2. coach	2. foam	2. sew
3. Paul	3. talk	3. call	3. fawn	3. sauce
4. putt	4. ton	4. come	4. fudge	4. some
5. pack	5. tab	5. cab	5. fad	5. sack
6. pace	6. tale	6. cage	6. face	6. safe
7. pair	7. tech	7. care	7. fair	7. said
8. palm	8. tart	8. card	8. fond	8. soft
9. poke	9. toast	9. cork	9. fork	9. sock
10. pause	10. tempt	10. cough	10. fate	10. Saul

/p/ words Set 2	/t/ words Set 2	/k/ words Set 2	/f/ words Set 2	/s/ words Set 2
1. pot	1. toss	1. car	1. farm	1. sob
2. pole	2. tote	2. coal	2. foe	2. soap
3. paw	3. taught	3. caught	3. fought	3. saw
4. puck	4. tongue	4. cub	4. fuss	4. such
5. pad	5. tack	5. calf	5. fan	5. sand
6. page	6. taste	6. cake	6. fade	6. saint
7. peck	7. ten	7. keg	7. fetch	7. self
8. pulp	8. tough	8. cuss	8. fund	8. suck
9. pal	9. tap	9. cash	9. fat	9. sash
10. paid	10. tang	10. came	10. phase	10. sale

/p/ words Set 3	/t/ words Set 3	/k/ words Set 3	/f/ words Set 3	/s/ words Set 3
1. parch	1. tot	1. cart	1. fog	1. sock
2. poll	2. toad	2. coast	2. four	2. sold
3. pawn	3. tock	3. cause	3. far	3. sought
4. pump	4. touch	4. cup	4. fun	4. sub
5. past	5. task	5. can't	5. fast	5. sap
6. pain	6. tape	6. case	6. faith	6. sail
7. peg	7. test	7. Ken	7. fell	7. sent
8. park	8. tall	8. carve	8. farce	8. song
9. pope	9. tore	9. cope	9. phone	9. sore
10. paste	10. take	10. cape	10. fake	10. same

APPENDIX F. PRACTICE STIMULI, RESTRICTED PHONETIC CONTEXT
For use during injection method for obstruents in esophageal speech.

LEVEL I: ONE-SYLLABLE WORDS BEGINNING WITH UNVOICED OBSTRUENTS PLUS MID AND LOW VOWELS (*continued*)

/ʃ/ words Set 1	/θ/ words Set 1	/tʃ/ words Set 1	/sp/ words Set 1	/st/ words Set 1
1. shark	1. thumb	1. charge	1. spa	1. start
2. shoal	2. thorn	2. choke	2. spoke	2. stole
3. Sean	3. thaw	3. chaw	3. spawn	3. stalk
4. shove	4. thud	4. chuck	4. spuds	4. stub
5. shack	5. Thad	5. champ	5. span	5. stab
6. shade	6. thanks	6. chafe	6. space	6. stage
7. chef	7. theft	7. chair	7. spare	7. stair
8. shop	8. thoughts	8. chum	8. Spock	8. stop
9. show	9. thatch	9. chased	9. spay	9. stove
10. shell	10. thong	10. chant	10. spend	10. stuff

/ʃ/ words Set 2	/θ/ words Set 2	/tʃ/ words Set 2	/sp/ words Set 2	/st/ words Set 2
1. sharp	1. thugs	1. chalk	1. spares	1. stall
2. shore	2. Thad	2. chore	2. spat	2. stone
3. shawl	3. thought	3. chest	3. sparse	3. stops
4. shunt	4. Thor	4. chump	4. spank	4. stud
5. shaft	5. theft	5. Chad	5. sports	5. stand
6. shake	6. thawed	6. chain	6. spawns	6. steak
7. share	7. thongs	7. check	7. spud	7. stead
8. shush	8. thump	8. chat	8. spade	8. starves
9. shone	9. thank	9. char	9. spell	9. stoke
10. shape	10. thatched	10. change	10. spends	10. stuck

/ʃ/ words Set 3	/θ/ words Set 3	/tʃ/ words Set 3	/sp/ words Set 3	/st/ words Set 3
1. shock	1. Thor	1. chop	1. spot	1. star
2. short	2. thumped	2. chose	2. sport	2. store
3. shod	3. thought	3. Chet	3. spares	3. starve
4. shut	4. thefts	4. chunk	4. spun	4. stung
5. shag	5. thanked	5. chance	5. sparks	5. staff
6. shame	6. Thad	6. chase	6. Spain	6. stale
7. shed	7. thumbs	7. charm	7. sped	7. step
8. shot	8. thug	8. chess	8. spas	8. stench
9. shall	9. thaws	9. chap	9. spar	9. stamp
10. shave	10. thorns	10. chomp	10. spells	10. stare

APPENDIX F. PRACTICE STIMULI, RESTRICTED PHONETIC CONTEXT
For use during injection method for obstruents in esophageal speech.

LEVEL I: ONE-SYLLABLE WORDS BEGINNING WITH UNVOICED OBSTRUENTS PLUS MID AND LOW VOWELS *(continued)*

/sk/ words Set 1	/h/ words Set 1	Mixed UV obstruents Set 1	Mixed UV obstruents Set 4	Mixed UV obstruents Set 7
1. scar	1. hard	1. parch	1. thaw	1. patch
2. scold	2. host	2. told	2. chuck	2. take
3. scotch	3. haunt	3. cost	3. span	3. care
4. scuff	4. hug	4. fuzz	4. stay	4. fall
5. scab	5. had	5. sack	5. sketch	5. soap
6. scale	6. hail	6. shave	6. halt	6. shawl
7. scarce	7. health	7. thug	7. post	7. thump
8. scant	8. honk	8. chalk	8. talk	8. chance
9. skunk	9. hose	9. sport	9. come	9. space
10. scope	10. hog	10. stalk	10. fat	10. step

/sk/ words Set 2	/h/ words Set 2	Mixed UV obstruents Set 2	Mixed UV obstruents Set 5	Mixed UV obstruents Set 8
1. scald	1. heart	1. scuff	1. save	1. scar
2. score	2. home	2. hash	2. share	2. hoax
3. Scot	3. haul	3. pace	3. thumb	3. pause
4. scum	4. hulk	4. test	4. chore	4. tough
5. scalp	5. half	5. card	5. spawn	5. catch
6. skate	6. hang	6. foam	6. stuck	6. fail
7. sketch	7. hair	7. sauce	7. scalp	7. said
8. skull	8. hush	8. shut	8. hail	8. sharp
9. scan	9. hatch	9. Thad	9. pest	9. thorn
10. skein	10. hate	10. chain	10. top	10. chaw

/sk/ words Set 3	/h/ words Set 3	Mixed UV obstruents Set 3	Mixed UV obstruents Set 6	Mixed UV obstruents Set 9
1. scarf	1. hot	1. spare	1. court	1. sponge
2. scorch	2. horse	2. stock	2. fought	2. stamp
3. scone	3. hawk	3. scold	3. such	3. scale
4. sculpt	4. hunch	4. haunt	4. shop	4. head
5. scamp	5. ham	5. pup	5. thanks	5. part
6. skates	6. haste	6. tack	6. chest	6. toast
7. scare	7. help	7. cage	7. spark	7. caught
8. scat	8. hunt	8. fare	8. stove	8. fun
9. scoff	9. hope	9. sod	9. scald	9. sash
10. scaled	10. hedge	10. short	10. hunch	10. shape

APPENDIX F. PRACTICE STIMULI, RESTRICTED PHONETIC CONTEXT
For use during injection method for obstruents in esophageal speech.

LEVEL I: ONE-SYLLABLE WORDS BEGINNING WITH UNVOICED OBSTRUENTS PLUS MID AND LOW VOWELS (continued)

Mixed UV obstruents Set 10	*Mixed UV obstruents Set 13*	*Mixed UV obstruents Set 16*	*Mixed UV obstruents Set 19*	*Mixed UV obstruents Set 22*
1. theft	1. pour	1. thud	1. paid	1. thaws
2. chart	2. taught	2. champ	2. ten	2. choke
3. spoke	3. cup	3. spank	3. carve	3. spar
4. stall	4. fast	4. stair	4. fork	4. stuff
5. skunk	5. sale	5. scarf	5. sought	5. scant
6. hand	6. shell	6. whole	6. shush	6. hang
7. paste	7. thought	7. Paul	7. Thad	7. pair
8. tempt	8. chose	8. touch	8. chase	8. tall
9. car	9. spot	9. cat	9. spend	9. coast
10. phone	10. stub	10. face	10. star	10. fog

Mixed UV obstruents Set 11	*Mixed UV obstruents Set 14*	*Mixed UV obstruents Set 17*	*Mixed UV obstruents Set 20*	*Mixed UV obstruents Set 23*
1. saw	1. scamp	1. safe	1. scorch	1. suck
2. shove	2. haste	2. shot	2. haul	2. shaft
3. thatch	3. pet	3. thorns	3. pump	3. thanked
4. change	4. talk	4. charge	4. tap	4. check
5. spell	5. coach	5. spud	5. case	5. spa
6. start	6. fawn	6. stand	6. fell	6. stone
7. scope	7. some	7. skate	7. sock	7. scoff
8. hog	8. shack	8. help	8. show	8. hush
9. puff	9. thank	9. pot	9. thawed	9. past
10. tapped	10. chair	10. torn	10. chump	10. tape

Mixed UV obstruents Set 12	*Mixed UV obstruents Set 15*	*Mixed UV obstruents Set 18*	*Mixed UV obstruents Set 21*	*Mixed UV obstruents Set 24*
1. cake	1. sparse	1. cause	1. spans	1. cared
2. fetch	2. store	2. fudge	2. stage	2. far
3. soft	3. scotch	3. sand	3. scarce	3. soul
4. shore	4. hunt	4. shame	4. heart	4. shock
5. thong	5. pass	5. thefts	5. poke	5. thud
6. chunk	6. tale	6. charm	6. toss	6. chant
7. spat	7. keg	7. sports	7. cut	7. Spain
8. steak	8. farm	8. starves	8. fan	8. stench
9. scare	9. sold	9. skull	9. same	9. Scott
10. hot	10. Sean	10. hat	10. shell	10. home

APPENDIX F. PRACTICE STIMULI, RESTRICTED PHONETIC CONTEXT
For use during injection method for obstruents in esophageal speech.

LEVEL II: ONE-SYLLABLE WORDS BEGINNING WITH UNVOICED (UV) OBSTRUENTS PLUS OTHER VOWELS

- Unvoiced obstruents /p/, /t/, /k/, /f/, /s/, /ʃ/, /θ/, /tʃ/, /sp/, /st/, /sk/, and /h/ as a "modified" /k/
- Vowels /u/, /ʊ/, /ɝ/, /i/, /ɪ/, /aɪ/, /aʊ/, and /ɔɪ/

/p/ words	/t/ words	/k/ words	/f/ words	/s/ words
Set 1	*Set 1*	*Set 1*	*Set 1*	*Set 1*
1. pooch	1. tomb	1. coins	1. food	1. soon
2. pea	2. took	2. kiss	2. foot	2. side
3. pierce	3. term	3. kind	3. firm	3. soil
4. pound	4. tea	4. keep	4. fee	4. cease
5. pull	5. tick	5. cool	5. fib	5. soot
6. peak	6. tube	6. curb	6. fight	6. search
7. pies	7. tight	7. cook	7. found	7. cyst
8. pearl	8. towel	8. coil	8. foil	8. sound
9. poise	9. toy	9. keen	9. fill	9. sip
10. pinch	10. tease	10. couch	10. fire	10. see

/p/ words	/t/ words	/k/ words	/f/ words	/s/ words
Set 2	*Set 2*	*Set 2*	*Set 2*	*Set 2*
1. peel	1. tool	1. coop	1. fool	1. soothe
2. pick	2. tour	2. kick	2. first	2. sigh
3. pile	3. terse	3. kite	3. feet	3. seal
4. perch	4. teach	4. Keith	4. fig	4. soiled
5. poof	5. till	5. curl	5. full	5. sour
6. peace	6. tune	6. key	6. fern	6. surge
7. pine	7. time	7. coy	7. fierce	7. scent
8. push	8. tip	8. kid	8. foiled	8. sign
9. perk	9. town	9. cowed	9. find	9. seed
10. pouch	10. toil	10. curt	10. fish	10. sue

/p/ words	/t/ words	/k/ words	/f/ words	/s/ words
Set 3	*Set 3*	*Set 3*	*Set 3*	*Set 3*
1. pink	1. tooth	1. kook	1. feast	1. soup
2. pool	2. turf	2. quiche	2. file	2. sight
3. pout	3. toiled	3. kill	3. fit	3. sir
4. peach	4. tin	4. king	4. fear	4. south
5. pig	5. tire	5. curve	5. foils	5. seat
6. puss	6. two	6. could	6. foods	6. sick
7. poised	7. team	7. kit	7. fur	7. soils
8. pipe	8. toured	8. coin	8. fifth	8. suit
9. purse	9. turn	9. cows	9. fowl	9. seek
10. pinch	10. towns	10. curse	10. fiend	10. sit

APPENDIX F. PRACTICE STIMULI, RESTRICTED PHONETIC CONTEXT
For use during injection method for obstruents in esophageal speech.

LEVEL II: ONE-SYLLABLE WORDS BEGINNING WITH UNVOICED OBSTRUENTS PLUS OTHER VOWELS (*continued*)

/ʃ/ words Set 1	/θ/ words Set 1	/tʃ/ words Set 1	/sp/ words Set 1	/st/ words Set 1
1. shoe	1. theme	1. cheap	1. speak	1. steal
2. shear	2. thin	2. cheer	2. spear	2. steer
3. shook	3. therm	3. chirp	3. spur	3. stern
4. ships	4. thigh	4. chew	4. spoof	4. stool
5. shout	5. thief	5. choice	5. spice	5. sty
6. sheet	6. thick	6. cheese	6. spouse	6. stout
7. shied	7. third	7. child	7. spoil	7. stilt
8. shirk	8. thieve	8. chow	8. speeds	8. Steve
9. she	9. thirst	9. chin	9. spite	9. stood
10. shines	10. think	10. chipped	10. spied	10. stooped

/ʃ/ words Set 2	/θ/ words Set 2	/tʃ/ words Set 2	/sp/ words Set 2	/st/ words Set 2
1. shoot	1. thieves	1. cheat	1. speech	1. steam
2. shirt	2. thing	2. chick	2. spill	2. stirs
3. ship	3. thinned	3. church	3. spurn	3. stick
4. sheet	4. thick	4. choose	4. spook	4. stewed
5. sheer	5. thirsts	5. chip	5. spike	5. style
6. should	6. thigh	6. chime	6. spout	6. stoic
7. shine	7. thinks	7. chief	7. speared	7. steered
8. shield	8. therm	8. chilled	8. spy	8. steep
9. shoed	9. third	9. chives	9. spit	9. still
10. sheik	10. themes	10. chinned	10. spoils	10. sties

/ʃ/ words Set 3	/θ/ words Set 3	/tʃ/ words Set 3	/sp/ words Set 3	/st/ words Set 3
1. sheep	1. thieved	1. cheek	1. speaks	1. steed
2. sure	2. therms	2. chimp	2. spin	2. stiff
3. shouts	3. things	3. churn	3. spurt	3. styles
4. shin	4. third	4. chewed	4. spool	4. sting
5. shoes	5. theme	5. chill	5. spine	5. stew
6. sheathe	6. thighs	6. cheats	6. spoiled	6. stirred
7. shy	7. thick	7. chows	7. spouts	7. stoop
8. chic	8. think	8. chide	8. speed	8. steel
9. sheared	9. thirst	9. cheered	9. spoon	9. stout
10. shined	10. thins	10. chiefs	10. spire	10. stitch

APPENDIX F. PRACTICE STIMULI, RESTRICTED PHONETIC CONTEXT
For use during injection method for obstruents in esophageal speech.

LEVEL II: ONE-SYLLABLE WORDS BEGINNING WITH UNVOICED OBSTRUENTS PLUS OTHER VOWELS (continued)

/sk/ words Set 1	/h/ words Set 1	Mixed UV obstruents Set 1	Mixed UV obstruents Set 4	Mixed UV obstruents Set 7
1. scheme	1. hoop	1. pooch	1. therm	1. pick
2. skeet	2. hood	2. took	2. cheap	2. tide
3. skid	3. heard	3. curb	3. spear	3. couch
4. skirt	4. hear	4. feast	4. sty	4. food
5. scalp	5. he	5. scent	5. scalp	5. soot
6. skied	6. height	6. shied	6. hoop	6. shirk
7. skin	7. hound	7. theme	7. poof	7. thieve
8. school	8. hoist	8. chew	8. term	8. cheer
9. sky	9. who'd	9. spoof	9. keel	9. spice
10. scoured	10. hip	10. stern	10. fear	10. stout

/sk/ words Set 2	/h/ words Set 2	Mixed UV obstruents Set 2	Mixed UV obstruents Set 5	Mixed UV obstruents Set 8
1. ski	1. who	1. skeet	1. side	1. school
2. skiff	2. hoof	2. hear	2. shout	2. hood
3. scoop	3. her	3. pies	3. thief	3. pearl
4. skilled	4. hinge	4. towel	4. choice	4. tea
5. scowl	5. heal	5. coo	5. spur	5. kick
6. skies	6. hide	6. foot	6. steal	6. fight
7. skinned	7. house	7. search	7. skid	7. sound
8. skimp	8. heed	8. she	8. height	8. shoe
9. scalps	9. Herb	9. thin	9. pouch	9. thick
10. scour	10. heist	10. chide	10. tomb	10. chirp

/sk/ words Set 3	/h/ words Set 3	Mixed UV obstruents Set 3	Mixed UV obstruents Set 6	Mixed UV obstruents Set 9
1. schemed	1. whose	1. spouse	1. cook	1. speak
2. skill	2. hook	2. stool	2. fern	2. steer
3. scoot	3. hurt	3. scoot	3. cease	3. skies
4. skirts	4. hit	4. hurt	4. ship	4. house
5. skip	5. heap	5. peace	5. thigh	5. pool
6. scalped	6. hike	6. tick	6. chow	6. toured
7. scout	7. how	7. kind	7. spoon	7. curl
8. skis	8. hoists	8. found	8. stood	8. fee
9. skim	9. hill	9. soil	9. skirts	9. sick
10. skeet	10. high	10. shook	10. he	10. shine

APPENDIX F. PRACTICE STIMULI, RESTRICTED PHONETIC CONTEXT
For use during injection method for obstruents in esophageal speech.

LEVEL II: ONE-SYLLABLE WORDS BEGINNING WITH UNVOICED OBSTRUENTS PLUS OTHER VOWELS *(continued)*

Mixed UV obstruents Set 10
1. third
2. chewed
3. spoil
4. stirred
5. scheme
6. here
7. pile
8. towns
9. cool
10. full

Mixed UV obstruents Set 13
1. pull
2. turn
3. keep
4. fit
5. sight
6. shouts
7. thing
8. cheese
9. spurt
10. steep

Mixed UV obstruents Set 16
1. think
2. chill
3. spied
4. stoic
5. coop
6. hoof
7. purse
8. tip
9. kiss
10. file

Mixed UV obstruents Set 19
1. pipe
2. town
3. coop
4. fooled
5. surge
6. sheath
7. thick
8. chime
9. spouts
10. stooped

Mixed UV obstruents Set 22
1. thing
2. chimp
3. spurn
4. steel
5. skim
6. hire
7. pound
8. tooth
9. curt
10. first

Mixed UV obstruents Set 11
1. sir
2. sheep
3. thinned
4. child
5. spout
6. stew
7. scour
8. herd
9. piece
10. tin

Mixed UV obstruents Set 14
1. skill
2. hide
3. pouch
4. tool
5. could
6. firm
7. see
8. sheer
9. thighs
10. chows

Mixed UV obstruents Set 17
1. sour
2. shoot
3. theme
4. church
5. speed
6. stick
7. sky
8. how
9. pool
10. tour

Mixed UV obstruents Set 20
1. skiff
2. hers
3. peach
4. tint
5. kites
6. foul
7. soup
8. shoes
9. third
10. chief

Mixed UV obstruents Set 23
1. seem
2. shin
3. thigh
4. chives
5. spoons
6. stood
7. skimp
8. heave
9. pit
10. time

Mixed UV obstruents Set 12
1. kite
2. fount
3. soon
4. should
5. thirst
6. cheat
7. spill
8. sties
9. scowl
10. who'd

Mixed UV obstruents Set 15
1. spook
2. team
3. skirts
4. heal
5. pinch
6. tight
7. cows
8. fool
9. seethe
10. shirt

Mixed UV obstruents Set 18
1. curve
2. feed
3. sent
4. shy
5. thief
6. choose
7. spool
8. stir
9. ski
10. hinge

Mixed UV obstruents Set 21
1. spin
2. tile
3. scout
4. whose
5. push
6. turf
7. keys
8. fill
9. sign
10. shout

Mixed UV obstruents Set 24
1. cowed
2. feet
3. soiled
4. sure
5. think
6. chip
7. spine
8. stout
9. scoops
10. hook

APPENDIX F. PRACTICE STIMULI, RESTRICTED PHONETIC CONTEXT
For use during injection method for obstruents in esophageal speech.

LEVEL III: ONE-SYLLABLE WORDS BEGINNING WITH VOICED (V) OBSTRUENTS PLUS MID AND LOW VOWELS

- Voiced obstruents /b/, /d/, /g/, /v/, /z/, /ð/, and /dʒ/ (Note: No words begin with /ʒ/)
- Mid and low vowels /ɑ/, /o/, /ɔ/, /ʌ/, /æ/, /e/, and /ɛ/

/b/ words Set 1	/d/ words Set 1	/g/ words Set 1	/v/ words Set 1	/z/ words Set 1
1. ball	1. dark	1. guard	1. vague	1. zone
2. board	2. dome	2. ghost	2. Val	2. zap
3. bus	3. dawn	3. gaunt	3. vault	3. zest
4. back	4. dad	4. gum	4. vast	4. Zack
5. babe	5. date	5. gap	5. vent	5. zag
6. bed	6. desk	6. gain	6. vogue	6. Zeb
7. bought	7. dodge	7. get	7. vales	7. zapped
8. boast	8. doll	8. gone	8. voted	8. Zen
9. buck	9. dove	9. goal	9. vans	9. zoned
10. badge	10. dose	10. gash	10. vase	10. zagged

/b/ words Set 2	/d/ words Set 2	/g/ words Set 2	/v/ words Set 2	/z/ words Set 2
1. bake	1. dart	1. got	1. vault	1. Zeb
2. best	2. door	2. go	2. vend	2. Zack
3. bark	3. dog	3. gauze	3. vamp	3. Zen
4. boat	4. dash	4. gun	4. Val's	4. zap
5. but	5. day	5. gas	5. volt	5. zoned
6. bath	6. deck	6. game	6. vat	6. zest
7. bear	7. dug	7. guest	7. veiled	7. zag
8. bomb	8. doze	8. gong	8. vet	8. zapped
9. bore	9. duck	9. gull	9. vote	9. Zack's
10. budge	10. Dave	10. gave	10. vast	10. zones

/b/ words Set 3	/d/ words Set 3	/g/ words Set 3	/v/ words Set 3	/z/ words Set 3
1. boss	1. dot	1. gosh	1. vale	1. zag
2. born	2. dough	2. goes	2. vest	2. zones
3. buff	3. Dan	3. gawk	3. veins	3. zap
4. batch	4. daze	4. gust	4. vamps	4. Zeb
5. bell	5. deaf	5. gab	5. vended	5. zest
6. box	6. dock	6. gate	6. votes	6. zoned
7. baste	7. dust	7. guess	7. van	7. Zen's
8. bowl	8. debt	8. garb	8. valve	8. zagged
9. bug	9. does	9. goat	9. vase	9. zaps
10. bay	10. dare	10. gaze	10. volt	10. Zack's

APPENDIX F. PRACTICE STIMULI, RESTRICTED PHONETIC CONTEXT
For use during injection method for obstruents in esophageal speech.

LEVEL III: ONE-SYLLABLE WORDS BEGINNING WITH VOICED OBSTRUENTS PLUS MID AND LOW VOWELS *(continued)*

/ð/ *words* Set 1	/dʒ/ *words* Set 1	*Mixed V obstruents* Set 1	*Mixed V obstruents* Set 4	*Mixed V obstruents* Set 7
1. those	1. jar	1. ball	1. garb	1. czar
2. the	2. George	2. dose	2. vote	2. those
3. than	3. jaw	3. gum	3. Zen	3. jump
4. their	4. Judd	4. Val	4. than	4. badge
5. them	5. jab	5. zone	5. jade	5. dale
6. they	6. jade	6. their	6. bed	6. guess
7. there	7. gem	7. jar	7. dark	7. vaults
8. they'll	8. jog	8. both	8. ghost	8. zoned
9. though	9. Joel	9. does	9. vet	9. the
10. thus	10. just	10. gab	10. zag	10. Jack

/ð/ *words* Set 2	/dʒ/ *words* Set 2	*Mixed V obstruents* Set 2	*Mixed V obstruents* Set 5	*Mixed V obstruents* Set 8
1. though	1. job	1. vague	1. they	1. bake
2. thus	2. Joe	2. Zen	2. gem	2. dead
3. that	3. judge	3. the	3. bar	3. gone
4. theirs	4. Jack	4. George	4. dome	4. vogue
5. they'd	5. jail	5. buck	5. gush	5. zag
6. then	6. gent	6. dab	6. vamps	6. than
7. they're	7. John	7. gain	7. Zane	7. jail
8. those	8. joke	8. vent	8. them	8. bear
9. than	9. jazz	9. zest	9. job	9. darn
10. them	10. Jane	10. those	10. bone	10. go

/ð/ *words* Set 3	/dʒ/ *words* Set 3	*Mixed V obstruents* Set 3	*Mixed V obstruents* Set 6	*Mixed V obstruents* Set 9
1. they	1. jock	1. Judd	1. done	1. vale
2. their	2. Job	2. back	2. gap	2. zapped
3. than	3. jug	3. daze	3. vain	3. they'll
4. the	4. jam	4. get	4. zest	4. gent
5. those	5. Jake	5. vault	5. theirs	5. bark
6. they'd	6. jet	6. zoned	6. Joe	6. door
7. them	7. josh	7. thus	7. budge	7. gust
8. that	8. Joan	8. jab	8. dad	8. valve
9. thus	9. jut	9. baste	9. game	9. Zen's
10. though	10. jest	10. dare	10. vend	10. them

APPENDIX F. PRACTICE STIMULI, RESTRICTED PHONETIC CONTEXT
For use during injection method for obstruents in esophageal speech.

LEVEL III: ONE-SYLLABLE WORDS BEGINNING WITH VOICED OBSTRUENTS PLUS MID AND LOW VOWELS (continued)

Mixed V obstruents Set 10	Mixed V obstruents Set 13	Mixed V obstruents Set 16	Mixed V obstruents Set 19	Mixed V obstruents Set 22
1. jock	1. dart	1. vats	1. than	1. bomb
2. board	2. goal	2. zone	2. jaw	2. dough
3. Doug	3. votes	3. there	3. bus	3. gun
4. gas	4. Zack	4. jazz	4. dads	4. valves
5. vane	5. they	5. bang	5. gauge	5. Zane
6. Zeb	6. jet	6. debt	6. vends	6. there
7. though	7. box	7. gosh	7. Zen	7. John
8. joke	8. dope	8. volts	8. though	8. born
9. bum	9. gut	9. zapped	9. jut	9. dug
10. dash	10. vast	10. than	10. batch	10. gad

Mixed V obstruents Set 11	Mixed V obstruents Set 14	Mixed V obstruents Set 17	Mixed V obstruents Set 20	Mixed V obstruents Set 23
1. gate	1. czar	1. Jane	1. date	1. vales
2. vest	2. theirs	2. beg	2. guests	2. zest
3. Zack's	3. jog	3. dock	3. Val's	3. they
4. those	4. boast	4. goes	4. zone	4. Job
5. judge	5. dove	5. vein	5. the	5. bed
6. bag	6. gal	6. zap	6. jam	6. Dan
7. dame	7. vase	7. they'd	7. bait	7. gaze
8. guest	8. Zen	8. Jeff	8. deck	8. vests
9. van	9. they'd	9. Bob	9. gorge	9. zap
10. zone	10. Joan	10. dorm	10. vote	10. those

Mixed V obstruents Set 12	Mixed V obstruents Set 15	Mixed V obstruents Set 18	Mixed V obstruents Set 21	Mixed V obstruents Set 24
1. the	1. buff	1. gull	1. zap	1. jug
2. jag	2. dam	2. vast	2. that	2. bat
3. base	3. gave	3. zagged	3. Jay	3. day
4. deaf	4. vents	4. then	4. best	4. get
5. gong	5. zag	5. josh	5. dodge	5. vague
6. volt	6. though	6. boat	6. goat	6. zoned
7. Zane's	7. just	7. duck	7. vault	7. thus
8. than	8. band	8. gash	8. Zack's	8. Jan
9. James	9. Deb	9. veil	9. they're	9. bet
10. Bess	10. gets	10. Zeb	10. jest	10. desk

APPENDIX F. PRACTICE STIMULI, RESTRICTED PHONETIC CONTEXT
For use during injection method for obstruents in esophageal speech.

LEVEL IV: ONE-SYLLABLE WORDS BEGINNING WITH VOICED (V) OBSTRUENTS PLUS OTHER VOWELS

- Voiced obstruents /b/, /d/, /g/, /v/, /z/, /ð/, and /dʒ/ (Note: No words begin with /ʒ/)
- Vowels /u/, /ʊ/, /ɝ/, /i/, /ɪ/, /aɪ/, /aʊ/, and /ɔɪ/

/b/ words Set 1	/d/ words Set 1	/g/ words Set 1	/v/ words Set 1	/z/ words Set 1
1. boot	1. due	1. ghoul	1. verse	1. Zeus
2. bull	2. dirt	2. good	2. veal	2. zeal
3. bird	3. deal	3. girl	3. veer	3. zip
4. beach	4. dear	4. geese	4. vial	4. zounds
5. bid	5. dice	5. gear	5. vouch	5. zinged
6. bike	6. doubt	6. guide	6. voice	6. zilch
7. bound	7. do	7. gouge	7. Vern	7. zoomed
8. boil	8. deed	8. goon	8. vie	8. Zeke
9. beak	9. dig	9. gowns	9. vows	9. zee
10. boom	10. dial	10. goosed	10. vine	10. zoo

/b/ words Set 2	/d/ words Set 2	/g/ words Set 2	/v/ words Set 2	/z/ words Set 2
1. boost	1. duel	1. goo	1. verb	1. -zyme
2. book	2. dearth	2. geek	2. veep	2. Zeke
3. burn	3. dean	3. gig	3. Vic	3. zinc
4. beat	4. dish	4. guys	4. vibes	4. zooms
5. big	5. dime	5. gout	5. vow	5. zings
6. bite	6. douse	6. goop	6. void	6. zounds
7. bow	7. dues	7. gill	7. verve	7. zipped
8. boy	8. deem	8. gives	8. vile	8. zees
9. bend	9. dip	9. geared	9. vouched	9. zoo
10. Butch	10. dike	10. gouged	10. versed	10. zeal

/b/ words Set 3	/d/ words Set 3	/g/ words Set 3	/v/ words Set 3	/z/ words Set 3
1. booth	1. duke	1. goof	1. verge	1. zoom
2. bush	2. Dirk	2. goods	2. vim	2. zing
3. burst	3. deep	3. girls	3. vice	3. zilch
4. bees	4. ditch	4. give	4. vowed	4. zounds
5. binge	5. dive	5. guy	5. vied	5. Zeus
6. buy	6. down	6. gown	6. veered	6. zeal
7. bowel	7. dune	7. goose	7. voiced	7. zinc
8. boys	8. deeds	8. guides	8. vials	8. Zeke's
9. birth	9. disk	9. ghouls	9. veeps	9. zips
10. bind	10. dine	10. guilt	10. Vic's	10. zoos

APPENDIX F. PRACTICE STIMULI, RESTRICTED PHONETIC CONTEXT
For use during injection method for obstruents in esophageal speech.

LEVEL IV: ONE-SYLLABLE WORDS BEGINNING WITH VOICED OBSTRUENTS PLUS OTHER VOWELS (continued)

/ð/ words Set 1	/dʒ/ words Set 1	Mixed V obstruents Set 1	Mixed V obstruents Set 4	Mixed V obstruents Set 7
1. the	1. jewel	1. boo	1. ghoul	1. Zeus
2. these	2. germ	2. dirt	2. verb	2. this
3. this	3. jeep	3. geese	3. zeal	3. gee
4. thine	4. Jim	4. veer	4. this	4. beard
5. thou	5. gibe	5. zip	5. gibe	5. dial
6. thy	6. joust	6. thou	6. bound	6. gouge
7. the	7. join	7. jewel	7. do	7. voice
8. this	8. Jude	8. bird	8. good	8. zoo
9. these	9. Gene	9. dean	9. veal	9. thee
10. thine	10. gyp	10. guilt	10. zinc	10. gin

/ð/ words Set 2	/dʒ/ words Set 2	Mixed V obstruents Set 2	Mixed V obstruents Set 5	Mixed V obstruents Set 8
1. thine	1. juice	1. vibes	1. thine	1. bide
2. these	2. jerk	2. zing	2. joust	2. doubt
3. this	3. Jean	3. the	3. boom	3. goo
4. the	4. gist	4. jerk	4. dearth	4. verge
5. thy	5. jive	5. beak	5. geek	5. zee
6. thou	6. joist	6. Dick	6. Vic	6. his
7. thine	7. Jew	7. guys	7. zilch	7. joy
8. this	8. jig	8. vow	8. thou	8. bow
9. these	9. joined	9. zoom	9. Jude	9. doom
10. the	10. jowl	10. this	10. birth	10. goods

/ð/ words Set 3	/dʒ/ words Set 3	Mixed V obstruents Set 3	Mixed V obstruents Set 6	Mixed V obstruents Set 9
1. these	1. June	1. Gene	1. deed	1. veep
2. thine	2. gee	2. bid	2. gig	2. zinc
3. thou	3. gym	3. dies	3. vice	3. thine
4. the	4. joy	4. gouged	4. Zeke	4. jowl
5. this	5. juke	5. void	5. these	5. boost
6. thy	6. germs	6. Zeus	6. germ	6. Dirk
7. thou	7. gin	7. these	7. beat	7. geese
8. the	8. joust	8. Jim	8. did	8. vim
9. this	9. jeeps	9. bite	9. guide	9. zip
10. thy	10. jived	10. down	10. vouch	10. thou

APPENDIX F. PRACTICE STIMULI, RESTRICTED PHONETIC CONTEXT
For use during injection method for obstruents in esophageal speech.

LEVEL IV: ONE-SYLLABLE WORDS BEGINNING WITH VOICED OBSTRUENTS PLUS OTHER VOWELS *(continued)*

Mixed V obstruents Set 10	*Mixed V obstruents Set 13*	*Mixed V obstruents Set 16*	*Mixed V obstruents Set 19*	*Mixed V obstruents Set 22*
1. Jew	1. dude	1. voice	1. the	1. boot
2. berg	2. girls	2. zoo	2. Joyce	2. dirt
3. deal	3. veal	3. the	3. bees	3. geese
4. gear	4. zilch	4. gym	4. dig	4. veered
5. vial	5. thine	5. buy	5. Guy	5. zipped
6. Zeke	6. joust	6. doubts	6. vouched	6. thou
7. the	7. booth	7. goop	7. Zeus	7. June
8. germ	8. dearth	8. verve	8. this	8. burn
9. beach	9. geek	9. zee	9. Gene	9. deem
10. dear	10. Vic's	10. this	10. big	10. gill

Mixed V obstruents Set 11	*Mixed V obstruents Set 14*	*Mixed V obstruents Set 17*	*Mixed V obstruents Set 20*	*Mixed V obstruents Set 23*
1. guide	1. zinc	1. join	1. dike	1. vice
2. vowed	2. thou	2. boys	2. gown	2. zinged
3. zoo	3. juice	3. duel	3. void	3. these
4. these	4. burp	4. girl	4. zoo	4. germs
5. jeep	5. deep	5. veep	5. these	5. beef
6. bend	6. give	6. zips	6. gyp	6. dill
7. dice	7. vied	7. thine	7. bind	7. guides
8. gout	8. zeal	8. joist	8. doused	8. vows
9. void	9. these	9. boon	9. goose	9. zoom
10. Zeus	10. germ	10. dim	10. verb	10. this

Mixed V obstruents Set 12	*Mixed V obstruents Set 15*	*Mixed V obstruents Set 18*	*Mixed V obstruents Set 21*	*Mixed V obstruents Set 24*
1. these	1. bean	1. geese	1. Zeke's	1. gee
2. gist	2. dish	2. veer	2. this	2. binge
3. bike	3. guide	3. zinc	3. join	3. dime
4. douse	4. vowed	4. thou	4. book	4. gouge
5. goof	5. Zeus	5. jute	5. dune	5. voiced
6. Vern	6. this	6. birch	6. goods	6. Zeus
7. zing	7. Jean	7. deals	7. veal	7. thee
8. this	8. bit	8. gear	8. zip	8. jeer
9. gibe	9. dive	9. vile	9. thine	9. bile
10. bowel	10. gown	10. zinged	10. jowl	10. down

APPENDIX F. PRACTICE STIMULI, RESTRICTED PHONETIC CONTEXT
For use during injection method for obstruents in esophageal speech.

LEVEL V: ONE-SYLLABLE WORDS BEGINNING WITH UNVOICED AND VOICED OBSTRUENT BLENDS

- Unvoiced obstruent blends /pl/, /pr/, /tr/, /tw/, /kl/, /kr/, /fl/, /fr/, /sl/, /sm/, /sn/, /sw/, /ʃr/, /θr/, /spl/, /spr/, /str/, and /skr/
- Voiced obstruent blends /bl/, /br/, /dr/, /gl/, and /gr/
- All vowels

Blends Set 1	Blends Set 4	Blends Set 7	Blends Set 10	Blends Set 13
1. plot	1. sprout	1. flesh	1. grade	1. prompt
2. blue	2. swan	2. scrounge	2. fright	2. bruise
3. troll	3. through	3. small	3. slept	3. twang
4. draw	4. probe	4. splotch	4. snout	4. claw
5. crunch	5. brook	5. stroke	5. sprang	5. glass
6. green	6. twirl	6. shrub	6. switch	6. flinch
7. France	7. club	7. plead	7. thread	7. scroll
8. slick	8. gleam	8. black	8. proud	8. smirk
9. snail	9. flag	9. trick	9. broil	9. splice
10. sprite	10. script	10. drain	10. tweak	10. struck

Blends Set 2	Blends Set 5	Blends Set 8	Blends Set 11	Blends Set 14
1. swear	1. smile	1. crime	1. close	1. shriek
2. proud	2. strength	2. grouch	2. glove	2. place
3. broil	3. shroud	3. frost	3. fleece	3. blind
4. clock	4. plus	4. slew	4. scratch	4. tread
5. gloom	5. bleach	5. snore	5. smear	5. drown
6. floor	6. track	6. sprawl	6. splint	6. cross
7. scrawl	7. drip	7. swirl	7. straight	7. group
8. smudge	8. crave	8. thrush	8. shred	8. froze
9. spleen	9. grind	9. breeze	9. plaid	9. slurp
10. strap	10. friend	10. class	10. blink	10. snug

Blends Set 3	Blends Set 6	Blends Set 9	Blends Set 12	Blends Set 15
1. shrimp	1. slouch	1. glimpse	1. train	1. sprain
2. plume	2. snarl	2. flake	2. drive	2. swine
3. blow	3. spruce	3. scribe	3. crest	3. throb
4. truck	4. swore	4. smell	4. groin	4. prove
5. dream	5. throng	5. strong	5. frown	5. broke
6. crack	6. preach	6. shrewd	6. slob	6. clerk
7. grip	7. branch	7. blurt	7. snooze	7. glum
8. Frank	8. twitch	8. treat	8. spring	8. fleet
9. slice	9. claim	9. drag	9. sway	9. scrap
10. snare	10. glide	10. crisp	10. throat	10. Smith

APPENDIX F. PRACTICE STIMULI, RESTRICTED PHONETIC CONTEXT
For use during injection method for obstruents in esophageal speech.

LEVEL V: ONE-SYLLABLE WORDS BEGINNING WITH UNVOICED AND VOICED OBSTRUENT BLENDS *(continued)*

Blends *Set 16*	*Blends* *Set 19*	*Blends* *Set 22*	*Blends* *Set 25*	*Blends* *Set 28*
1. splash	1. sleep	1. flight	1. blouse	1. snoop
2. strike	2. snack	2. scrape	2. tromp	2. sprawl
3. stretch	3. swift	3. smooth	3. drove	3. swarm
4. plow	4. thrash	4. splurge	4. crook	4. throng
5. Troy	5. prince	5. street	5. grand	5. priest
6. drop	6. brave	6. shrill	6. freeze	6. brush
7. cruise	7. twice	7. plop	7. slap	7. clay
8. grown	8. cleanse	8. bloom	8. sniff	8. globe
9. fraud	9. flour	9. trust	9. sprain	9. flat
10. slump	10. scrub	10. drank	10. swipe	10. scribe

Blends *Set 17*	*Blends* *Set 20*	*Blends* *Set 23*	*Blends* *Set 26*	*Blends* *Set 29*
1. sneak	1. smart	1. crash	1. thread	1. strand
2. swam	2. stroll	2. grill	2. prowl	2. plane
3. thrift	3. shrunk	3. frame	3. bronze	3. blimp
4. praise	4. please	4. slide	4. twirl	4. tree
5. bright	5. blast	5. snare	5. clove	5. dry
6. twelve	6. trip	6. sprout	6. glad	6. crush
7. cloud	7. drape	7. swap	7. flirt	7. fruit
8. gloss	8. crowd	8. through	8. scrounge	8. slow
9. flute	9. greet	9. probe	9. smear	9. snort
10. smoke	10. frisk	10. brought	10. splice	10. swerve

Blends *Set 18*	*Blends* *Set 21*	*Blends* *Set 24*	*Blends* *Set 27*	*Blends* *Set 30*
1. splurge	1. slay	1. twin	1. straw	1. three
2. strut	2. snake	2. clear	2. shriek	2. prawn
3. shrank	3. spread	3. glare	3. plunge	3. brown
4. plight	4. sweat	4. flame	4. bloat	4. climb
5. blend	5. three	5. screen	5. truth	5. float
6. trout	6. prize	6. smug	6. drum	6. smack
7. droop	7. bread	7. splash	7. cream	7. strange
8. crow	8. tweeze	8. string	8. grape	8. ploy
9. grudge	9. clam	9. shrine	9. fright	9. block
10. front	10. glaze	10. pledge	10. sled	10. trend

APPENDIX F. PRACTICE STIMULI, RESTRICTED PHONETIC CONTEXT
For use during injection method for obstruents in esophageal speech.

LEVEL VI: TWO-SYLLABLE WORDS AND PHRASES: UNVOICED (UV) OBSTRUENTS

- Unvoiced obstruents /p/, /t/, /k/, /f/, /s/, /ʃ/, /θ/, /tʃ/, /sp/, /st/, and /sk/ occurring in the releasing positions

/p/ plus UV
Set 1
1. pop top
2. poop deck
3. post card
4. push cart
5. pauper
6. percent
7. pucker
8. peace pipe
9. pack sack
10. pitch dark

/t/ plus UV
Set 1
1. taco
2. too soon
3. toaster
4. took on
5. talker
6. turkey
7. touch up
8. tea cake
9. tattoo
10. tickle

/k/ plus UV
Set 1
1. carpool
2. coupon
3. coating
4. cook out
5. coffee
6. curfew
7. cocoon
8. keep out
9. castle
10. kick off

/f/ plus UV
Set 1
1. fossil
2. futon
3. focus
4. footage
5. faucet
6. fur coat
7. fatigue
8. fee paid
9. fattest
10. filter

/p/ plus UV
Set 2
1. paste up
2. pipe fish
3. pep talk
4. pouches
5. poi paste
6. pot shot
7. poochie
8. poke fun
9. put down
10. paw paw

/t/ plus UV
Set 2
1. take time
2. tight end
3. test tube
4. toss up
5. toy shop
6. topic
7. toothy
8. topaz
9. took off
10. toffee

/k/ plus UV
Set 2
1. caper
2. kite tail
3. ketchup
4. counter
5. coy pooch
6. coffee
7. cuckoo
8. kosher
9. cushion
10. coffin

/f/ plus UV
Set 2
1. facial
2. fighter
3. fencing
4. fountain
5. foil it
6. foster
7. fool Tom
8. fortune
9. fulfill
10. faulty

/p/ plus UV
Set 3
1. perfect
2. puppet
3. peach pit
4. patch test
5. pig pen
6. pale star
7. pie time
8. pet shop
9. pouting
10. poetess

/t/ plus UV
Set 3
1. turtle
2. tough kid
3. teacher
4. tactful
5. tick tack
6. taste test
7. typhoon
8. tester
9. tissue
10. toy car

/k/ plus UV
Set 3
1. curtain
2. compute
3. keystone
4. cafe
5. kitchen
6. kapok
7. kite check
8. kettle
9. cowpoke
10. coy Sue

/f/ plus UV
Set 3
1. first kiss
2. fussy
3. feel pain
4. fashion
5. fisher
6. facial
7. fireside
8. fetch it
9. foul scent
10. foil sheet

APPENDIX F. PRACTICE STIMULI, RESTRICTED PHONETIC CONTEXT
For use during injection method for obstruents in esophageal speech.

LEVEL VI: TWO-SYLLABLE WORDS AND PHRASES: UNVOICED OBSTRUENTS (*continued*)

/s/ plus UV Set 1	/ʃ/ plus UV Set 1	/θ/ plus UV Set 1	/tʃ/ plus UV Set 1
1. soft cap	1. shopper	1. thanking	1. chart it
2. soup's on	2. shoot pool	2. thicken	2. chew stick
3. soak socks	3. short stuff	3. thorn stick	3. choke up
4. soot stain	4. shook out	4. thirty	4. chafing
5. sought care	5. Sean came	5. thought fun	5. chaw pack
6. sir Scott	6. sure thing	6. thirsty	6. church pew
7. such stuff	7. shuck corn	7. thump fast	7. chuck it
8. seated	8. sheepskin	8. theme park	8. cheap suit
9. sack out	9. shack house	9. thatch care	9. Chap Stick
10. sip it	10. ship sail	10. thin chips	10. chicken

/s/ plus UV Set 2	/ʃ/ plus UV Set 2	/θ/ plus UV Set 2	/tʃ/ plus UV Set 2
1. safe space	1. shake shack	1. thankful	1. chase cars
2. sightsee	2. shy cat	2. thigh patch	2. chime ten
3. self start	3. chef sauce	3. theft score	3. chess champ
4. south paw	4. shout out	4. thistle	4. chow time
5. soy sauce	5. shut up	5. thesis	5. choice spot
6. sock hop	6. shark cage	6. thicket	6. chop off
7. suit coat	7. shoe tongue	7. thin-skinned	7. chew fat
8. soap scum	8. show time	8. thorny	8. choke up
9. soot ash	9. shook up	9. thinking	9. chant song
10. saw Ted	10. Shaw spoke	10. thaw fish	10. chalk up

/s/ plus UV Set 3	/ʃ/ plus UV Set 3	/θ/ plus UV Set 3	/tʃ/ plus UV Set 3
1. search out	1. shirt tail	1. thirteen	1. chirping
2. sup sauce	2. shush Pam	2. thumb tip	2. chunky
3. seek out	3. she passed	3. think fast	3. cheat cards
4. sat still	4. shall come	4. thatch stack	4. chance call
5. sit up	5. sheer fear	5. thick soup	5. chipped tooth
6. Saint Paul	6. shape sand	6. thank Carl	6. chain saw
7. siphon	7. shine shoes	7. thigh pain	7. child star
8. sent cash	8. share thoughts	8. theft shock	8. check stub
9. sour puss	9. shower	9. theme song	9. chow chow
10. soil test	10. short change	10. thought through	10. choice cut

APPENDIX F. PRACTICE STIMULI, RESTRICTED PHONETIC CONTEXT
For use during injection method for obstruents in esophageal speech.

LEVEL VI: TWO-SYLLABLE WORDS AND PHRASES: UNVOICED OBSTRUENTS *(continued)*

/sp/ plus UV
Set 1
1. spot check
2. spoof of
3. spoke out
4. spell check
5. spawn fish
6. spurt oil
7. spun silk
8. speak for
9. spastic
10. spear fish

/st/ plus UV
Set 1
1. start up
2. stew pot
3. stone cold
4. stood tall
5. stalking
6. stir food
7. stuck in
8. steep hill
9. stash cash
10. stick shift

/sk/ plus UV
Set 1
1. scotch all
2. scoop up
3. scorched shirt
4. skeptic
5. scared stiff
6. skirt hem
7. skunk in
8. skeet shoot
9. scampi
10. skin tone

Mixed UV plus UV
Set 1
1. pop top
2. too soon
3. coating
4. footage
5. sought care
6. sure thing
7. thump fast
8. cheap suit
9. spastic
10. stick shift

/sp/ plus UV
Set 2
1. space suit
2. spy ship
3. spare tire
4. spout off
5. spoiler
6. sparkle
7. spoon feed
8. sport shirt
9. speech aid
10. spa pool

/st/ plus UV
Set 2
1. stake out
2. style type
3. staircase
4. stout pig
5. stoic Ken
6. stop at
7. stoop to
8. stove top
9. stood for
10. station

/sk/ plus UV
Set 2
1. skate key
2. sky king
3. sketch pad
4. scour tub
5. skipper
6. Scottish
7. scoot off
8. scone cake
9. schemer
10. skim fat

Mixed UV plus UV
Set 2
1. skate key
2. pipe fish
3. test tube
4. counter
5. foil it
6. sock hop
7. shoe tongue
8. thorny
9. chant song
10. spa pool

/sp/ plus UV
Set 3
1. spur track
2. sputter
3. speed trap
4. spatter
5. spinster
6. spacious
7. spicy
8. special
9. spouting
10. spoil sport

/st/ plus UV
Set 3
1. stern talk
2. stunt at
3. steal cars
4. status
5. stiff arm
6. stay tuned
7. stipend
8. step up
9. stoutest
10. steep curve

/sk/ plus UV
Set 3
1. scurry
2. scuff shoes
3. ski shoes
4. scaffold
5. skip it
6. scapegoat
7. sky cap
8. scarecrow
9. scout camp
10. score card

Mixed UV plus UV
Set 3
1. stern talk
2. scuff shoes
3. peach pit
4. tactful
5. kitchen
6. facial
7. siphon
8. share thoughts
9. theme song
10. choice cut

APPENDIX F. PRACTICE STIMULI, RESTRICTED PHONETIC CONTEXT
For use during injection method for obstruents in esophageal speech.

LEVEL VI: TWO-SYLLABLE WORDS AND PHRASES: UNVOICED OBSTRUENTS (continued)

Mixed UV plus UV Set 4
1. spot check
2. stew pot
3. scorched shirt
4. push cart
5. talker
6. curfew
7. fatigue
8. seated
9. shack house
10. thin chips

Mixed UV plus UV Set 5
1. chase cars
2. spy ship
3. staircase
4. scour tub
5. poi paste
6. topic
7. cuckoo
8. fortune
9. soot ash
10. Shaw spoke

Mixed UV plus UV Set 6
1. thirteen
2. chunky
3. speed trap
4. status
5. skip it
6. pale star
7. typhoon
8. kettle
9. foul scent
10. soil test

Mixed UV plus UV Set 7
1. shopper
2. thicken
3. choke up
4. spell check
5. stalking
6. skirt hem
7. pucker
8. tea cake
9. castle
10. filter

Mixed UV plus UV Set 8
1. safe space
2. shy cat
3. theft score
4. chow time
5. spoiler
6. stop at
7. scoot off
8. poke fun
9. took off
10. coffin

Mixed UV plus UV Set 9
1. first kiss
2. sup sauce
3. she passed
4. thatch stack
5. chipped tooth
6. spacious
7. stipend
8. scarecrow
9. pouting
10. toy car

Mixed UV plus UV Set 10
1. carpool
2. futon
3. soak socks
4. shook out
5. thought fun
6. church pew
7. spun silk
8. steep hill
9. scampi
10. pitch dark

Mixed UV plus UV Set 11
1. take time
2. kite tail
3. fencing
4. south paw
5. shut up
6. thicket
7. chew fat
8. sport shirt
9. stood for
10. skim fat

Mixed UV plus UV Set 12
1. perfect
2. tough kid
3. keystone
4. fashion
5. sit up
6. shape sand
7. thigh pain
8. check stub
9. spouting
10. steep curve

Mixed UV plus UV Set 13
1. scotch all
2. poop deck
3. toaster
4. cook out
5. faucet
6. Sir Scott
7. shuck corn
8. theme park
9. Chap Stick
10. spear fish

Mixed UV plus UV Set 14
1. stake out
2. sky king
3. pep talk
4. toss up
5. coy pooch
6. foster
7. suit coat
8. show time
9. thinking
10. chalk up

Mixed UV plus UV Set 15
1. spur track
2. stunt at
3. ski shoes
4. patch test
5. tick tack
6. kapok
7. fireside
8. sent cash
9. shower
10. thought through

APPENDIX F. PRACTICE STIMULI, RESTRICTED PHONETIC CONTEXT
For use during injection method for obstruents in esophageal speech.

LEVEL VI: TWO-SYLLABLE WORDS AND PHRASES: UNVOICED OBSTRUENTS (continued)

Mixed UV plus UV
Set 16
1. chart it
2. spoof of
3. stone cold
4. skeptic
5. pauper
6. turkey
7. cocoon
8. fee paid
9. sack out
10. ship sail

Mixed UV plus UV
Set 17
1. thankful
2. chime ten
3. spare tire
4. stout pig
5. skipper
6. pot shot
7. toothy
8. kosher
9. fulfill
10. saw Ted

Mixed UV plus UV
Set 18
1. shirt tail
2. thumb tip
3. cheat cards
4. spatter
5. stiff arm
6. scapegoat
7. pie time
8. tester
9. cowpoke
10. foil sheet

Mixed UV plus UV
Set 19
1. soft cap
2. shoot pool
3. thorn stick
4. chafing
5. spawn fish
6. stir food
7. skunk in
8. peace pipe
9. tattoo
10. kick off

Mixed UV plus UV
Set 20
1. facial
2. sightsee
3. chef sauce
4. thistle
5. choice spot
6. sparkle
7. stoop to
8. scone cake
9. put down
10. toffee

Mixed UV plus UV
Set 21
1. curtain
2. fussy
3. seek out
4. shall come
5. thick soup
6. chain saw
7. spicy
8. step up
9. scout camp
10. poetess

Mixed UV plus UV
Set 22
1. taco
2. coupon
3. focus
4. soot stain
5. Sean came
6. thirsty
7. chuck it
8. speak for
9. stash cash
10. skin tone

Mixed UV plus UV
Set 23
1. paste up
2. tight end
3. ketchup
4. fountain
5. soy sauce
6. shark cage
7. thin-skinned
8. choke up
9. speech aid
10. station

Mixed UV plus UV
Set 24
1. scurry
2. puppet
3. teacher
4. cafe
5. fisher
6. Saint Paul
7. shine shoes
8. theft shock
9. chow chow
10. spoil sport

Mixed UV plus UV
Set 25
1. start up
2. scoop up
3. post card
4. took on
5. coffee
6. fur coat
7. such stuff
8. sheepskin
9. thatch care
10. chicken

Mixed UV plus UV
Set 26
1. space suit
2. style type
3. sketch pad
4. pouches
5. toy shop
6. coffee
7. fool Tom
8. soap scum
9. shook up
10. thaw out

Mixed UV plus UV
Set 27
1. chirping
2. sputter
3. steal cars
4. scaffold
5. pig pen
6. taste test
7. kite check
8. fetch it
9. sour puss
10. short change

APPENDIX F. PRACTICE STIMULI, RESTRICTED PHONETIC CONTEXT
For use during injection method for obstruents in esophageal speech.

LEVEL VII: TWO-SYLLABLE WORDS AND PHRASES: UNVOICED (UV) AND VOICED (V) OBSTRUENTS

- Unvoiced obstruents /p/, /t/, /k/, /f/, /s/, /ʃ/, /θ/, /tʃ/, /sp/, /st/, and /sk/ occurring in releasing position of first word or syllable
- Voiced obstruents /b/, /d/, /g/, /v/, /z/, /ʒ/, /ð/, and /dʒ/ occurring in releasing position of second word or syllable

/p/ plus V Set 1	*/t/ plus V* Set 1	*/k/ plus V* Set 1	*/f/ plus V* Set 1
1. pot boil	1. target	1. combo	1. father
2. poodle	2. today	2. cougar	2. Fuji
3. posies	3. tollgate	3. cozy	3. folder
4. put down	4. tomboy	4. could use	4. football
5. pauses	5. talk big	5. call back	5. fought them
6. pervert	6. turbine	6. curvy	6. fervor
7. puddle	7. tug boat	7. caboose	7. fungus
8. pea bean	8. teething	8. keyboard	8. feedbag
9. pageant	9. tangle	9. cash box	9. faddish
10. pitch dark	10. tid bit	10. kidding	10. fish bone

/p/ plus V Set 2	*/t/ plus V* Set 2	*/k/ plus V* Set 2	*/f/ plus V* Set 2
1. peace dove	1. tailgate	1. case book	1. face down
2. piebald	2. tidal	2. kindest	2. find out
3. pedal	3. text book	3. Kevin	3. feather
4. powder	4. town judge	4. cowboy	4. found out
5. poi juice	5. toys are	5. coin booth	5. foil badge
6. pardon	6. tardy	6. carbon	6. foggy
7. pool deck	7. tool box	7. kudos	7. fool's gold
8. pole jump	8. toed in	8. colder	8. forgave
9. push back	9. tour bus	9. cool deal	9. fullback
10. Pa's dog	10. talk back	10. cough drop	10. fawn dog

/p/ plus V Set 3	*/t/ plus V* Set 3	*/k/ plus V* Set 3	*/f/ plus V* Set 3
1. per day	1. turban	1. curdle	1. further
2. puzzle	2. touch base	2. cupboard	2. fuzzy
3. pink zone	3. teal duck	3. King Gus	3. feel good
4. paddle	4. tabby	4. cabbage	4. fast ball
5. pigeon	5. timber	5. killjoy	5. fidget
6. page boy	6. taste bud	6. cable	6. favor
7. pie dish	7. tiger	7. kite zone	7. fight back
8. pegboard	8. Teddy	8. Ken votes	8. pheasant
9. pounder	9. towel dry	9. cowbell	9. founder
10. poison	10. toy van	10. coy Deb	10. phone bill

APPENDIX F. PRACTICE STIMULI, RESTRICTED PHONETIC CONTEXT
For use during injection method for obstruents in esophageal speech.

LEVEL VII: TWO-SYLLABLE WORDS AND PHRASES: UNVOICED AND VOICED OBSTRUENTS *(continued)*

/s/ plus V Set 1	/ʃ/ plus V Set 1	/θ/ plus V Set 1	/tʃ/ plus V Set 1
1. sergeant	1. shop door	1. thought deep	1. charging
2. soothe it	2. shoe dye	2. third base	2. choose it
3. sold it	3. shogun	3. Thor's zest	3. chores done
4. same day	4. should do	4. thick beads	4. change jeeps
5. sawdust	5. Sean's van	5. thawed out	5. chaw beef
6. servant	6. shirt box	6. Thursday	6. church door
7. sunbeam	7. shovel	7. thunder	7. chubby
8. seething	8. shielded	8. think big	8. cheese ball
9. savage	9. shadow	9. Thad dared	9. chance guess
10. single	10. shingle	10. thimble	10. chip dip

/s/ plus V Set 2	/ʃ/ plus V Set 2	/θ/ plus V Set 2	/tʃ/ plus V Set 2
1. savings	1. shaded	1. thank God	1. chain gang
2. side dish	2. shy bear	2. thigh bone	2. children
3. seldom	3. shedder	3. theft game	3. chair back
4. sour bread	4. shout zone	4. thousand	4. chowder
5. soybean	5. showed up	5. thin dime	5. choice gems
6. sobbing	6. shot gun	6. third base	6. chalkboard
7. sue them	7. shoot darts	7. thudding	7. chew gum
8. sorbet	8. shoulder	8. thorn bush	8. chosen
9. soldier	9. should go	9. thought vague	9. cheap zoo
10. sauce boat	10. Shaw gave	10. thaw juice	10. chaw veal

/s/ plus V Set 3	/ʃ/ plus V Set 3	/θ/ plus V Set 3	/tʃ/ plus V Set 3
1. service	1. sure does	1. third boy	1. chirp birds
2. southern	2. shudder	2. thumbs up	2. chugging
3. season	3. sheep dog	3. theme jazz	3. cheekbone
4. sandbar	4. shampoo	4. thieving	4. champ boasts
5. sizzle	5. shiver	5. thin girl	5. chisel
6. safeguard	6. shake down	6. thank Zack	6. chamber
7. sizes	7. sugar	7. thigh joint	7. chided
8. seltzer	8. shelving	8. think dough	8. cheddar
9. sounded	9. shabby	9. thousandth	9. chow down
10. soil them	10. shindig	10. thick bag	10. choice beef

APPENDIX F. PRACTICE STIMULI, RESTRICTED PHONETIC CONTEXT
For use during injection method for obstruents in esophageal speech.

LEVEL VII: TWO-SYLLABLE WORDS AND PHRASES: UNVOICED AND VOICED OBSTRUENTS *(continued)*

/sp/ plus V Set 1	*/st/ plus V* Set 1	*/sk/ plus V* Set 1	*Mixed UV plus V* Set 1
1. spot Bob	1. stop gap	1. scarf down	1. pot boil
2. spooked duck	2. stew game	2. school book	2. today
3. sports dial	3. storm's eye	3. scolded	3. cozy
4. spoon bread	4. stood there	4. scale back	4. football
5. spawned in	5. stalk bent	5. skip dues	5. sawdust
6. spurred on	6. stirred up	6. skirt gores	6. shirt box
7. sponge bath	7. stuck them	7. scum bag	7. thunder
8. speed boat	8. steamboat	8. ski gear	8. cheese ball
9. spasm	9. standard	9. scandal	9. spasm
10. spindle	10. stick gum	10. skidded	10. stick gum

/sp/ plus V Set 2	*/st/ plus V* Set 2	*/sk/ plus V* Set 2	*Mixed UV plus V* Set 2
1. space game	1. stage hand	1. scathing	1. scale back
2. spied Zeb	2. style guide	2. sky bird	2. pie-bald
3. sped off	3. stare back	3. schedule	3. text book
4. spouses	4. stout bull	4. scour van	4. cowboy
5. spoiled brat	5. stoic Dave	5. scoop jellies	5. foil badge
6. spark gap	6. starched jeans	6. Scotch bowl	6. sobbing
7. spoof joke	7. stooped vet	7. scuba	7. shoot darts
8. spoke there	8. store bought	8. scone dough	8. thorn bush
9. spill beans	9. steel guard	9. scuff those	9. cheap zoo
10. spite Val	10. stalk those	10. scorn booze	10. spite Val

/sp/ plus V Set 3	*/st/ plus V* Set 3	*/sk/ plus V* Set 3	*Mixed UV plus V* Set 3
1. spurt blood	1. stern boss	1. scare Vern	1. stern boss
2. spud bake	2. stuff bag	2. skunk bite	2. skunk bite
3. speed bump	3. steel bolts	3. ski bum	3. pink zone
4. Spandex	4. stabbing	4. scavenge	4. tabby
5. spigot	5. stiff back	5. skivvy	5. killjoy
6. Spain dame	6. stale bread	6. skateboard	6. favor
7. spider	7. sty gate	7. sky blue	7. sizes
8. spare bed	8. step down	8. sketch Bess	8. shelving
9. spout juice	9. stout geese	9. scout badge	9. thousandth
10. spoil Judd	10. still dark	10. Scotch jail	10. choice beef

APPENDIX F. PRACTICE STIMULI, RESTRICTED PHONETIC CONTEXT
For use during injection method for obstruents in esophageal speech.

LEVEL VII: TWO-SYLLABLE WORDS AND PHRASES: UNVOICED AND VOICED OBSTRUENTS (continued)

Mixed UV plus V
Set 4
1. spot Bob
2. stew game
3. scolded
4. put down
5. talk big
6. curvy
7. fungus
8. seething
9. shadow
10. thimble

Mixed UV plus V
Set 5
1. chain gang
2. spied Zeb
3. stare back
4. scour van
5. poi juice
6. tardy
7. kudos
8. forgave
9. soldier
10. Shaw gave

Mixed UV plus V
Set 6
1. third boy
2. chugging
3. speed bump
4. stabbing
5. skivvy
6. page boy
7. tiger
8. Ken votes
9. founder
10. soil them

Mixed UV plus V
Set 7
1. shop door
2. third base
3. chores done
4. spoon bread
5. stalk bent
6. skirt gores
7. puddle
8. teething
9. cash box
10. fish bone

Mixed UV plus V
Set 8
1. savings
2. shy bear
3. theft game
4. chowder
5. spoiled brat
6. starched jeans
7. scuba
8. pole jump
9. tour bus
10. cough drop

Mixed UV plus V
Set 9
1. further
2. southern
3. sheep dog
4. thieving
5. chisel
6. Spain dame
7. sty gate
8. sketch Bess
9. pounder
10. toy van

Mixed UV plus V
Set 10
1. combo
2. Fuji
3. sold it
4. should do
5. thawed out
6. church door
7. sponge bath
8. steamboat
9. scandal
10. pitch dark

Mixed UV plus V
Set 11
1. tailgate
2. kindest
3. feather
4. sour milk
5. showed up
6. third base
7. chew gum
8. spoke there
9. steel guard
10. scorn booze

Mixed UV plus V
Set 12
1. per day
2. touch base
3. King Gus
4. fast ball
5. sizzle
6. shake down
7. thigh joint
8. cheddar
9. spout juice
10. still dark

Mixed UV plus V
Set 13
1. scarf down
2. poodle
3. toll gate
4. could use
5. fought them
6. servant
7. shovel
8. think big
9. chance guess
10. spindle

Mixed UV plus V
Set 14
1. stage hand
2. sky bird
3. pedal
4. town judge
5. coin booth
6. foggy
7. sue them
8. shoulder
9. thought vague
10. chaw veal

Mixed UV plus V
Set 15
1. spurt blood
2. stuff bag
3. ski bum
4. paddle
5. timber
6. cable
7. fight back
8. seltzer
9. shabby
10. thick bag

APPENDIX F. PRACTICE STIMULI, RESTRICTED PHONETIC CONTEXT
For use during injection method for obstruents in esophageal speech.

LEVEL VII: TWO-SYLLABLE WORDS AND PHRASES: UNVOICED AND VOICED OBSTRUENTS *(continued)*

Mixed UV plus V
Set 16
1. charging
2. spooked duck
3. storm's eye
4. scale back
5. pauses
6. turbine
7. caboose
8. feedbag
9. savage
10. shingle

Mixed UV plus V
Set 17
1. thank God
2. children
3. sped off
4. stout bull
5. scoop jellies
6. pardon
7. tool box
8. colder
9. fullback
10. sauce boat

Mixed UV plus V
Set 18
1. sure does
2. thumbs up
3. cheekbone
4. Spandex
5. stiff back
6. skateboard
7. pie dish
8. Teddy
9. cowbell
10. phone bill

Mixed UV plus V
Set 19
1. sergeant
2. shoe dye
3. Thor's zest
4. change jeeps
5. spawned in
6. stirred up
7. scum bag
8. pea bean
9. tangle
10. kidding

Mixed UV plus V
Set 20
1. face down
2. side dish
3. shedder
4. thousand
5. choice gems
6. spark gap
7. stooped vet
8. scone dough
9. push back
10. talk back

Mixed UV plus V
Set 21
1. curdle
2. fuzzy
3. season
4. shampoo
5. thin girl
6. chamber
7. spider
8. step down
9. scout badge
10. poison

Mixed UV plus V
Set 22
1. target
2. cougar
3. folder
4. same day
5. Sean's van
6. Thursday
7. chubby
8. speed boat
9. standard
10. skidded

Mixed UV plus V
Set 23
1. peace dove
2. tidal
3. Kevin
4. found out
5. soybean
6. shot gun
7. thudding
8. chosen
9. spill beans
10. stalk those

Mixed UV plus V
Set 24
1. scare Vern
2. puzzle
3. teal duck
4. cabbage
5. fidget
6. safeguard
7. sideburns
8. think dough
9. chow down
10. spoil Judd

Mixed UV plus V
Set 25
1. stop gap
2. school book
3. posies
4. tomboy
5. call back
6. fervor
7. sunbeam
8. shielded
9. Thad dared
10. chip dip

Mixed UV plus V
Set 26
1. space game
2. style guide
3. schedule
4. powder
5. toys are
6. carbon
7. fool's gold
8. sorbet
9. should go
10. thaw juice

Mixed UV plus V
Set 27
1. chirp birds
2. spud bake
3. steel bolts
4. scavenge
5. pigeon
6. taste bud
7. kite zone
8. pheasant
9. sounded
10. shindig

APPENDIX F. PRACTICE STIMULI, RESTRICTED PHONETIC CONTEXT
For use during injection method for obstruents in esophageal speech.

LEVEL VIII: TWO-SYLLABLE WORDS AND PHRASES: VOICED (V) OBSTRUENTS

- Voiced obstruents /b/, /d/, /g/, /v/, /z/, /ð/, and /dʒ/ occurring in releasing position of second word or syllable

/b/ plus V
Set 1
1. bargain
2. bruises
3. boarder
4. book bag
5. bondage
6. birthday
7. bazaar
8. beaver
9. backbone
10. builder

/d/ plus V
Set 1
1. dodge ball
2. doodle
3. doughboy
4. date book
5. dog days
6. dirt bike
7. done that
8. deejay
9. dragon
10. disguise

/g/ plus V
Set 1
1. garbage
2. goober
3. goes down
4. goodies
5. gaudy
6. girdle
7. govern
8. greedy
9. gather
10. griddle

/v/ plus V
Set 1
1. vendor
2. vaguest
3. Vote Dan!
4. Val's eyes
5. vast beach
6. verbal
7. vulgar
8. veal dish
9. valving
10. vigil

/b/ plus V
Set 2
1. baby
2. binder
3. bedding
4. blouses
5. boy Jack
6. bother
7. bluebird
8. boredom
9. back door
10. boggle

/d/ plus V
Set 2
1. daisy
2. digest
3. desert
4. drowsy
5. daddy
6. dauber
7. doomsday
8. dove in
9. double
10. Dodger

/g/ plus V
Set 2
1. grapevine
2. guided
3. gelding
4. ground ball
5. gumbo
6. garden
7. goof ball
8. golden
9. good-bye
10. gorgeous

/v/ plus V
Set 2
1. vaguest
2. visors
3. veggie
4. Vault this!
5. vision
6. vend eggs
7. verging
8. vogue doll
9. version
10. vandal

/b/ plus V
Set 3
1. birth date
2. brother
3. beach bum
4. Band-Aid
5. bridges
6. baseball
7. buy back
8. beggar
9. browses
10. budget

/d/ plus V
Set 3
1. dirt bike
2. dozen
3. diva
4. dandy
5. drip dry
6. day bed
7. diver
8. dead bolt
9. downbeat
10. doghouse

/g/ plus V
Set 3
1. gurgle
2. grumble
3. green bean
4. grab bag
5. give back
6. glazes
7. glider
8. get dry
9. grounded
10. gear box

/v/ plus V
Set 3
1. verdant
2. virgin
3. vet's dog
4. van Gogh
5. vigor
6. vase box
7. visor
8. vent gas
9. vows dashed
10. vivid

APPENDIX F. PRACTICE STIMULI, RESTRICTED PHONETIC CONTEXT
For use during injection method for obstruents in esophageal speech.

LEVEL VIII: TWO-SYLLABLE WORDS AND PHRASES: VOICED OBSTRUENTS *(continued)*

/z/ plus V Set 1	/ð/ plus V Set 1	/dʒ/ plus V Set 1	Mixed V plus V Set 1
1. zip gun	1. those jewels	1. jar broke	1. bargain
2. zoo bird	2. the boot	2. George goofed	2. doodle
3. zoned bus	3. than Dirk	3. jawbone	3. goes down
4. zing zing	4. their gowns	4. Judd biked	4. Val's eyes
5. zibet	5. the verse	5. job done	5. zibet
6. zygote	6. they jumped	6. gem booth	6. they jumped
7. zapped bees	7. those bells	7. jet black	7. jet black
8. "zee" dial	8. they'll doze	8. Joel gained	8. boredom
9. Zack's badge	9. though gone	9. just bathed	9. double
10. zip boots	10. these vans	10. jade doll	10. gorgeous

/z/ plus V Set 2	/ð/ plus V Set 2	/dʒ/ plus V Set 2	Mixed V plus V Set 2
1. zebu	1. those eyes	1. jewel box	1. vaguest
2. zither	2. these are	2. Jude dined	2. zither
3. Zeb's girl	3. this jar	3. jerk back	3. this jar
4. zap gun	4. the beach	4. June bride	4. June bride
5. zinged Joel	5. thy deed	5. jail bound	5. bridges
6. Zeb gave	6. those girls	6. join them	6. day bed
7. zoomed down	7. than Vern	7. judge deeds	7. glider
8. zilch desks	8. these bowls	8. gym ball	8. vent gas
9. zinc blend	9. this day	9. juice bowl	9. Zounds, Butch!
10. zigzag	10. the guard	10. Jim gave	10. they'll bake

/z/ plus V Set 3	/ð/ plus V Set 3	/dʒ/ plus V Set 3	Mixed V plus V Set 3
1. Zack votes	1. those eggs	1. jeep door	1. jeep door
2. zoo jeep	2. than Zack	2. joy that	2. bruises
3. zebra	3. this deal	3. germs boiled	3. doughboy
4. zag dash	4. their jobs	4. gin glass	4. goodies
5. Zen book	5. these eight	5. Gene dove	5. vast beach
6. zip this	6. the booth	6. gents' boast	6. zygote
7. zwieback	7. this goes	7. joke book	7. those bells
8. zest go	8. they ducked	8. jazz band	8. Joel gained
9. Zounds, Butch!	9. though dark	9. jaw gum	9. back door
10. Zeke gained	10. they'll bake	10. juke box	10. Dodger

APPENDIX F. PRACTICE STIMULI, RESTRICTED PHONETIC CONTEXT
For use during injection method for obstruents in esophageal speech.

LEVEL VIII: TWO-SYLLABLE WORDS AND PHRASES: VOICED OBSTRUENTS (continued)

Mixed V plus V
Set 4
1. grapevine
2. visors
3. Zeb's girl
4. the beach
5. jail bound
6. baseball
7. diver
8. get dry
9. vows dashed
10. Zeke gained

Mixed V plus V
Set 5
1. those eggs
2. joy that
3. boarder
4. date book
5. gaudy
6. verbal
7. zapped bees
8. they'll doze
9. just bathed
10. boggle

Mixed V plus V
Set 6
1. daisy
2. guided
3. veggie
4. zap gun
5. thy deed
6. join them
7. buy back
8. dead bolt
9. grounded
10. vivid

Mixed V plus V
Set 7
1. Zack votes
2. this deal
3. germs boiled
4. book bag
5. dog days
6. girdle
7. vulgar
8. "zee" dial
9. though gone
10. jade doll

Mixed V plus V
Set 8
1. baby
2. digest
3. gelding
4. vault this
5. zinged Joel
6. those girls
7. judge deeds
8. beggar
9. down beat
10. gear box

Mixed V plus V
Set 9
1. verdant
2. zoo jeep
3. than Jack
4. gin glass
5. bondage
6. dirt bike
7. govern
8. veal dish
9. Zack's badge
10. these vans

Mixed V plus V
Set 10
1. jar broke
2. binder
3. desert
4. ground ball
5. vision
6. Zeb gave
7. than Vern
8. juice bowl
9. browses
10. doghouse

Mixed V plus V
Set 11
1. gurgle
2. virgin
3. zebra
4. their jobs
5. Gene drove
6. birthday
7. done that
8. greedy
9. valving
10. zip boots

Mixed V plus V
Set 12
1. those jewels
2. George goofed
3. bedding
4. drowsy
5. gumbo
6. vend eggs
7. zoomed down
8. these bowls
9. gym ball
10. budget

Mixed V plus V
Set 13
1. dirt bike
2. grumble
3. vet's dog
4. zag dash
5. these eight
6. gent's boast
7. bazaar
8. dee jay
9. gather
10. vigil

Mixed V plus V
Set 14
1. zip gun
2. the boot
3. jawbone
4. blouses
5. daddy
6. garden
7. verging
8. zilch desks
9. this day
10. Jim gave

Mixed V plus V
Set 15
1. birth date
2. dozen
3. green bean
4. van Gogh
5. Zen book
6. the booth
7. jazz band
8. beaver
9. dragon
10. griddle

APPENDIX F. PRACTICE STIMULI, RESTRICTED PHONETIC CONTEXT
For use during injection method for obstruents in esophageal speech.

LEVEL VIII: TWO-SYLLABLE WORDS AND PHRASES: VOICED OBSTRUENTS *(continued)*

Mixed V plus V
Set 16
1. vendor
2. zoo bird
3. than Dirk
4. Judd biked
5. boy Jack
6. dauber
7. goof ball
8. vogue doll
9. zinc blend
10. the guard

Mixed V plus V
Set 17
1. jewel box
2. brother
3. diva
4. grab bag
5. vigor
6. zip this
7. this goes
8. joke book
9. backbone
10. disguise

Mixed V plus V
Set 18
1. garbage
2. vaguest
3. zoned bus
4. their gowns
5. job done
6. bother
7. doomsday
8. golden
9. version
10. zigzag

Mixed V plus V
Set 19
1. those eyes
2. Jude dined
3. beach bum
4. dandy
5. give back
6. vase box
7. zwieback
8. they ducked
9. jaw gum
10. builder

Mixed V plus V
Set 20
1. dodgeball
2. goober
3. vote Dan
4. zing zing
5. the verse
6. gym booth
7. bluebird
8. dove in
9. good-bye
10. vandal

Mixed V plus V
Set 21
1. zebu
2. these are
3. jerk back
4. Band-Aid
5. drip dry
6. glazes
7. visor
8. zest go
9. though dark
10. juke box

Mixed V plus V
Set 22
1. bruises
2. date book
3. girdle
4. veal dish
5. zip boots
6. than Dirk
7. Judd biked
8. bother
9. dove in
10. gorgeous

Mixed V plus V
Set 23
1. visors
2. zap gun
3. those girls
4. gym ball
5. budget
6. dozen
7. grab bag
8. vase box
9. zest go
10. they'll bake

Mixed V plus V
Set 24
1. joy that
2. book bag
3. dirt bike
4. greedy
5. vigil
6. zoo bird
7. their gowns
8. gem booth
9. boredom
10. Dodger

Mixed V plus V
Set 25
1. guided
2. vault this
3. Zeb gave
4. these bowls
5. jail bound
6. brother
7. dandy
8. glazes
9. vent gas
10. Zeke gained

Mixed V plus V
Set 26
1. this deal
2. gin glass
3. birthday
4. deejay
5. griddle
6. vaguest
7. zing zing
8. they jumped
9. jet black
10. boggle

Mixed V plus V
Set 27
1. digest
2. ground ball
3. vend eggs
4. zilch desks
5. the guard
6. Jude dined
7. Band-Aid
8. day bed
9. get dry
10. vivid

APPENDIX F. PRACTICE STIMULI, RESTRICTED PHONETIC CONTEXT
For use during injection method for obstruents in esophageal speech.

LEVEL IX: THREE- TO FOUR-SYLLABLE PHRASES AND SENTENCES WITH UNVOICED AND VOICED OBSTRUENTS IN THE RELEASING POSITIONS

Set 1
1. sugar cookies
2. done that before
3. Stop and go.
4. quick and easy
5. Get started.
6. Vacuum carpets.
7. Keep on truckin'.
8. Forget it.
9. because of Ted
10. Pocket some cash.

Set 2
1. Start up the car.
2. first to fight
3. just a kid
4. Keep off the grass.
5. buttered popcorn
6. savage beast
7. Smell the coffee.
8. ghost of a chance
9. church on Sunday
10. poodle fuzz

Set 3
1. dirty dozen
2. through thick and thin
3. Block the pass.
4. Sign the contract.
5. can't talk today
6. Take two tablets.
7. Join the club.
8. for Pete's sake
9. postcard from France
10. gastric juices

Set 4
1. Suck a cough drop.
2. That's good thinking.
3. fifteen seconds
4. gone fishing
5. Compare prices.
6. Shop and save.
7. baked potato
8. Close the door.
9. veggie burger
10. Pocket the cash.

Set 5
1. Bring a friend.
2. Flip that pancake.
3. Sit in the shade.
4. Chop up coleslaw.
5. deep friendship
6. took a break
7. good company
8. Put out the cat.
9. vice president
10. time to stop by

Set 6
1. Don't count on Bill.
2. Three's a crowd.
3. Feed a fever.
4. zebra's stripes
5. Stop the paper.
6. vegetable soup
7. Strike a deal.
8. first at the scene
9. Go south two blocks.
10. Patience pays off.

Set 7
1. Pay the piper.
2. Just sit tight.
3. soup and sandwich
4. Keep it simple.
5. by the back door
6. Check up on Bob.
7. decaf coffee
8. shirked his duty
9. Father Time
10. vice squad captain

Set 8
1. Take up the fight.
2. pet shop supplies
3. Jump ship at port.
4. smart as a fox
5. bird in the bush
6. Don't count on it.
7. Flip a coin.
8. Catch the first bus.
9. Greet the day.
10. Stretch the truth.

APPENDIX F. PRACTICE STIMULI, RESTRICTED PHONETIC CONTEXT
For use during injection method for obstruents in esophageal speech.

LEVEL IX: THREE- TO FOUR-SYLLABLE PHRASES AND SENTENCES WITH UNVOICED AND VOICED OBSTRUENTS IN THE RELEASING POSITIONS *(continued)*

Set 9
1. Pick a time.
2. got the flu
3. Check out that car!
4. Saturday job
5. Collect back pay.
6. doeskin slippers
7. back to school
8. friend or foe
9. Take a picture.
10. Zip it up.

Set 10
1. Pass the salt.
2. from the garden
3. Going, going, gone!
4. three free tickets
5. Visit often.
6. Slow down, Peg.
7. between two streets
8. certain people
9. chicken pot pie
10. dry-cleaned jacket

Set 11
1. Set the table.
2. gained ten pounds
3. Take on the day.
4. point of view
5. down the street
6. Build confidence.
7. kitchen sink
8. Choose a time.
9. fishing boats
10. zoned for school

Set 12
1. bread and butter
2. seven days
3. cup of bleach
4. jewel box contents
5. Take time to talk.
6. drip dry clothes
7. good bargains
8. spoke too soon
9. visa to France
10. through the grapevine

Set 13
1. Stop for gas.
2. just between them
3. too tired to sleep
4. detour sign
5. by the book
6. pretty good biscuits
7. caught a cold
8. Sample the cheese.
9. good-bye Charlie
10. Feed the dog.

Set 14
1. Beat the system.
2. Cross the street.
3. good as gold
4. taught a class
5. vivid dreams
6. pots and pans
7. far to travel
8. dessert tray
9. Don't slip and fall.
10. stick-on Band-Aid

Set 15
1. pickup truck
2. jumped the gun
3. Third floor, please.
4. deep blue background
5. shade-tree swing
6. Keep a secret.
7. fruit basket
8. gospel songs
9. black and blue
10. sliding glass doors

Set 16
1. Give to the poor.
2. day is done
3. past her bedtime
4. salt and pepper
5. bought out the store
6. Tow the car.
7. cold outside
8. three blocks to go
9. because she cried
10. glossy photos

APPENDIX F. PRACTICE STIMULI, RESTRICTED PHONETIC CONTEXT
For use during injection method for obstruents in esophageal speech.

LEVEL IX: THREE- TO FOUR-SYLLABLE PHRASES AND SENTENCES WITH UNVOICED AND VOICED OBSTRUENTS IN THE RELEASING POSITIONS *(continued)*

Set 17
1. public servant
2. joke's on George
3. Bring a sweater.
4. Keep two copies.
5. Steep the tea.
6. drowsy driver
7. sunken gardens
8. prescription drug
9. futon bed
10. greetings from Spain

Set 18
1. time to quit
2. passport photo
3. salty pretzel
4. bed and breakfast
5. third broken vase
6. vintage cars
7. shop door key
8. goldfish bowl
9. spray gun paint
10. diesel fuel

Set 19
1. snap green beans
2. jazz combo
3. Soothe it over.
4. baby powder
5. Plan a trip.
6. Dodger fans
7. sloppy joes
8. frighten to death
9. table for two
10. getting better

Set 20
1. fragile package
2. choice-cut beef
3. Devise a plan.
4. quarter pounder
5. too bad for Jack
6. Pull some strings.
7. Bill chewed gum.
8. thin shirt box
9. sergeant Bilko
10. Zeb's feet toed in.

Set 21
1. Go to bed.
2. perfect timing
3. treasure trove
4. charge account
5. busy day
6. blue sweat suit
7. flagpole sitter
8. divine guidance
9. stick-shift car
10. dozen posies

Set 22
1. basic floor plan
2. piece of cake
3. That's a put-down.
4. close call for Jeff
5. Depart at three.
6. frozen pot pies
7. slumber party
8. grand pageantry
9. cheese and crackers
10. shovel snow

Set 23
1. Don't talk back.
2. pancake griddle
3. Join the club.
4. too far to go
5. dove of peace
6. sold it cheap
7. church founder
8. buddy system
9. gravy boat
10. springtime sunshine

Set 24
1. chalkboard dust
2. Sean came too soon.
3. Beg his pardon.
4. Just kidding!
5. bag of fool's gold
6. Predict success.
7. frantic phone call
8. double trouble
9. stool pigeon
10. thawed out today

APPENDIX F. PRACTICE STIMULI, RESTRICTED PHONETIC CONTEXT
For use during injection method for obstruents in esophageal speech.

LEVEL IX: THREE- TO FOUR-SYLLABLE PHRASES AND SENTENCES WITH UNVOICED AND VOICED OBSTRUENTS IN THE RELEASING POSITIONS
(continued)

Set 25
1. chosen few
2. Beat the clock.
3. sports banter
4. decaf coffee
5. scuba diver
6. guilty thieves
7. pleasure trip
8. zip-up jacket
9. taxi for two
10. veto bill

Set 26
1. job to do
2. creature comforts
3. goes down fast
4. Fuji peaches
5. cheap zoo prices
6. barber shop
7. sawdust cloud
8. deserve a break
9. Think about it.
10. garbage pail

Set 27
1. voted for Gus
2. Starve a cold.
3. germ-free bottle
4. skunk bite fever
5. dimpled cheeks
6. pool deck chairs
7. beat-up old car
8. today's paper
9. kindest person
10. Bypass our place.

Set 28
1. Pass out the cards.
2. spare bed for guests
3. bother to tell
4. thimble sized
5. charging bull
6. become stronger
7. golfer's tees
8. servant's quarters
9. downtown shopping
10. foggy coast

Set 29
1. spied Zeb sleeping
2. duty calls
3. puddle jumper
4. Begin to smile.
5. vapor trail
6. teddy bear
7. frequent pauses
8. defense team
9. classic car show
10. showed up to play

Set 30
1. scuff those shoes
2. goes down fast
3. cold sponge bath
4. beaded jacket
5. spoke there before
6. Push back the time.
7. tailgate party
8. vampire bats
9. became king
10. Call the doctor.

Set 31
1. bruised cheekbone
2. Scare Vern to death.
3. duffel bag
4. golden pond
5. Pass the cough drops.
6. beaver dam
7. guitar strings
8. carbon copy
9. tour bus crowd
10. shudder to think

Set 32
1. jockey's saddle
2. barking dogs
3. cold side dish
4. single father
5. pop top drink
6. Scavenge for food.
7. Disarm the bomb.
8. goes out for sports
9. Take it easy.
10. thumbs up sign

APPENDIX F. PRACTICE STIMULI, RESTRICTED PHONETIC CONTEXT
For use during injection method for obstruents in esophageal speech.

LEVEL IX: THREE- TO FOUR-SYLLABLE PHRASES AND SENTENCES WITH UNVOICED AND VOICED OBSTRUENTS IN THE RELEASING POSITIONS
(continued)

Set 33
1. Thank God for bread.
2. beagle boys
3. Defeat that team!
4. paddle boat
5. tollgate person
6. darkened skies
7. Ken votes often.
8. Depend on Stan.
9. shampoo bottle
10. sobbing child

Set 34
1. Defer to dad.
2. faddish clothes
3. Take advantage.
4. gutter talk
5. cabbage patch
6. That's in style.
7. van Gogh painting
8. thieving bus boy
9. bitter cold
10. stirred up a fight

Set 35
1. vaguest thoughts
2. boxer shorts
3. shoot darts for fun
4. Take a chance.
5. gaping jaw
6. thousandth driver
7. feather duster
8. just for today
9. cable vision
10. big talk for Sam

Set 36
1. Buy back the books.
2. guzzle beer
3. thighbone pain
4. savings account
5. this book case
6. should sue them
7. fish gumbo
8. Call the doctor.
9. bedside vigil
10. dental plan

Set 37
1. The diva sang.
2. body builder
3. garden grown
4. tardy to school
5. pauses to breathe
6. daughter's phone
7. shadow boxing
8. cheddar cheese
9. biker bags
10. gothic spire

Set 38
1. goober peas
2. seconds to go
3. tomboy jeans
4. stood there shaking
5. Keep it coming.
6. Boycott the store.
7. pitch-dark attic
8. Sunday service
9. bright beacon
10. dissolve sugar

Set 39
1. Steamboat Springs
2. dishonored soldier
3. quite a few
4. peach sorbet
5. vouched for Susan
6. shampoo bottle
7. for the best
8. these apple pies
9. tangle up
10. cozy fireplace

Set 40
1. football team
2. verbal contract
3. frequent guests
4. go fish game
5. taste bud pleaser
6. pea bean soup
7. They'll find out soon.
8. could use some cash
9. better than cake
10. tabby cat

APPENDIX F. PRACTICE STIMULI, RESTRICTED PHONETIC CONTEXT
For use during injection method for obstruents in esophageal speech.

LEVEL IX: THREE- TO FOUR-SYLLABLE PHRASES AND SENTENCES WITH UNVOICED AND VOICED OBSTRUENTS IN THE RELEASING POSITIONS (*continued*)

Set 41
1. Thursday chores done
2. fuzzy sweater
3. stabbing back pain
4. Bible study
5. Pa's dog, Spot
6. before they came
7. test tube baby
8. detest scrubbing
9. seldom seen
10. They took off.

Set 42
1. Stare back at her!
2. cougar country
3. Devour the pie.
4. got it done
5. season to cheer
6. forgave Zack
7. guided tour
8. Pick out a shirt.
9. butcher paper
10. Check the schedule.

Set 43
1. belt beeper
2. guppy food
3. saved by the bell
4. Pay taxes.
5. zoomed down the track
6. banker box
7. kudos to Paul
8. sleet or snow
9. decayed teeth
10. text book case

Set 44
1. frisky puppy
2. poison darts
3. baker's dozen
4. steel guardrail
5. dainty daisies
6. street car fare
7. target bull's-eye
8. crystal ball
9. dented fender
10. bathtub cleanser

Set 45
1. Take that bus.
2. Stalk those deer.
3. vantage point
4. Cheer the team.
5. then check it out
6. shaded figure
7. Tell the truth.
8. Defog the glass.
9. soldier boy
10. Block the door.

Set 46
1. cowboy saddle
2. devoted to Bess
3. Zoos are for bears.
4. southern belle
5. foot fungus
6. garter belt
7. beside the point
8. too tough to cry
9. downtown fair
10. sketch pad pen

Set 47
1. before they came
2. gobble turkey
3. Close the door.
4. Step aside.
5. gopher digs
6. buckle seatbelts
7. credit card
8. shrimp boat catch
9. Detect fraud.
10. seething fighter

Set 48
1. denture cleanser
2. between Peg and Bob
3. their tool box
4. kitchen chores
5. Davy Crockett
6. Take it easy.
7. sizes too small
8. daytime soaps
9. busiest day
10. store-bought jeans

APPENDIX F. PRACTICE STIMULI, RESTRICTED PHONETIC CONTEXT
For use during injection method for obstruents in esophageal speech.

LEVEL X: FIVE- TO SIX-SYLLABLE PHRASES AND SENTENCES WITH UNVOICED AND VOICED OBSTRUENTS IN THE RELEASING POSITIONS

Set 1
1. back in the saddle
2. decent cup of coffee
3. face-down position
4. vision for the future
5. Put the car top down.
6. Schedule time to rest.
7. Table for two, please.
8. That is a good show.
9. Gail's blind as a bat.
10. fifty-fifty chance

Set 2
1. back to back classes
2. Spend time together.
3. tall pink snapdragons
4. vital statistics
5. That dog should stop barking!
6. Zoos are for tigers.
7. Cut it in three pieces.
8. stitch in time saves nine
9. Don't cross the sagging bridge.
10. put out of action

Set 3
1. productive session
2. The car keys are gone.
3. Take two copies for Fred.
4. shot footage of the play
5. duty to country
6. goes out for pizza
7. Bake a dozen cookies.
8. credit card debit
9. started to paint the door
10. Fight a speeding ticket.

Set 4
1. Cut Betty some slack.
2. Go to church on Sunday.
3. spot Bob in the truck
4. skipped to the back page
5. down the bridle path
6. built by three carpenters
7. checkbook in Sue's purse
8. Vote for president.
9. The show begins at eight.
10. critical to the case

Set 5
1. Call the fire station.
2. best time to stop by
3. Get it together.
4. snapshots from vacation
5. Fred, pull down the shades.
6. practice 'til perfect
7. George said, "Talk is cheap."
8. Strike three, Thompson's out!
9. fast as a speeding train
10. Children can play games.

Set 6
1. cream for the coffee
2. don't understand it
3. The frozen food thawed.
4. sunset at six-fifteen
5. Purchase a pound of beef.
6. Get it together.
7. Count sheep at bedtime.
8. Shut down the computer.
9. backed against the door
10. special gratitude

Set 7
1. can't stand the constant pain
2. Give us a good clue.
3. chunky football players
4. two sides to the problem
5. fireflies in the dark
6. The price tag is too steep.
7. Prepare to be stopped.
8. bathing suit in June
9. vegetable garden
10. Thursday's garbage pick up

Set 8
1. Peter got shortchanged.
2. pheasant under glass
3. shook out the bedding
4. credit card purchase
5. seventy-six trombones
6. basis for quitting
7. Press the button twice.
8. Talk to the doctor.
9. Thanksgiving turkey
10. dry clean by Friday

APPENDIX F. PRACTICE STIMULI, RESTRICTED PHONETIC CONTEXT
For use during injection method for obstruents in esophageal speech.

LEVEL X: FIVE- TO SIX-SYLLABLE PHRASES AND SENTENCES WITH UNVOICED AND VOICED OBSTRUENTS IN THE RELEASING POSITIONS (*continued*)

Set 9
1. beautiful butterfly
2. gone to Glacier Gorge
3. critical condition
4. question for the teacher
5. The show begins soon.
6. packed for a trip
7. calm before the storm
8. dawdled in the bathtub
9. Supreme Court decision
10. tiger by the tail

Set 10
1. prime time TV shows
2. That's a good approach.
3. Pay by the due date.
4. Beeping foiled the car thief.
5. took a pot shot at Jane
6. Sit in the first church pew.
7. could change two flat tires
8. Smart shoppers skip junk.
9. Don't fight gravity.
10. found it in the closet

Set 11
1. public transportation
2. Green grapes are the best.
3. Stop for the stop sign.
4. zebras at the zoo
5. car seat belts fastened
6. film for the projector
7. Don't be so depressed.
8. the best I can do
9. thirteen chirping birds
10. better take a chance

Set 12
1. This compass points south.
2. Go to the dentist.
3. slice of pumpkin pie
4. black-eyed peas in the pot
5. Camp David for three days
6. Drive the car for pleasure.
7. two dogs and two cats
8. jars of pickled corn
9. Flights depart at twelve.
10. thirty cents postage due

Set 13
1. Fill the prescription.
2. Come to the party.
3. paid five traffic tickets
4. because of the storm
5. Put gas in the truck.
6. Toast is a breakfast food.
7. They put out the fire.
8. vacation schedule
9. dropped the shoes by the store
10. grandfather's old chair

Set 14
1. Take a bus or taxi.
2. snipped the buttercups
3. green beans and potatoes
4. boxes of photos
5. divorce proceedings
6. Gas up the four-by-four.
7. The tattoos tickled.
8. service station tow truck
9. Consider the source.
10. swayed to the dance tunes

Set 15
1. Those scissors are too sharp.
2. glided down the slope
3. Keep up the good job.
4. tiptoed up the stairs
5. changes in the clouds
6. juice from the blender
7. smidgen of pepper
8. birthday cake and ice cream
9. panned for flakes of gold
10. Drunk drivers should be stopped.

Set 16
1. black and blue bruises
2. cows in the clover
3. This is Saturday.
4. detect a burglar
5. She can bake a pie.
6. gone too far to stop
7. box cars and cabooses
8. Plug in the TV.
9. took Sam's blood pressure
10. jumped up and gave his seat

APPENDIX F. PRACTICE STIMULI, RESTRICTED PHONETIC CONTEXT
For use during injection method for obstruents in esophageal speech.

LEVEL X: FIVE- TO SIX-SYLLABLE PHRASES AND SENTENCES WITH UNVOICED AND VOICED OBSTRUENTS IN THE RELEASING POSITIONS *(continued)*

Set 17
1. Defy the system.
2. tripped over the door jamb
3. spurted blood on the floor
4. predicted sunshine
5. Becky's birthday party
6. Flapjacks or pancakes?
7. Scotch tape it to the door.
8. This is too difficult.
9. coffee, juice, or tea
10. Buy back-to-school clothes.

Set 18
1. Good things come to those folks.
2. took us to the store
3. Pick seven daffodils.
4. Don't cross the train tracks.
5. six-foot jumper cables
6. Come prepared to jog.
7. blanket on the sand
8. The shops and stores are closed.
9. found a parking space
10. plastic ketchup bottle

Set 19
1. threw the ball to third base
2. get into trouble
3. blinded by the sun
4. too soon to cook out
5. pork chops or chicken
6. stunned the crowd by quitting
7. disguised as the devil
8. conductor said "tickets!"
9. These gloves are too tight.
10. broken glass on the floor

Set 20
1. copper pots and pans
2. substitute teacher
3. Don't give it a thought.
4. protected her babies
5. blast off in ten seconds
6. The soldier played taps.
7. toothbrush and toothpaste
8. fragile crystal goblets
9. Please print two copies.
10. gulped the drink and belched

Set 21
1. things to do Tuesday
2. colder by the door
3. gave Jerrod a present
4. splinter in this finger
5. The sculptor shaped the clay.
6. bad tempered traffic cop
7. Victor quit his job.
8. Scrape off the burned crust.
9. Put it in the trash can.
10. too good to be true

Set 22
1. preside over the group
2. beautiful June bride
3. deposit cans here
4. The porter toted bags.
5. frequent visitor
6. Stretch out on the couch.
7. Crushed grapes become Chablis.
8. They posted bail for Jack.
9. peeled potatoes for stew
10. checkout at the dime store

Set 23
1. potatoes and gravy
2. drip dry seersucker
3. The bulb is burned out.
4. green carpet for sale
5. Tom's billfold's too full.
6. sought care for thigh pain
7. spare pocket change
8. Barbra crawled to safety.
9. prefer to play cards
10. shot tin cans off the fence

Set 24
1. bronze statue for the park
2. three steps to good speech
3. stumbled on the stairs
4. put in jail for speeding
5. crowded circus tent
6. Saint Patrick's Day green
7. Drive the car to Texas.
8. Bake at three hundred fifty degrees.
9. twelve-foot bridal train
10. caused a plane disaster

APPENDIX F. PRACTICE STIMULI, RESTRICTED PHONETIC CONTEXT
For use during injection method for obstruents in esophageal speech.

LEVEL X: FIVE- TO SIX-SYLLABLE PHRASES AND SENTENCES WITH UNVOICED AND VOICED OBSTRUENTS IN THE RELEASING POSITIONS *(continued)*

Set 25
1. prescribed thirty tablets
2. She plays chess and checkers.
3. portrait of Saint Paul
4. then call the doctor
5. Cover the vegetables.
6. Someone pays the bill.
7. classical concert
8. top Pentagon brass
9. bent the chrome fenders
10. the group's biggest problem

Set 26
1. three full plastic bags
2. did it on purpose
3. Children chew bubble gum.
4. prefer fact or fiction
5. bought a fluffy kitten
6. coffee, cream, sugar
7. standing by the goal post
8. five o'clock, quitting time
9. shortest path to freedom
10. pleased as punch to speak

Set 27
1. three days in the car
2. Time to take a pill.
3. shoulder to shoulder
4. Simply complete the form.
5. Please clean the table.
6. faulty product complaint
7. Jim's a school crossing guard.
8. bucket of fried chicken
9. sobered by sad thoughts
10. quick to take offense

Set 28
1. They jogged for three blocks.
2. fur coat in the closet
3. Don't bother to call.
4. box of cotton balls
5. cashew-filled cookies
6. sand castles at the beach
7. pagodas from Japan
8. cry crocodile tears
9. cheeseburger special
10. Sing the praises of Joe.

Set 29
1. sweat suit for jogging
2. David and his slingshot
3. blistered by the sun
4. pledged to be truthful
5. tough kid to baby-sit
6. sip from the teaspoon
7. five-and-ten bargains
8. cookie crumbs in bed
9. set off the blasting caps
10. cheat on their taxes

Set 30
1. flash photography
2. Govern the people.
3. kitchen countertop
4. Divulge a secret.
5. pecan pie for dessert
6. suit coat or best jacket
7. These crackers are stale.
8. tackled the quarterback
9. spooky campfire tales
10. Forgive each other.

Set 31
1. Snack on cheese crackers.
2. cowboy's silver buckle
3. Pick up a dozen.
4. Call poison control.
5. days in September
6. turned off the gas stove
7. The split pea soup is cold.
8. sailed the seven seas
9. bound and blindfolded
10. crystal clear to Bobbie

Set 32
1. turned to say good-bye
2. swept the cabin's dirt floor
3. box and tissue paper
4. trespass against us
5. They played Parcheesi.
6. Soldiers guarded the tomb.
7. drugstore prescription
8. pulled back the curtains
9. Boil the freshest eggs.
10. Check their ticket dates.

APPENDIX F. PRACTICE STIMULI, RESTRICTED PHONETIC CONTEXT
For use during injection method for obstruents in esophageal speech.

LEVEL X: FIVE- TO SIX-SYLLABLE PHRASES AND SENTENCES WITH UNVOICED AND VOICED OBSTRUENTS IN THE RELEASING POSITIONS (*continued*)

Set 33
1. The dentist filled the tooth.
2. greetings from Boston
3. Pass the salt and pepper.
4. second grade teacher
5. Too bad Jack has a cold.
6. Discuss the problems.
7. flexible schedule
8. Practice the guitar.
9. Beat Fred at checkers.
10. should get a bandage

Set 34
1. pumpkin pie sliver
2. Thad dared to think big.
3. Send a check to David.
4. Shut off dripping faucets.
5. Take that as a friend.
6. propane fuel for the tank
7. The car's safety features.
8. Divide and conquer.
9. corned beef and cabbage
10. Clark saw Field of Dreams.

Set 35
1. set a good example
2. Princess Diana
3. twinkle, twinkle star
4. three tea bags in the pot
5. butterscotch pudding
6. tiger by the tail
7. dental floss or toothpick
8. Find a cure for cancer.
9. Sean got a fair trial.
10. Keep peace in the country.

Set 36
1. Chop up the cabbage.
2. pancakes on the griddle
3. Scour the tub and sink.
4. See the bucking bronco.
5. canceled because of snow
6. joined before she did
7. tea bag in the cup
8. Zip up the cloth jacket.
9. Buy some pretzels and beer.
10. poodle fuzz on the couch

Set 37
1. breakable dishes
2. Predict the future.
3. pocket protector
4. That's the best I can do.
5. gave it to brother
6. Stop at the pet shop.
7. Find dark sunglasses.
8. Chicago's skyscrapers
9. truck driver stopped to sleep
10. found it in the kitchen

Set 38
1. Black Jack or poker?
2. San Francisco crabs
3. pasted in the scrapbook
4. cheesy spaghetti
5. film festival program
6. Don should be sleeping.
7. too few station breaks
8. cockatiel bird cage
9. Begin practicing.
10. tribute to George Burns

Set 39
1. Grease the cake pan first.
2. percent of the profits
3. They think it's downstairs.
4. basket of baked chicken
5. Subtract three from ten.
6. Decrease shoulder tension.
7. confessed to the crime
8. private property
9. teal duck on the pond
10. thankful to be chosen

Set 40
1. trick or treat costume
2. cheek-to-cheek dancing
3. Swiss apple strudel
4. barns in the countryside
5. shuddered to think of it
6. Chicago's skyscrapers
7. Teasing can be cruel.
8. study group on Thursday
9. too cheap to buy tickets
10. flip-flop decision

APPENDIX F. PRACTICE STIMULI, RESTRICTED PHONETIC CONTEXT
For use during injection method for obstruents in esophageal speech.

LEVEL X: FIVE- TO SIX-SYLLABLE PHRASES AND SENTENCES WITH UNVOICED AND VOICED OBSTRUENTS IN THE RELEASING POSITIONS *(continued)*

Set 41
1. Seek out good company.
2. That's what friends are for.
3. prefers swivel-backed chairs
4. She's a graceful dancer.
5. Sleep in Saturday.
6. Take close up photos.
7. French fried potatoes
8. Don't slip up and fall.
9. percent of the profits
10. Buy the charcoal gray suit.

Set 42
1. better than baked bread
2. sales clerk at the store
3. Think positive thoughts.
4. carrot cake for dessert
5. butterscotch flavored
6. proud as a peacock
7. Divide twelve by six.
8. quick and easy to solve
9. steam-driven paddle boat
10. toured the city by bus

Set 43
1. six striped candy canes
2. visited Steamboat Springs
3. served peaches and cream
4. before they said it
5. dark skies before the storm
6. father's touch-tone phone
7. Cucumbers are green.
8. That's in style today.
9. detest scrubbing the tub
10. bought back all the books

Set 44
1. Sunshine dried the puddle.
2. bright beacon for ships
3. They should provide this form.
4. blue grass of Kentucky
5. can't take it to school
6. jockey's position
7. covered by dental plans
8. Put on boxing gloves.
9. fruity popsicle
10. Steve strummed the banjo.

Set 45
1. Pass the potatoes, please.
2. between those two people
3. forced to sell the car
4. Soothe the savage beast.
5. tempting dessert tray
6. the jet's vapor trail
7. Cash a check for food.
8. Smell the perking coffee.
9. tamed the bucking bronco
10. Build up confidence.

Set 46
1. cut grapefruit sections
2. Denver string quartet
3. sun-faded curtains
4. freshen the bedding
5. Keep it a secret.
6. bought pewter bookends
7. stop-and-go traffic
8. two pounds of boiled shrimp
9. black-and-blue cheekbone
10. cold cuts as a side dish

Set 47
1. Send a greeting card.
2. canned goods for the pantry
3. Bitter cold drove Tim back.
4. They took off for Kansas.
5. crashed through the steel guardrail
6. bean sprouts in the stir fry
7. Subscribe to cable.
8. vouched for Vickie's birth date
9. That's beside the point.
10. kept a bedside vigil

Set 48
1. comfortable sweater
2. Turn back the covers.
3. sorted through the tool box
4. paper clips and thumb tacks
5. The bugler played taps.
6. took a guided tour
7. president Jackson
8. Buzzing bees swarmed the tent.
9. sunshine through the sheer drapes
10. barber shop quartet

Practice Stimuli, Restricted Phonetic Context

APPENDIX G: PRACTICE STIMULI, RESTRICTED PHONETIC CONTEXT

For use during
- Injection method for sonorants and vowels in esophageal speech
- Inhalation method in esophageal speech

LEVEL I: ONE-SYLLABLE WORDS BEGINNING WITH MID AND LOW VOWELS
- Mid and low vowels /a/, /o/, /ɔ/, /ʌ/, /æ/, /e/, and /ɛ/

Mixed vowels Set 1	Mixed vowels Set 4	Mixed vowels Set 7	Mixed vowels Set 10	Mixed vowels Set 13
1. a	1. awed	1. ash	1. ebbs	1. owes
2. oaf	2. ughs	2. ape	2. ought	2. awe
3. all	3. an	3. etch	3. oats	3. un-
4. of	4. aid	4. arts	4. off	4. aunt
5. act	5. egg	5. own	5. us	5. aimed
6. Abe	6. art	6. awl	6. Ann's	6. erred
7. air	7. oh	7. upped	7. aches	7. aren't
8. arch	8. ought	8. ask	8. edged	8. owns
9. oak	9. ump	9. ate	9. Oz	9. auk
10. awl	10. and	10. aired	10. oaths	10. ups

Mixed vowels Set 2	Mixed vowels Set 5	Mixed vowels Set 8	Mixed vowels Set 11	Mixed vowels Set 14
1. ugh	1. ail	1. odd	1. alms	1. ax
2. ad	2. elm	2. oafs	2. ughs	2. apes
3. ace	3. arched	3. awe	3. asked	3. etched
4. ebb	4. old	4. of	4. ached	4. arm
5. are	5. off	5. acts	5. eggs	5. oast
6. oar	6. um	6. eight	6. a	6. awed
7. awe	7. Ann	7. airs	7. ohs	7. upped
8. up	8. aim	8. off	8. all	8. abs
9. Al	9. else	9. oaks	9. ump	9. aims
10. ache	10. arms	10. auk	10. asks	10. el

Mixed vowels Set 3	Mixed vowels Set 6	Mixed vowels Set 9	Mixed vowels Set 12	Mixed vowels Set 15
1. Ed	1. or	1. ugh	1. aids	1. art
2. aren't	2. alms	2. ads	2. elms	2. owed
3. oat	3. un-	3. eighth	3. arch	3. ought
4. auk	4. as	4. ebbed	4. Olds	4. of
5. us	5. ale	5. on	5. awl	5. aunts
6. am	6. err	6. oared	6. um	6. eights
7. age	7. armed	7. awed	7. at	7. air
8. edge	8. owe	8. up	8. ailed	8. arched
9. arm	9. all	9. Al's	9. errs	9. owned
10. oath	10. ups	10. aide	10. are	10. off

APPENDIX G: PRACTICE STIMULI, RESTRICTED PHONETIC CONTEXT

For use during
- Injection method for sonorants and vowels in esophageal speech
- Inhalation method in esophageal speech

LEVEL I: ONE-SYLLABLE WORDS BEGINNING WITH MID AND LOW VOWELS
(continued)

Mixed vowels Set 16	Mixed vowels Set 19	Mixed vowels Set 22	Mixed vowels Set 25	Mixed vowels Set 28
1. ugh	1. an	1. aired	1. oars	1. un-
2. act	2. age	2. a	2. awed	2. aunt
3. aped	3. elm	3. owe	3. us	3. aimed
4. ebb	4. off	4. all	4. Ann's	4. air
5. arms	5. oath	5. uh	5. aches	5. odd
6. oaf	6. auk	6. ask	6. egged	6. owes
7. alms	7. um	7. ape	7. art	7. awl
8. up	8. and	8. ebbed	8. oats	8. ups
9. ad	9. aid	9. arch	9. ought	9. ax
10. Abe	10. else	10. own	10. ughs	10. apes

Mixed vowels Set 17	Mixed vowels Set 20	Mixed vowels Set 23	Mixed vowels Set 26	Mixed vowels Set 29
1. Ed	1. on	1. awl	1. asked	1. ebb
2. arts	2. oh	2. of	2. ached	2. off
3. oak	3. awed	3. acts	3. errs	3. owns
4. all	4. un-	4. ate	4. arched	4. awe
5. us	5. Ann	5. edged	5. oaths	5. uh
6. Al	6. ail	6. are	6. off	6. abs
7. ace	7. err	7. oafs	7. ump	7. eights
8. edge	8. ought	8. awe	8. asks	8. Ed
9. odd	9. old	9. ugh	9. aids	9. on
10. oar	10. off	10. ads	10. etched	10. ohms

Mixed vowels Set 18	Mixed vowels Set 21	Mixed vowels Set 24	Mixed vowels Set 27	Mixed vowels Set 30
1. awl	1. ups	1. eight	1. arms	1. auk
2. poll	2. as	2. eggs	2. ohs	2. of
3. ughs	3. aim	3. aren't	3. alms	3. act
4. am	4. etch	4. oaks	4. um	4. Abe
5. ache	5. Oz	5. auk	5. at	5. edge
6. egg	6. or	6. up	6. ailed	6. Oz
7. odds	7. alms	7. Al's	7. el	7. oast
8. oat	8. upped	8. aide	8. arts	8. awed
9. awe	9. ash	9. elms	9. Olds	9. ugh
10. ump	10. ale	10. arms	10. all	10. ad

APPENDIX G: PRACTICE STIMULI, RESTRICTED PHONETIC CONTEXT

For use during
- Injection method for sonorants and vowels in esophageal speech
- Inhalation method in esophageal speech

LEVEL II: ONE-SYLLABLE WORDS BEGINNING WITH OTHER VOWELS
- Vowels /u/, /ʊ/, /ɝ/, /i/, /ɪ/, /aɪ/, /aʊ/, and /ɔɪ/

Mixed vowels Set 1	Mixed vowels Set 4	Mixed vowels Set 7	Mixed vowels Set 10	Mixed vowels Set 13
1. ooze	1. oust	1. eke	1. oomph	1. oiled
2. oops	2. oinks	2. eared	2. ergs	2. ooze
3. earl	3. ooze	3. ire	3. eeks	3. oomph
4. each	4. oops	4. ousts	4. ears	4. irked
5. ear	5. urn	5. oink	5. iced	5. each
6. aisle	6. eek	6. oozed	6. ounce	6. its
7. ouch	7. ill	7. oops	7. oinked	7. eyes
8. oil	8. ice	8. urns	8. ooze	8. owl
9. oozed	9. out	9. eased	9. oops	9. oinks
10. oomph	10. oils	10. is	10. Irv	10. oozed

Mixed vowels Set 2	Mixed vowels Set 5	Mixed vowels Set 8	Mixed vowels Set 11	Mixed vowels Set 14
1. earn	1. oozed	1. aisles	1. eve	1. oops
2. ease	2. oomph	2. outs	2. ifs	2. Earl
3. ick	3. Earp	3. oiled	3. ires	3. ease
4. eyes	4. eel	4. ooh'd	4. our	4. itched
5. ounce	5. off	5. oomph	5. oil	5. I
6. oink	6. imp	6. Earps	6. oozed	6. ours
7. ooze	7. Ike	7. eels	7. oomph	7. oils
8. oops	8. owl	8. it	8. Erse	8. ooh'd
9. earth	9. oinked	9. I'm	9. eked	9. oomph
10. east	10. ooh'd	10. owls	10. imps	10. earn

Mixed vowels Set 3	Mixed vowels Set 6	Mixed vowels Set 9	Mixed vowels Set 12	Mixed vowels Set 15
1. id	1. oops	1. oinks	1. I've	1. East
2. I	2. Earl's	2. ooze	2. oust	2. inch
3. our	3. eve	3. oops	3. oink	3. I'd
4. oiled	4. in	4. irk	4. ooh'd	4. ousts
5. oozed	5. I'll	5. eats	5. oops	5. oinked
6. oomph	6. ours	6. itch	6. Ernst	6. ooze
7. urge	7. oil	7. eye	7. eaves	7. oops
8. eat	8. ooze	8. ouch	8. inns	8. Earth
9. if	9. oomph	9. oils	9. aisle	9. eat
10. I'd	10. urged	10. oozed	10. out	10. ear

APPENDIX G: PRACTICE STIMULI, RESTRICTED PHONETIC CONTEXT

For use during
- Injection method for sonorants and vowels in esophageal speech
- Inhalation method in esophageal speech

LEVEL III: ONE-SYLLABLE WORDS BEGINNING WITH SONORANTS PLUS MID AND LOW VOWELS

- Sonorants /w/, /l/, /r/, /j/, /m/, and /n/ (Note: No words begin with /ng/)
- Mid and low vowels /ɑ/, /o/, /ɔ/, /ʌ/, /æ/, /e/, and /ɛ/

/w/ words Set 1	/l/ words Set 1	/r/ words Set 1	/j/ words Set 1	/m/ words Set 1
1. wad	1. large	1. rob	1. yacht	1. mall
2. wore	2. lone	2. road	2. York	2. moan
3. wasp	3. launch	3. raw	3. yaw	3. Maude
4. once	4. love	4. rough	4. young	4. much
5. wag	5. lab	5. rat	5. yak	5. Mack
6. wade	6. lace	6. raise	6. Yale	6. made
7. ware	7. lair	7. wreck	7. yells	7. mare
8. walk	8. lock	8. rock	8. yard	8. march
9. wove	9. loaf	9. roast	9. yoke	9. most
10. wharf	10. law	10. wrong	10. yawn	10. maul

/w/ words Set 2	/l/ words Set 2	/r/ words Set 2	/j/ words Set 2	/m/ words Set 2
1. was	1. luck	1. rush	1. yum	1. must
2. whack	2. lamb	2. wrap	2. yams	2. man
3. wage	3. lake	3. raid	3. Yank	3. make
4. wealth	4. less	4. rest	4. yes	4. mess
5. want	5. long	5. Ron	5. yarn	5. mom
6. woke	6. lore	6. rode	6. your	6. more
7. war	7. lawn	7. raw	7. y'all	7. mauve
8. one	8. lunch	8. rug	8. yuck	8. mud
9. wham	9. last	9. rack	9. yap	9. mask
10. waist	10. late	10. rain	10. Yale	10. mail

/w/ words Set 3	/l/ words Set 3	/r/ words Set 3	/j/ words Set 3	/m/ words Set 3
1. west	1. left	1. rare	1. yet	1. met
2. wash	2. lost	2. rot	2. yachts	2. mop
3. won't	3. load	3. rose	3. yokes	3. mow
4. wart	4. launched	4. wronged	4. yawl	4. Maude's
5. won	5. lung	5. rust	5. young	5. mug
6. wag	6. land	6. ran	6. yaks	6. match
7. weight	7. lane	7. race	7. yanked	7. may
8. went	8. let	8. wrench	8. yell	8. mesh
9. watch	9. loss	9. rod	9. yards	9. Mars
10. woe	10. low	10. rope	10. yours	10. mole

APPENDIX G: PRACTICE STIMULI, RESTRICTED PHONETIC CONTEXT

For use during
- Injection method for sonorants and vowels in esophageal speech
- Inhalation method in esophageal speech

LEVEL III: ONE-SYLLABLE WORDS BEGINNING WITH SONORANTS PLUS MID AND LOW VOWELS (continued)

/n/ words Set 1	Mixed sonorants Set 1	Mixed sonorants Set 4	Mixed sonorants Set 7	Mixed sonorants Set 10
1. knob	1. wad	1. west	1. waist	1. wharf
2. nope	2. lone	2. lost	2. luck	2. large
3. naught	3. raw	3. rose	3. wrap	3. road
4. none	4. young	4. yawl	4. Yank	4. yaw
5. nap	5. Mack	5. mug	5. mess	5. much
6. nail	6. nail	6. nabbed	6. knock	6. nap
7. nest	7. war	7. ware	7. wag	7. woke
8. not	8. lunch	8. lock	8. lane	8. lawn
9. know	9. rack	9. roast	9. wrench	9. rug
10. nosh	10. Yale	10. yawn	10. yards	10. yap

/n/ words Set 2	Mixed sonorants Set 2	Mixed sonorants Set 5	Mixed sonorants Set 8	Mixed sonorants Set 11
1. numb	1. must	1. maul	1. mole	1. mail
2. nagged	2. nagged	2. knob	2. net	2. numb
3. name	3. won't	3. whack	3. wore	3. wash
4. neck	4. launched	4. lake	4. launch	4. load
5. knock	5. rust	5. rest	5. rough	5. wronged
6. nose	6. yaks	6. yarn	6. yak	6. young
7. naught	7. may	7. more	7. made	7. match
8. nudge	8. nest	8. naught	8. nest	8. names
9. gnat	9. wove	9. went	9. one	9. walk
10. nailed	10. law	10. loss	10. last	10. loaf

/n/ words Set 3	Mixed sonorants Set 3	Mixed sonorants Set 6	Mixed sonorants Set 9	Mixed sonorants Set 12
1. net	1. rob	1. rope	1. rain	1. wrong
2. notch	2. York	2. yet	2. yum	2. yacht
3. known	3. Maude	3. mop	3. man	3. moan
4. nog	4. none	4. known	4. name	4. naught
5. nuts	5. want	5. once	5. wart	5. wealth
6. nabbed	6. lore	6. lab	6. lung	6. long
7. names	7. raw	7. raise	7. ran	7. rode
8. nests	8. yuck	8. yells	8. yanked	8. y'all
9. knot	9. mask	9. march	9. mesh	9. mud
10. note	10. nailed	10. no	10. knot	10. gnat

APPENDIX G: PRACTICE STIMULI, RESTRICTED PHONETIC CONTEXT

For use during
- **Injection method for sonorants and vowels in esophageal speech**
- **Inhalation method in esophageal speech**

LEVEL III: ONE-SYLLABLE WORDS BEGINNING WITH SONORANTS PLUS MID AND LOW VOWELS *(continued)*

Mixed sonorants Set 13	*Mixed sonorants Set 16*	*Mixed sonorants Set 19*	*Mixed sonorants Set 22*	*Mixed sonorants Set 25*
1. woe	1. was	1. wall	1. wet	1. way
2. left	2. lamb	2. loathe	2. lodge	2. lush
3. rot	3. raid	3. raw	3. wrote	3. razz
4. yokes	4. yes	4. young	4. yawp	4. Yank
5. Maude's	5. mom	5. mad	5. muff	5. men
6. nuts	6. nose	6. nails	6. nabbed	6. knocked
7. wade	7. won	7. warred	7. where	7. wag
8. lair	8. land	8. lump	8. log	8. laid
9. rock	9. race	9. rag	9. roar	9. retch
10. yoke	10. yell	10. Yale	10. yawn	10. yards

Mixed sonorants Set 14	*Mixed sonorants Set 17*	*Mixed sonorants Set 20*	*Mixed sonorants Set 23*	*Mixed sonorants Set 26*
1. most	1. Mars	1. muck	1. maul	1. mode
2. nope	2. note	2. knack	2. nod	2. Ned
3. wage	3. wasp	3. won't	3. whack	3. wore
4. less	4. love	4. launched	4. lame	4. launch
5. Ron	5. rat	5. rub	5. red	5. run
6. your	6. Yale	6. yap	6. yarn	6. yak
7. mauve	7. mall	7. main	7. mope	7. mate
8. nudge	8. not	8. Nell	8. naught	8. nets
9. watch	9. wham	9. wove	9. wedge	9. one
10. low	10. late	10. laws	10. lard	10. lamp

Mixed sonorants Set 15	*Mixed sonorants Set 18*	*Mixed sonorants Set 21*	*Mixed sonorants Set 24*	*Mixed sonorants Set 27*
1. rare	1. rush	1. robbed	1. roll	1. rate
2. yachts	2. yams	2. York	2. yet	2. yum
3. mow	3. make	3. mauve	3. mock	3. mash
4. nog	4. neck	4. nub	4. knoll	4. name
5. wag	5. weight	5. warn	5. once	5. wart
6. lace	6. let	6. lobe	6. latch	6. lust
7. wreck	7. rod	7. raw	7. rake	7. rash
8. yard	8. yours	8. yuck	8. yells	8. yanked
9. mare	9. met	9. map	9. Mark	9. med
10. nosh	10. notch	10. nailed	10. notes	10. notched

APPENDIX G: PRACTICE STIMULI, RESTRICTED PHONETIC CONTEXT

For use during
- Injection method for sonorants and vowels in esophageal speech
- Inhalation method in esophageal speech

LEVEL IV: ONE-SYLLABLE WORDS BEGINNING WITH SONORANTS PLUS OTHER VOWELS

- Sonorants /w/, /l/, /r/, /j/, /m/, and /n/
- Vowels /u/, /ʊ/, /ɝ/, /i/, /ɪ/, /aɪ/, /aʊ/, and /ɔɪ/

/w/ words Set 1	/l/ words Set 1	/r/ words Set 1	/j/ words Set 1	/m/ words Set 1
1. wounds	1. lewd	1. roof	1. uke	1. move
2. wolf	2. look	2. rook	2. you'll	2. meek
3. were	3. learn	3. rhyme	3. yearned	3. merge
4. we	4. lead	4. reach	4. yeast	4. me
5. which	5. lick	5. rear	5. year	5. mill
6. while	6. light	6. ripe	6. yikes	6. mice
7. wow	7. loud	7. round	7. yowl	7. mound
8. whiff	8. Lloyd	8. Roy	8. you're	8. moist
9. whoosh	9. loose	9. room	9. use	9. mood
10. wood	10. looked	10. root	10. yeek	10. meet

/w/ words Set 2	/l/ words Set 2	/r/ words Set 2	/j/ words Set 2	/m/ words Set 2
1. weren't	1. lurch	1. rice	1. yearns	1. Merv's
2. weed	2. league	2. ring	2. yeeks	2. meal
3. whim	3. lift	3. rich	3. yip	3. miss
4. whine	4. lied	4. rise	4. yipes	4. mile
5. we'll	5. lounge	5. rouse	5. you've	5. mouse
6. whip	6. loin	6. royal	6. years	6. moist
7. wound	7. lure	7. roost	7. you	7. ming
8. woods	8. looks	8. rooks	8. yule	8. moon
9. whirl	9. lurk	9. ride	9. yearn	9. Mick
10. we're	10. leaves	10. read	10. yield	10. mirth

/w/ words Set 3	/l/ words Set 3	/r/ words Set 3	/j/ words Set 3	/m/ words Set 3
1. whisk	1. list	1. ridge	1. years	1. mean
2. white	2. life	2. write	2. yikes	2. myth
3. weed	3. louse	3. roust	3. yowl	3. mine
4. wince	4. loyal	4. Royce	4. Ute	4. mouth
5. word	5. loop	5. route	5. used	5. mist
6. woof	6. look	6. rook	6. youth	6. moose
7. work	7. learned	7. right	7. you'd	7. might
8. wheat	8. least	8. real	8. yearned	8. Merle
9. wing	9. limp	9. rip	9. yeasts	9. meat
10. wipe	10. like	10. rind	10. yipped	10. mid

APPENDIX G: PRACTICE STIMULI, RESTRICTED PHONETIC CONTEXT

For use during
- Injection method for sonorants and vowels in esophageal speech
- Inhalation method in esophageal speech

LEVEL IV: ONE-SYLLABLE WORDS BEGINNING WITH SONORANTS PLUS OTHER VOWELS *(continued)*

/n/ words Set 1	Mixed sonorants Set 1	Mixed sonorants Set 4	Mixed sonorants Set 7	Mixed sonorants Set 10
1. new	1. wounds	1. wipe	1. we're	1. wood
2. nook	2. look	2. list	2. lurch	2. lewd
3. nerve	3. rhyme	3. write	3. ring	3. rook
4. knead	4. yeast	4. yowl	4. yip	4. yearned
5. knit	5. mill	5. mouth	5. mile	5. me
6. knife	6. knife	6. news	6. now	6. knit
7. noun	7. wound	7. while	7. woof	7. whip
8. noise	8. looks	8. loud	8. learned	8. lure
9. nude	9. ride	9. Roy	9. real	9. rooks
10. kneel	10. yield	10. use	10. yeasts	10. yearn

/n/ words Set 2	Mixed sonorants Set 2	Mixed sonorants Set 5	Mixed sonorants Set 8	Mixed sonorants Set 11
1. nurse	1. Merv's	1. meet	1. mid	1. mirth
2. knee	2. knee	2. new	2. niche	2. nurse
3. near	3. white	3. weed	3. wolf	3. whisk
4. nice	4. louse	4. lift	4. learn	4. life
5. now	5. Royce	5. rise	5. reach	5. roust
6. Nick	6. used	6. you've	6. year	6. Ute
7. noon	7. moose	7. moist	7. mice	7. mist
8. niece	8. nerves	8. noon	8. noun	8. noose
9. nerd	9. whiff	9. wheat	9. woods	9. wow
10. neat	10. loose	10. limp	10. lurk	10. Lloyd

/n/ words Set 3	Mixed sonorants Set 3	Mixed sonorants Set 6	Mixed sonorants Set 9	Mixed sonorants Set 12
1. niche	1. root	1. rind	1. read	1. room
2. night	2. uke	2. years	2. yearns	2. yeek
3. nouns	3. meek	3. myth	3. meal	3. move
4. noise	4. nerve	4. nouns	4. near	4. nook
5. news	5. whine	5. we	5. wince	5. whim
6. noose	6. lounge	6. lick	6. loop	6. lied
7. nerves	7. royal	7. ripe	7. rook	7. rouse
8. need	8. you	8. yowl	8. you'd	8. years
9. nip	9. moon	9. moist	9. Merle	9. ming
10. nine	10. nerd	10. nude	10. nip	10. niece

APPENDIX G: PRACTICE STIMULI, RESTRICTED PHONETIC CONTEXT

For use during
- Injection method for sonorants and vowels in esophageal speech
- Inhalation method in esophageal speech

LEVEL IV: ONE-SYLLABLE WORDS BEGINNING WITH SONORANTS PLUS OTHER VOWELS *(continued)*

Mixed sonorants Set 13	*Mixed sonorants Set 16*	*Mixed sonorants Set 19*	*Mixed sonorants Set 22*	*Mixed sonorants Set 25*
1. wing	1. whirl	1. wounds	1. wife	1. weave
2. like	2. leaves	2. look	2. lint	2. lurched
3. ridge	3. rice	3. rhyme	3. rye	3. wreath
4. yikes	4. yeeks	4. yeast	4. yowl	4. yip
5. mine	5. miss	5. mill	5. mouthed	5. mime
6. noise	6. nice	6. knife	6. nuke	6. now
7. which	7. word	7. wound	7. why	7. wool
8. light	8. look	8. looks	8. loud	8. learned
9. round	9. right	9. ride	9. Roy's	9. reap
10. you're	10. yearned	10. yield	10. used	10. yeasts

Mixed sonorants Set 14	*Mixed sonorants Set 17*	*Mixed sonorants Set 20*	*Mixed sonorants Set 23*	*Mixed sonorants Set 26*
1. mood	1. meat	1. Merv's	1. meet	1. mitt
2. kneel	2. nine	2. knee	2. newt	2. nil
3. weren't	3. whoosh	3. white	3. week	3. would
4. league	4. looked	4. louse	4. lid	4. learns
5. rich	5. roof	5. Royce	5. rile	5. reed
6. yipes	6. you'll	6. used	6. you've	6. year
7. mouse	7. merge	7. moose	7. moist	7. mite
8. Nick	8. knead	8. nerves	8. noon	8. noun
9. work	9. we'll	9. whiff	9. wheel	9. wolves
10. least	10. loin	10. loose	10. lip	10. lurked

Mixed sonorants Set 15	*Mixed sonorants Set 18*	*Mixed sonorants Set 21*	*Mixed sonorants Set 24*	*Mixed sonorants Set 27*
1. rip	1. roost	1. root	1. writhe	1. wring
2. yipped	2. yule	2. uke	2. years	2. yearns
3. mean	3. Mick	3. meek	3. Mitch	3. meals
4. night	4. neat	4. nerve	4. nouns	4. nears
5. were	5. weed	5. whine	5. wheeze	5. weird
6. lead	6. loyal	6. lounge	6. limb	6. loot
7. rear	7. route	7. royal	7. rife	7. rooks
8. yikes	8. youth	8. you	8. yowled	8. you'd
9. mound	9. might	9. moon	9. moist	9. merged
10. noise	10. need	10. nerd	10. noon	10. nib

APPENDIX G: PRACTICE STIMULI, RESTRICTED PHONETIC CONTEXT

For use during
- Injection method for sonorants and vowels in esophageal speech
- Inhalation method in esophageal speech

LEVEL V: TWO-SYLLABLE WORDS: SONORANTS AND VOWELS
- Sonorants and vowels occurring in the releasing position of both syllables

Set 1
1. awning
2. oolong
3. way out
4. omit
5. early
6. lay off
7. alert
8. Eli
9. really
10. Alan

Set 2
1. ear lobe
2. yawning
3. aiming
4. Eileen
5. mainline
6. air raid
7. our room
8. mail in
9. orange
10. align

Set 3
1. wary
2. only
3. ermine
4. lemon
5. amount
6. emu
7. remain
8. aloe
9. eerie
10. Eunice

Set 4
1. A-one
2. I know.
3. marriage
4. air mail
5. oil well
6. none are
7. all night
8. amuse
9. wore out
10. Owen

Set 5
1. earn it
2. Le Mans
3. around
4. Enid
5. room rates
6. an edge
7. enough
8. unit
9. annex
10. eyelash

Set 6
1. manner
2. arrow
3. owl eggs
4. no match
5. army
6. announce
7. one night
8. owner
9. urn rack
10. lone man

Set 7
1. amaze
2. eon
3. rhyming
4. Anna
5. image
6. You rang?
7. aim at
8. I will
9. money
10. errand

Set 8
1. oiler
2. numb ears
3. almost
4. awhile
5. warning
6. Oh, no!
7. earnest
8. llama
9. arrive
10. eely

Set 9
1. renew
2. Alice
3. inlaid
4. Yale man
5. ailing
6. eyelet
7. more ice
8. error
9. hour walk
10. name it

Set 10
1. are made
2. alike
3. we were
4. oral
5. earn much
6. lawyer
7. awake
8. Elaine
9. Roy was
10. an egg

Set 11
1. in use
2. unite
3. aerate
4. I won't.
5. meaning
6. Aaron
7. our eyes
8. no way
9. all out
10. unleash

Set 12
1. winner
2. ornate
3. ermine
4. Lima
5. onion
6. eland
7. rear end
8. alley
9. ill will
10. yellow

Set 13
1. emir
2. eyelid
3. minute
4. airless
5. oily
6. new moon
7. on-line
8. unwind
9. woolen
10. or else

Set 14
1. urn lost
2. Leonard
3. unwise
4. elite
5. railroad
6. Annette
7. inmate
8. union
9. a road
10. Ireland

Set 15
1. mammal
2. Arab
3. our age
4. nine hours
5. all right
6. onyx
7. Why me?
8. Oh, well.
9. Ernest
10. lament

Set 16
1. arrest
2. elapse
3. rainy
4. allied
5. elope
6. you'll need
7. in on
8. eyewash
9. minor
10. Ellen

APPENDIX G: PRACTICE STIMULI, RESTRICTED PHONETIC CONTEXT

For use during
- Injection method for sonorants and vowels in esophageal speech
- Inhalation method in esophageal speech

LEVEL V: TWO-SYLLABLE WORDS: SONORANTS AND VOWELS (continued)

Set 17
1. our all
2. no one
3. olive
4. aware
5. worry
6. own name
7. earn wealth
8. lonely
9. among
10. erase

Set 18
1. rare meat
2. Alma
3. earache
4. yummy
5. elude
6. iris
7. mail run
8. enroll
9. owl mess
10. now look

Set 19
1. on one
2. amend
3. whaler
4. omen
5. earnings
6. Leon
7. alarm
8. eeler
9. ran on
10. Alan's

Set 20
1. emerge
2. You're out.
3. earring
4. iron works
5. more air
6. enrich
7. our lunch
8. near miss
9. aura
10. allow

Set 21
1. well-known
2. orate
3. Earl rode.
4. limit
5. arrange
6. emit
7. real men
8. ally
9. erect
10. Europe

Set 22
1. immense
2. Irene
3. may rain
4. enrage
5. oil wars
6. gnaw loose
7. almond
8. annoy
9. one more
10. owing

Set 23
1. early
2. lu-lu
3. award
4. erupt
5. railway
6. Anna's
7. erode
8. yell out
9. inland
10. I woke.

Set 24
1. mower
2. enlarge
3. owl young
4. Know me?
5. onward
6. along
7. woman
8. omits
9. Irwin
10. lurid

Set 25
1. alone
2. elate
3. run off
4. alleys
5. in-law
6. You're right.
7. inning
8. Irish
9. marry
10. arid

Set 26
1. hour ride
2. none known
3. armrest
4. arise
5. wallet
6. onus
7. ermine
8. lion
9. away
10. elect

Set 27
1. Ron ran.
2. allies
3. inner
4. yo-yo
5. airy
6. I made
7. mail man
8. any
9. our mom
10. Nan read.

Set 28
1. awning
2. align
3. wore out
4. owner
5. earnest
6. lawyer
7. onion
8. elapse
9. rare meat
10. Alan

Set 29
1. erect
2. yell out
3. inning
4. I made
5. way out
6. only
7. earn it
8. lone man
9. arrive
10. Elaine

Set 30
1. rear end
2. allied
3. earache
4. You're out.
5. immense
6. awoke
7. marry
8. any
9. alert
10. emu

Set 31
1. room rates
2. Anna
3. inlaid
4. unite
5. emir
6. eyewash
7. mail run
8. enrich
9. oil wars
10. normal

Set 32
1. aiming
2. I know.
3. manner
4. errand
5. our eyes
6. no way
7. all out
8. onyx
9. worry
10. lemon

APPENDIX G: PRACTICE STIMULI, RESTRICTED PHONETIC CONTEXT

For use during
- Injection method for sonorants and vowels in esophageal speech
- Inhalation method in esophageal speech

LEVEL VI: THREE- TO FOUR-SYLLABLE PHRASES AND SENTENCES: SONORANTS AND VOWELS

- Sonorants and vowels occurring in the releasing positions of syllables

Set 1
1. A roan mare neighed.
2. early alarm
3. hour on hour
4. I'm all out.
5. lanolin
6. Many are nice.
7. None are known.
8. on a walk
9. roll away
10. unaware

Set 2
1. wary ermine
2. Who are you?
3. You were wrong.
4. a minor wound
5. Earn more money.
6. IOU
7. Know your weight.
8. lemon ice
9. new wire wheels
10. real lemons

Set 3
1. Ohio
2. ran a mile
3. union railroad
4. will run our lives
5. yellow awning
6. a well-known law
7. army ant
8. emulate
9. I'll mail it.
10. Lie in wait.

Set 4
1. Marry Elaine.
2. No one ran.
3. our noon meal
4. rare moment
5. wallaroo
6. You were right.
7. airiness
8. emery
9. immoral
10. lemon yellow

Set 5
1. à la mode
2. eliminate
3. I am ill.
4. knew no one
5. lemonade
6. Name your lamb.
7. memory lane
8. remain in Europe
9. none in our eyes
10. unroll a map

Set 6
1. Renew your will.
2. yearly raise
3. a lame leg
4. all right
5. enormous
6. I am married.
7. lariat
8. Many are rude.
9. no rhyme or rule
10. unerring

Set 7
1. We are alone.
2. yell or roar
3. Align my wheels.
4. Are you armed?
5. Eleanor
6. I am well.
7. lawn mower
8. may win a role
9. No, I won't.
10. oriole nest

Set 8
1. ran an ad
2. unruly
3. Where are you?
4. yellow onion
5. almanac
6. element
7. I am warm.
8. Learn all your lines.
9. more aware
10. no way out

APPENDIX G: PRACTICE STIMULI, RESTRICTED PHONETIC CONTEXT

For use during
- Injection method for sonorants and vowels in esophageal speech
- Inhalation method in esophageal speech

LEVEL VI: THREE- TO FOUR-SYLLABLE PHRASES AND SENTENCES: SONORANTS AND VOWELS *(continued)*

Set 9
1. mirror image
2. new airline
3. None were early.
4. only one way
5. roll along
6. unwary mole
7. We will write.
8. You are right.
9. alleyway
10. early or late

Set 10
1. I'm in all year.
2. limerick
3. minor error
4. No one knows.
5. orient
6. raw onion
7. We're early.
8. You're a woman.
9. all around
10. emerald

Set 11
1. I mean it!
2. lemon or lime
3. mom or me
4. no way out
5. on a roll
6. remain loyal
7. well-mannered man
8. You are mine.
9. a rainy year
10. enrollment

Set 12
1. ill or well
2. lemon oil
3. more alike
4. None was amused.
5. on your own
6. Renew your oath.
7. unknown winner
8. Were you worried?
9. You're willing?
10. all in one

Set 13
1. oleo
2. rain on me
3. unwilling
4. weenie roast
5. yell aloud
6. Alan laughed.
7. Eloise
8. ill-mannered
9. Lie awake.
10. Men unite!

Set 14
1. neon lights
2. one on one
3. really early
4. unanimous
5. We were worn out.
6. You are my wife.
7. Am I awake?
8. Eileen enrolled.
9. Illinois
10. linoleum

Set 15
1. money winner
2. None remain.
3. on a railway
4. really low
5. when men roam
6. yellow lab
7. an earache
8. enamored
9. in a minute
10. Lean on me.

Set 16
1. Men are mammals.
2. None was early.
3. on all airlines
4. run away
5. unerring mom
6. well-meaning
7. yellow yams
8. a lion roar
9. Eileen wheezed.
10. I will lie low.

APPENDIX G: PRACTICE STIMULI, RESTRICTED PHONETIC CONTEXT

For use during
- Injection method for sonorants and vowels in esophageal speech
- Inhalation method in esophageal speech

LEVEL VI: THREE- TO FOUR-SYLLABLE PHRASES AND SENTENCES: SONORANTS AND VOWELS (*continued*)

Set 17
1. enema
2. I'm unarmed.
3. known in Rio
4. lily white
5. my yearnings
6. new meal menus
7. only worn once
8. really awake
9. unearth nine urns
10. will whinny

Set 18
1. year around
2. aluminum
3. Eliot knew.
4. I will unload.
5. lineage
6. my rare rock
7. near our woods
8. one more minute
9. run along
10. when you whine

Set 19
1. yowling wolves
2. Alamo
3. early up
4. I will ride.
5. lie awhile
6. main name list
7. nine new menus
8. only one
9. rain alert
10. unruly

Set 20
1. well-mannered
2. year-round lake
3. All were late.
4. enamel
5. I will race.
6. Lean on Maude.
7. more lemonade
8. Nell worked nights.
9. oily wharf
10. run errands

Set 21
1. lenient
2. many errands
3. new moon image
4. ornament
5. rhyming nouns
6. unused meat
7. wire wheels
8. You'll learn more.
9. aerial
10. enemy land

Set 22
1. I am alone.
2. Learn Ute lore.
3. mine or yours
4. new knee lifts
5. only one hour
6. roam all night
7. unaware
8. win an Emmy
9. Y'all lost?
10. am willing

Set 23
1. area rug
2. eerie knock
3. I am wronged.
4. Loan me money.
5. minor war
6. no more wolves
7. on our yacht
8. Write new lists.
9. Who worries?
10. yellow lemons

Set 24
1. Any more milk?
2. Eliminate nuts.
3. I will roast.
4. lunar launch
5. many mice
6. no warning
7. oral news
8. rare woman
9. unwilling
10. Where else?

APPENDIX G: PRACTICE STIMULI, RESTRICTED PHONETIC CONTEXT

For use during
- Injection method for sonorants and vowels in esophageal speech
- Inhalation method in esophageal speech

LEVEL VI: THREE- TO FOUR-SYLLABLE PHRASES AND SENTENCES: SONORANTS AND VOWELS (continued)

Set 25
1. Where will we meet?
2. Use my knife.
3. animal
4. enemy
5. I am washed.
6. lie in need
7. many walk
8. Name your niece.
9. oil well wealth
10. run enough

Set 26
1. We are lonely.
2. yearly rains
3. a whole onion
4. early image
5. in May or March
6. lowermost
7. move my lunch
8. No one knew.
9. Orion
10. run away

Set 27
1. unwary moose
2. woolen rug
3. yell or roar
4. Are we alike?
5. Eleanor wept.
6. in our lives
7. Lean on Mack.
8. Marry in May.
9. No one yawned.
10. rare onyx

Set 28
1. Our mare neighed.
2. enumerate
3. an hour early
4. I am not!
5. lone man running
6. more moist
7. None were known.
8. on a lark
9. roll in nuts
10. unearned money

Set 29
1. You're really late.
2. Are you yawning?
3. Earn your way out.
4. in a rush
5. lone mailman
6. money made
7. neon lights
8. on-line news
9. royal march
10. union railroad

Set 30
1. Women unite!
2. yell aloud
3. alumni
4. early art
5. I am wrong.
6. lioness
7. Meet now or noon?
8. No, I went.
9. Owen lied.
10. running on

Set 31
1. while rhyming
2. a mile away
3. Eliot
4. I am awake.
5. loan you my watch
6. mail my mom
7. annual rains
8. in your room
9. wire rimmed wheels
10. your army

Set 32
1. à la mode
2. eminent
3. Iowa lambs
4. knew nine women
5. lone warrior
6. nail in once
7. memory loss
8. Remain in York.
9. nine, in our minds
10. unroll a rug

APPENDIX G: PRACTICE STIMULI, RESTRICTED PHONETIC CONTEXT

For use during • **Injection method for sonorants and vowels in esophageal speech**
• **Inhalation method in esophageal speech**

LEVEL VI: THREE- TO FOUR-SYLLABLE PHRASES AND SENTENCES: SONORANTS AND VOWELS *(continued)*

Set 33
1. wooly lamb
2. Worm your way in.
3. You were late.
4. airless room
5. Earn your lunch.
6. in our yard
7. nine-naught-nine
8. lunar ice
9. new main line
10. real orange

Set 34
1. a large reward
2. e-mail your work
3. Iowa
4. lowermost
5. monologue
6. only one rinse
7. rural railroad
8. Were we early?
9. You've met my mom.
10. menial work

Set 35
1. new in-laws
2. rain run-off
3. When will you learn?
4. your worst nightmare
5. a well-known league
6. Earn one or more.
7. in name only
8. lean, mean mule
9. Mark my words.
10. on all wounds

Set 36
1. nine-year-old
2. owe or own
3. unwise remark
4. will weigh more
5. all alone
6. earned more money
7. loudmouth liar
8. mineral oil
9. ornate mummy
10. well-meaning nurse

Set 37
1. Renew room rates.
2. year-end rush
3. all or none
4. arena
5. emollient
6. irony
7. loyalist
8. more money
9. no rule on winning
10. up near us

Set 38
1. when Lonnie laughed
2. an hour or more
3. eerie mirage
4. I won't marry.
5. large monument
6. man who owes rent
7. narrow road
8. once released
9. royal eye wear
10. We are all out.

Set 39
1. young romance
2. a million eggs
3. elated mood
4. lame Mayan
5. meet my needs
6. on-line remark
7. reap my reward
8. Why will you miss?
9. Are we allies?
10. I will manage.

Set 40
1. late night arrests
2. Mail in your names.
3. one moose limit
4. renew or else
5. Watch reruns.
6. ammonia
7. early morning
8. immense melon
9. linear
10. You are low ranked.

APPENDIX G: PRACTICE STIMULI, RESTRICTED PHONETIC CONTEXT

For use during
- Injection method for sonorants and vowels in esophageal speech
- Inhalation method in esophageal speech

LEVEL VI: THREE- TO FOUR-SYLLABLE PHRASES AND SENTENCES: SONORANTS AND VOWELS *(continued)*

Set 41
1. a merit raise
2. early release
3. in our room
4. Lenny yawned.
5. minelayer
6. no ill will meant
7. runny eggs
8. Where are our meals?
9. all night long
10. enumerate

Set 42
1. Learn my name.
2. manly yell
3. neon orange
4. Roman army
5. Were you asked?
6. any age
7. illuminate
8. looked normal
9. memory loss
10. nine minors

Set 43
1. renewed marriage
2. Use my nine iron.
3. wooly mammoth
4. arrow released
5. lower room rates
6. minor leagues
7. run around
8. wore out my name
9. Your remarks?
10. all I need

Set 44
1. lowland mammals
2. main menu
3. no one munched
4. Roman relic
5. Women are near.
6. anymore
7. mail room layoffs
8. mourn Aunt Mary
9. We will wait.
10. area rug

Set 45
1. annual rematch
2. I will relax.
3. Learn all nine rules.
4. Mars mania
5. nary a moose
6. raw remark
7. Were you ill?
8. Wyoming
9. any more rain
10. imminent

Set 46
1. lost memo
2. minimum wage
3. ran a mile
4. wary mermaid
5. wore a ring
6. Are you warm?
7. in or out
8. lunar month
9. minus nine minutes
10. rare emeralds

Set 47
1. war relic
2. Were you in Maine?
3. anywhere
4. lone male inmate
5. Mel raised lambs.
6. No one will wait.
7. roaming nomads
8. wrong yacht launched
9. alimony
10. early remarks

Set 48
1. lowly mouse
2. mirror image
3. no one remains
4. rural ranch
5. will weigh less
6. analyze
7. mellow yellow
8. When will we learn?
9. enemy lines
10. I owe Ernest.

APPENDIX G: PRACTICE STIMULI, RESTRICTED PHONETIC CONTEXT

For use during
- Injection method for sonorants and vowels in esophageal speech
- Inhalation method in esophageal speech

LEVEL VII: FIVE- TO SIX-SYLLABLE PHRASES AND SENTENCES: SONORANTS AND VOWELS

- Sonorants and vowels occur in the releasing positions of syllables

Set 1
1. a lenient nun
2. Elaine will run our lives.
3. Know your enemies.
4. Loan me your lawn mower.
5. My mare will whinny.
6. on area rugs
7. really low on money
8. way out maniac
9. You are in an army.
10. Amelia Earhart

Set 2
1. early one morning
2. in a rare moment
3. Lenny wore orange.
4. moonlit night means romance
5. rich Roman ruins
6. We remain loyal.
7. You must remind me.
8. any way you earn it
9. I am a loner.
10. Lower our limit.

Set 3
1. Miller annoyed Mack.
2. not many relics
3. Our mule ran away
4. union railroad man
5. Were any men maimed?
6. an early lawn mower
7. enemy alert
8. Leonard married Molly.
9. money in my wallet
10. Norway or Ireland

Set 4
1. only one monarch
2. raw onion on a roast
3. Women wear a ring.
4. Annoy Eleanor.
5. in an alleyway
6. lemon or lime oil
7. mirror on a wall
8. noon meal on a ranch
9. Read my manual.
10. We meant no malice.

Set 5
1. e-mail anywhere
2. Illinois laws
3. lemon marinade
4. minus neon lights
5. numerous remarks
6. Owen or Leonard?
7. Ron may win an award.
8. When I'm lonely, I walk.
9. Airlines rely on you.
10. layer on layer

Set 6
1. Merv won't manage long.
2. nine-minute monologue
3. only a minor
4. Relate your yearnings.
5. warm rain on my nose
6. yellow Halloween moon
7. Aaron ran a mile.
8. Elaine knew our mom well.
9. llama in Lima
10. minor error in math

Set 7
1. nightmare at midnight
2. Only enroll once.
3. roam an area
4. We are more aware.
5. You are my main man.
6. Aim at renewal.
7. I owe you a meal.
8. mailman on a route
9. No way are you early!
10. old Mayor Miller

Set 8
1. war memorial
2. yellow runny eggs
3. a well-known airline
4. early morning noise
5. know my enemy
6. Mary wore an ermine.
7. nearly won a race
8. only nine more minutes
9. remained monarch nine years
10. Wean a wooly lamb.

APPENDIX G: PRACTICE STIMULI, RESTRICTED PHONETIC CONTEXT

For use during
- Injection method for sonorants and vowels in esophageal speech
- Inhalation method in esophageal speech

LEVEL VII: FIVE- TO SIX-SYLLABLE PHRASES AND SENTENCES: SONORANTS AND VOWELS (*continued*)

Set 9
1. An airline ran an ad.
2. eerie Halloween moon
3. Loan Ron your mower.
4. my mirror or yours
5. oil well in Omaha
6. warrior ran away
7. You'll need nine more wheels.
8. Alan may row alone.
9. I knew all along.
10. Many men are married.

Set 10
1. Nell won an award.
2. only one way out
3. Warn your airmen away!
4. You've met my in-laws.
5. annual winner
6. lemon yellow awning
7. mild-mannered Lola
8. No one knew our name.
9. We knew we were early.
10. Am I in Wyoming?

Set 11
1. anywhere you reach
2. early morning yawn
3. large area rug
4. many more rare whales
5. nine-year-old niece, Millie
6. old mayor Miller
7. removed minor rules
8. We are all alike.
9. You are my main man.
10. an hour or more wait

Set 12
1. earned more mad money
2. I will manage all right.
3. Know your enemy.
4. Leon knocked young romance.
5. minor error in math
6. No one knew our name.
7. owes me a large reward
8. rare royal emeralds
9. way in or way out
10. an aerial ride

Set 13
1. in only a moment
2. Linoleum will yellow.
3. many more in-laws
4. No men are allowed.
5. really in a rush
6. We will rely on you.
7. You're on your own, Louise.
8. an hour or a minute
9. Loan me your remote.
10. marooned mariner

Set 14
1. only a minnow
2. real men in our army
3. We're near a railroad.
4. a lot more rain
5. I rely on rumors.
6. Lynn ran a mile alone.
7. Mom won a new ermine.
8. We are all alike.
9. won money in rummy
10. almost memorized

Set 15
1. earned my merit raise
2. I owe you a meal.
3. lemon marinade
4. mineral oil relief
5. No one remains relaxed.
6. only one way out
7. Roy, would you wait?
8. Where are your manners?
9. yellow Halloween moon
10. A mare will whinny.

Set 16
1. eerie moonlit night
2. Ian used my nine iron.
3. Laurie raised mellow lambs.
4. mailman on a route
5. nearly won a race
6. only a minnow
7. Read my manual.
8. warm rain on my nose
9. You are in an army.
10. Aunt Mary's monument

APPENDIX G: PRACTICE STIMULI, RESTRICTED PHONETIC CONTEXT

For use during
- Injection method for sonorants and vowels in esophageal speech
- Inhalation method in esophageal speech

LEVEL VII: FIVE- TO SIX-SYLLABLE PHRASES AND SENTENCES: SONORANTS AND VOWELS *(continued)*

Set 17
1. Ernest owes me rent.
2. I ran off my legs.
3. Leanne wore a ring.
4. Many men are married.
5. nightmare at midnight
6. only nine more minutes
7. ran on narrow roads
8. war memorial
9. Why won't Mona relent?
10. Amelia's wreck lost

Set 18
1. early one morning
2. I rely on rumors.
3. Laurie meant no ill will.
4. money in my mail
5. neon orange ornament
6. only one way in
7. really in a rush
8. union railroad man
9. woman on an errand
10. Any more winners?

Set 19
1. early morning noise
2. immense yellow melons
3. lemon yellow awning
4. Men are in an army.
5. No one ran a mile.
6. only a mirage
7. Roy in Wyoming
8. When will we mourn our loss?
9. alien lunar map
10. Lorraine knew our mom well.

Set 20
1. Mark my warning words.
2. No men are allowed.
3. Only enroll once.
4. remained monarch nine years
5. warrior ran away
6. won money in rummy
7. yowling lowland wolves
8. An owl will weigh less.
9. Eliminate layoffs.
10. I am a loner.

Set 21
1. Elaine will run our lives.
2. Illinois laws
3. like roaming nomads
4. mild-mannered Lola
5. noon meal on a ranch
6. Owen or Leonard?
7. really low on money
8. We knew we were early.
9. You are all I need.
10. Are you warm enough?

Set 22
1. enemy alert
2. in only a moment
3. Loan me your remote.
4. Mom won a new ermine.
5. Norway or Ireland
6. Our mule ran away.
7. Ron may win an award.
8. Will you wear a warm muff?
9. You're on your own, Louise.
10. at least minimum wage

Set 23
1. eminent monarch
2. I knew all along.
3. llama in Lima
4. minus nine minutes
5. numerous remarks
6. raw onion on a roast
7. way out maniac
8. You must remind me.
9. annual yacht launch
10. memorized moments

Set 24
1. I won't marry Wally.
2. Merrill watched reruns.
3. not my mirror image
4. on area rugs
5. Rarely will Maude relax.
6. war memorial
7. women on our list
8. Anyway, you lied.
9. Earn one or more rewards.
10. in a rare moment

APPENDIX G: PRACTICE STIMULI, RESTRICTED PHONETIC CONTEXT

For use during
- **Injection method for sonorants and vowels in esophageal speech**
- **Inhalation method in esophageal speech**

LEVEL VII: FIVE- TO SIX-SYLLABLE PHRASES AND SENTENCES: SONORANTS AND VOWELS *(continued)*

Set 25
1. large war monument
2. midnight monologue
3. nine weary warriors
4. only a mirror
5. ran a mile with no limp
6. Warn your airmen away.
7. when you relieve Mark
8. An airline ran an ad.
9. early news release
10. I reaped my reward.

Set 26
1. know my enemy
2. My mare will whinny.
3. no, not in our room
4. Relate your yearnings.
5. We are more aware.
6. You may release Raymond.
7. Am I in Wyoming?
8. e-mail your rewrite
9. in your name only
10. lemon or lime oil

Set 27
1. Miller annoyed Mack.
2. Nell won an award.
3. Renew your will or else.
4. roam an area
5. when Anarose laughed
6. yearly almanac
7. any more airmen
8. early morning rematch
9. Iowa run off
10. Loan me your lawn mower.

Set 28
1. Merv won't manage long.
2. Name all who remain.
3. rain on our immense yard
4. We will lie low all night.
5. all alone in Norway
6. Enid, learn all nine rules.
7. Leonard married Molly.
8. marooned mariner
9. No way are you early!
10. one-way Eloise

Set 29
1. Learn our inland roads.
2. minus neon lights
3. normal memory loss
4. oil well in Omaha
5. real men in our army
6. We meant no malice.
7. yellow, runny eggs
8. a lenient nun
9. eerie Halloween moon
10. layer on layer

Set 30
1. minutemen alert
2. nine-minute monologue
3. only one monarch
4. War relics need names.
5. Win or earn money.
6. You are our relay man.
7. Amelia Earhart
8. early inmate release
9. Laurie, are you warm?
10. mirror on a wall

Set 31
1. nine arrows released
2. oily omelet
3. rich Roman ruins
4. We remain loyal.
5. Write new manuals.
6. Aaron ran a mile.
7. e-mail anywhere
8. in an alleyway
9. Lenny wore orange.
10. Marilyn Monroe

Set 32
1. not many relics
2. unerring monarch
3. rare new mineral
4. When were you last launched?
5. an early yellow moon
6. emerald lake woods
7. I am on a walk.
8. lonely wooly mammoth
9. money in a wallet
10. numerous arias

APPENDIX G: PRACTICE STIMULI, RESTRICTED PHONETIC CONTEXT

For use during
- Injection method for sonorants and vowels in esophageal speech
- Inhalation method in esophageal speech

LEVEL VII: FIVE- TO SIX-SYLLABLE PHRASES AND SENTENCES: SONORANTS AND VOWELS *(continued)*

Set 33
1. unlike minor wounds
2. really low errors
3. Wean a wooly lamb.
4. your enemy's rank
5. Al wore a yellow robe.
6. Elude marriage, not Mel!
7. I owe you my life.
8. Loan Ron your mower.
9. men or women Marines
10. No one likes relish?

Set 34
1. only one rainy year
2. Read your enrollment list.
3. Were you in Europe?
4. a million nest eggs
5. Emmy-winning rerun
6. Are we ironing lace?
7. looked normal in manner
8. Merv or Eileen will wait.
9. Noel knew no one.
10. unanimous "yes!"

Set 35
1. Reward your yearnings.
2. We're near a railroad.
3. Unload your memories.
4. alimony owed
5. Eat more Oreos.
6. I'll erase your work.
7. lower our limit
8. made late night arrests
9. no rule on winning money
10. Why aren't you enraged?

Set 36
1. We will rely on you.
2. You were always mild.
3. A whale will weigh more.
4. enlist nine enrollees
5. Illinois yell
6. Lynn ran a mile alone.
7. moonlit night means romance
8. narrow road near my ranch
9. rare orange minnows
10. Why alarm your mom?

Set 37
1. oleo on rye
2. ran a relay race
3. Where are my minerals?
4. Yes, Nan may win an iron.
5. any age you want
6. unwilling mayor
7. I am unwilling.
8. lone woman athlete
9. many more in-laws
10. new oriole nest

Set 38
1. one way on all airlines
2. Ronnie relies on you.
3. Why are you renewing?
4. a lot more rain
5. each error in math
6. Alan laughed; Max murmured.
7. loudmouthed maniac
8. Meet your worst nightmare.
9. In no way were we robbed!
10. Orion in May

Set 39
1. really low on milk
2. Why will you miss Ronald?
3. Your mule ate my rye.
4. Alan may row alone.
5. We knew we were roaming.
6. I owe you an onion.
7. Linoleum will yellow.
8. made my minnow lure
9. Nurse, relieve my aches.
10. Reap my own reward.

Set 40
1. When I'm lonely, I walk.
2. Aunt Arlene liked North Mall.
3. a lean, mean Marine
4. Elect me your mayor.
5. in an old limerick
6. Lionel was right.
7. my mirror or yours
8. Know your way around.
9. Ruth read you and me.
10. Were you really ill?

APPENDIX G: PRACTICE STIMULI, RESTRICTED PHONETIC CONTEXT

For use during
- Injection method for sonorants and vowels in esophageal speech
- Inhalation method in esophageal speech

LEVEL VII: FIVE- TO SIX-SYLLABLE PHRASES AND SENTENCES: SONORANTS AND VOWELS (continued)

Set 41
1. Win or earn money.
2. a well-known airline
3. early morning alarm
4. ill-mannered young man
5. linoleum unrolled
6. might remain all night
7. No one was released.
8. rinsed lily white lace
9. Were any men maimed?
10. annual Marine march

Set 42
1. Alamo unearthed
2. when you relieve Mark
3. Leanna worked nights.
4. In May, you are where?
5. Now I am more awake.
6. unmanned lunar launch
7. Are you warm enough?
8. Were we always rich?
9. yet Amy looked normal
10. aim at renewal

Set 43
1. well known in Yuma
2. It may rain at midnight.
3. alumni reunion
4. More men were unmasked.
5. noon winner at rummy
6. "Oops," remarked Nina.
7. Aren't you a loyalist?
8. Why rely on me?
9. Yawning won't make me end.
10. a mile on a railway

Set 44
1. Ellen will run your life.
2. Who were Iron Age men?
3. Lock your money away.
4. Must you read my mail?
5. new one-way mirror
6. one-on-one rematch
7. Rowland meant no malice.
8. when your lion roared
9. our army en route
10. an unwise remark

Set 45
1. an early rumor
2. We are unarmed men.
3. I meant my remark.
4. low on oleo
5. Mine was removed neatly.
6. unleashed malamute
7. rooming with my in-laws
8. Why are we all out?
9. Use my reward money.
10. an hour or a minute

Set 46
1. Erin or Eileen
2. unless Ruth elopes
3. loaned Leon war relics
4. warm mineral oil
5. on our well-known list
6. our enormous ranch
7. remote memory loss
8. Were we early enough?
9. your army in Europe
10. alias Ron Miller

Set 47
1. Lake Erie run-off
2. Why alarm your mom?
3. Lou annoyed Laura.
4. Marilyn wore lace.
5. No one wore a warm muff.
6. Oh, Ruth won an Emmy!
7. rhyme almost memorized
8. When will you walk more miles?
9. uranium mine
10. a yellow lemon

Set 48
1. Yes, remain in Yuma.
2. Enroll with Mario.
3. Were you really ill?
4. Meet Lonnie at noon.
5. nor were you yourself
6. Oona asked when you'll move.
7. roaring lion unleashed
8. women or men in line
9. unwary young yaks
10. Airlines rely on you.

Stimuli for the Evaluation of Alaryngeal Speech

APPENDIX H: STIMULI FOR THE EVALUATION OF ALARYNGEAL SPEECH

EVALUATION OF THE ARTIFICIAL LARYNX

Client Name _____   Date _____

I. Two- to four-syllable phrases and sentences	Placement		"On" control		Articulation		Phrasing		Rate		Nonverbal behaviors
Unrestricted phonetic context	OK	Not OK	OK	Not OK	OK	Not OK	OK	Not OK	OK	Not OK	Describe
1. Stop the paper.											
2. last to be served											
3. choice garage space											
4. mashed potatoes											
5. Close the door.											
6. all together											
7. Judge for yourself.											
8. What's new with you?											
9. vitamin B											
10. Empty the trash.											
Total											
Percentage											

APPENDIX H: STIMULI FOR THE EVALUATION OF ALARYNGEAL SPEECH

EVALUATION OF THE ARTIFICIAL LARYNX (continued)

Client Name _____   Date _____

II. Five- to seven-syllable phrases and sentences	Placement		"On" control		Articulation		Phrasing		Rate		Nonverbal behaviors
Unrestricted phonetic context	OK	Not OK	OK	Not OK	OK	Not OK	OK	Not OK	OK	Not OK	Describe
1. age before beauty											
2. time off for good behavior											
3. How long will we have to wait?											
4. That's what friends are for.											
5. Mail the letter to Boston.											
6. Paul is taller than Jim.											
7. Read the instructions.											
8. Don't talk with your mouth full.											
9. I'll pick you up at eight.											
10. She had a good cry.											
Total											
Percentage											

APPENDIX H: STIMULI FOR THE EVALUATION OF ALARYNGEAL SPEECH

EVALUATION OF THE ARTIFICIAL LARYNX

Client Name _____ Date _____

III. Eight-syllable or more phrases and sentences	Placement		"On" control		Articulation		Phrasing		Rate		Nonverbal behaviors
Unrestricted phonetic context	OK	Not OK	OK	Not OK	OK	Not OK	OK	Not OK	OK	Not OK	Describe
1. A good start is an early morning walk.											
2. He is on a low salt, fat-free diet.											
3. Just the person I wanted to see!											
4. One for the money and two for the show.											
5. Take off your coat and have some tea.											
6. You can go, or you can stay right here.											
7. more than anything else in the world											
8. Give credit where credit is due.											
9. Take as many samples as you want.											
10. I told you that a hundred times.											
Total											
Percentage											

APPENDIX H: STIMULI FOR THE EVALUATION OF ALARYNGEAL SPEECH

EVALUATION OF THE ARTIFICIAL LARYNX (continued)

Client Name _____   Date _____

IV. Oral reading of paragraphs Unrestricted phonetic context	Placement		"On" control		Articulation		Phrasing		Rate		Nonverbal behaviors
	OK	Not OK	OK	Not OK	OK	Not OK	OK	Not OK	OK	Not OK	Describe
1. Headlights have been a standard feature on automobiles for many years.											
2. The accepted rules for use of headlights include turning your lights on between the hours of dusk and dawn.											
3. Special weather conditions, such as fog and rain, may also require use of the vehicle's headlights.											
4. Generally, the use of high beams is reserved for night driving on dark roads when there are no other cars around.											
5. Recently, you may have noticed more cars than usual with their headlights on during the daytime.											

Form continued on next page.

APPENDIX H: STIMULI FOR THE EVALUATION OF ALARYNGEAL SPEECH

EVALUATION OF THE ARTIFICIAL LARYNX (continued)

IV. Oral reading of paragraphs Unrestricted phonetic context	Placement		"On" control		Articulation		Phrasing		Rate		Nonverbal behaviors
	OK	Not OK	OK	Not OK	OK	Not OK	OK	Not OK	OK	Not OK	Describe
6. The reason is that, as of 1995, General Motors has made daytime headlights a standard feature on several of their new models.											
7. These "running lights" do not have as much glare as regular headlights and are designed to come on automatically when the car is started.											
8. The idea is to alert oncoming drivers of the car's presence.											
9. Running lights have already been in use in Canada and Scandinavian countries for a number of years.											

	Placement		"On" control		Articulation		Phrasing		Rate		Nonverbal behaviors
	OK	Not OK	OK	Not OK	OK	Not OK	OK	Not OK	OK	Not OK	Describe
IV. Oral reading of paragraphs Unrestricted phonetic context											
10. Only time will tell whether the use of running lights will reduce traffic accidents in the daylight hours.											
Total											
Percentage											

Note: These stimuli appear in paragraph form in Appendix D, "Oral Reading of Paragraphs," Paragraph 1.

APPENDIX H: STIMULI FOR THE EVALUATION OF ALARYNGEAL SPEECH

EVALUATION OF THE ARTIFICIAL LARYNX (continued)

Client Name _____   Date _____

V. Structured conversation. (Respond in 2–3 sentences) Unrestricted phonetic context	Placement		"On" control		Articulation		Phrasing		Rate		Nonverbal behaviors
	OK	Not OK	OK	Not OK	OK	Not OK	OK	Not OK	OK	Not OK	Describe
1. Describe how to change the batteries in the artificial larynx.											
2. Think of four tourist spots to visit with out-of-town guests in a weekend.											
3. Would it be a good idea to be able to "see" the future?											
4. If you could have dinner with a famous person, what would you talk about?											
5. What television show do you enjoy and why?											
6. How do you use a mail order catalogue?											
7. True or false: Large doses of vitamin C are worthless against the common cold.											
8. How would winning a $1 million lottery change your life?											

	Placement		"On" control		Articulation		Phrasing		Rate		Nonverbal behaviors
V. Structured conversation.	OK	Not OK	OK	Not OK	OK	Not OK	OK	Not OK	OK	Not OK	Describe
(Respond in 2–3 sentences) Unrestricted phonetic context											
9. What is the difference between a letter and a postcard?											
10. "A woman's place is in the home." Is this a valid statement today?											
Total											
Percentage											

APPENDIX H: STIMULI FOR THE EVALUATION OF ALARYNGEAL SPEECH

EVALUATION OF THE ARTIFICIAL LARYNX (continued)

Client Name _____   Date _____

VI. Spontaneous and extended conversation	Placement		"On" control		Articulation		Phrasing		Rate		Nonverbal behaviors
Unrestricted phonetic context	OK	Not OK	OK	Not OK	OK	Not OK	OK	Not OK	OK	Not OK	Describe
1. Discuss a recently read book or journal article.											
2. What year of your life would you like to repeat? Why?											
3. Describe the most exotic vacation you've ever taken.											
4. Debate political issues surrounding an upcoming election.											
5. Tell about your first car: make and model, cost, performance, "fun" value.											
6. Describe the teacher who had the most influence on you during your school years.											
7. Go through your wallet or purse and talk about some of the items.											

VI. Spontaneous and extended conversation Unrestricted phonetic context	Placement		"On" control		Articulation		Phrasing		Rate		Nonverbal behaviors
	OK	Not OK	OK	Not OK	OK	Not OK	OK	Not OK	OK	Not OK	Describe
8. Teach stoma hygiene care to a new laryngectomee in the group.											
9. Make a phone call to a local airline to inquire about rates to a certain city.											
10. Recommend a good pet and tell about the care and feeding involved.											
Total											
Percentage											

APPENDIX H: STIMULI FOR THE EVALUATION OF ALARYNGEAL SPEECH

EVALUATION OF THE INJECTION METHOD FOR OBSTRUENTS IN ESOPHAGEAL SPEECH

Client Name _____   Date _____

I. One-syllable words	Voicing							Intelligibility				Nonverbal behaviors
	Consistency		Quality		Latency			Articulation		Rate		
Unvoiced obstruents plus mid and low vowels	Yes	No	Esoph-ageal	Pharyn-geal	OK	Not OK		OK	Not OK	OK	Not OK	Describe
1. pop												
2. taupe												
3. call												
4. fudge												
5. shack												
6. thanks												
7. chair												
8. Spock												
9. stove												
10. stalk												
Total												
Percentage												

APPENDIX H: STIMULI FOR THE EVALUATION OF ALARYNGEAL SPEECH

EVALUATION OF THE INJECTION METHOD FOR OBSTRUENTS IN ESOPHAGEAL SPEECH *(continued)*

Client Name _____   Date _____

II. One-syllable words	Voicing				Latency		Intelligibility				Nonverbal behaviors
	Consistency		Quality				Articulation		Rate		Describe
Unvoiced obstruents plus other vowels	Yes	No	Esoph-ageal	Pharyn-geal	OK	Not OK	OK	Not OK	OK	Not OK	
1. pooch											
2. took											
3. curb											
4. feet											
5. sip											
6. shine											
7. chow											
8. spoil											
9. stood											
10. theme											
Total											
Percentage											

APPENDIX H: STIMULI FOR THE EVALUATION OF ALARYNGEAL SPEECH

EVALUATION OF THE INJECTION METHOD FOR OBSTRUENTS IN ESOPHAGEAL SPEECH (continued)

Client Name _____   Date _____

III. One-syllable words	Voicing								Intelligibility						Nonverbal behaviors
Voiced obstruents plus mid and low vowels	Consistency		Quality		Latency		Articulation		Rate		Describe
	Yes	No	Esoph-ageal	Pharyn-geal	OK	Not OK	OK	Not OK	OK	Not OK	
1. ball											
2. dome											
3. gaunt											
4. vast											
5. zapped											
6. they											
7. gem											
8. boast											
9. dog											
10. gum											
Total											
Percentage											

APPENDIX H: STIMULI FOR THE EVALUATION OF ALARYNGEAL SPEECH

EVALUATION OF THE INJECTION METHOD FOR OBSTRUENTS IN ESOPHAGEAL SPEECH (continued)

Client Name _____ Date _____

IV. One-syllable words	Voicing						Intelligibility				Nonverbal behaviors
	Consistency		Quality		Latency		Articulation		Rate		Describe
Voiced obstruents plus other vowels	Yes	No	Esoph-ageal	Pharyn-geal	OK	Not OK	OK	Not OK	OK	Not OK	
1. boot											
2. dirt											
3. good											
4. veal											
5. zip											
6. thine											
7. joust											
8. boy											
9. duke											
10. girl											
Total											
Percentage											

APPENDIX H: STIMULI FOR THE EVALUATION OF ALARYNGEAL SPEECH

EVALUATION OF THE INJECTION METHOD FOR OBSTRUENTS IN ESOPHAGEAL SPEECH (continued)

Client Name _____   Date _____

| V. One-syllable words | Voicing | | | | | | | Intelligibility | | | | Nonverbal behaviors |
| | Consistency | | Quality | | Latency | | Articulation | | Rate | | Describe |
Unvoiced and voiced obstruent blends	Yes	No	Esoph-ageal	Pharyn-geal	OK	Not OK	OK	Not OK	OK	Not OK	Describe
1. plot											
2. troll											
3. clay											
4. France											
5. smear											
6. shriek											
7. thrush											
8. blue											
9. draw											
10. glide											
Total											
Percentage											

APPENDIX H: STIMULI FOR THE EVALUATION OF ALARYNGEAL SPEECH

EVALUATION OF THE INJECTION METHOD FOR OBSTRUENTS IN ESOPHAGEAL SPEECH (continued)

Client Name _____   Date _____

VI. Two-syllable words	Voicing				Intelligibility			Nonverbal behaviors
	Consistency		Quality		Latency	Articulation	Rate	Describe
Unvoiced obstruents plus any vowel	Yes	No	Esoph-ageal	Pharyn-geal	OK / Not OK	OK / Not OK	OK / Not OK	
1. pop top								
2. too soon								
3. coating								
4. footage								
5. sought care								
6. sure thing								
7. thump fast								
8. cheap suit								
9. spastic								
10. stick shift								
Total								
Percentage								

APPENDIX H: STIMULI FOR THE EVALUATION OF ALARYNGEAL SPEECH

EVALUATION OF THE INJECTION METHOD FOR OBSTRUENTS IN ESOPHAGEAL SPEECH (continued)

Client Name _____ Date _____

| VII. Two-syllable words | Voicing | | | | | | Intelligibility | | | | Nonverbal behaviors |
| | Consistency | | Quality | | Latency | | Articulation | | Rate | | Describe |
Unvoiced and voiced obstruents plus any vowel	Yes	No	Esoph-ageal	Pharyn-geal	OK	Not OK	OK	Not OK	OK	Not OK	
1. pot boil											
2. today											
3. cozy											
4. football											
5. sawdust											
6. shirt box											
7. thunder											
8. cheeseball											
9. spasm											
10. stick gum											
Total											
Percentage											

APPENDIX H: STIMULI FOR THE EVALUATION OF ALARYNGEAL SPEECH

EVALUATION OF THE INJECTION METHOD FOR OBSTRUENTS IN ESOPHAGEAL SPEECH (continued)

Client Name _____   Date _____

VIII. Two-syllable words	Voicing						Intelligibility						Nonverbal behaviors
	Consistency		Quality		Latency		Articulation		Rate				Describe
Voiced obstruents plus any vowel	Yes	No	Esoph-ageal	Pharyn-geal	OK	Not OK	OK	Not OK	OK	Not OK			
1. bargain													
2. doodle													
3. goes down													
4. Val's eyes													
5. zibet													
6. They jumped.													
7. jet black													
8. boredom													
9. double													
10. gorgeous													
Total													
Percentage													

APPENDIX H: STIMULI FOR THE EVALUATION OF ALARYNGEAL SPEECH

EVALUATION OF THE INJECTION METHOD FOR OBSTRUENTS IN ESOPHAGEAL SPEECH (continued)

Client Name _____   Date _____

IX. Three- to four-syllable phrases	Voicing							Intelligibility					Nonverbal behaviors
	Consistency		Quality		Latency			Articulation		Rate		Describe
Voiced and unvoiced obstruents in the releasing positions	Yes	No	Esoph-ageal	Pharyn-geal	OK	Not OK		OK	Not OK	OK	Not OK	
1. sugar cookies												
2. done that before												
3. Stop and go.												
4. quick and easy												
5. Get started.												
6. Vacuum carpets.												
7. Keep on truckin'.												
8. Forget it.												
9. because of Ted												
10. Pocket some cash.												
Total												
Percentage												

APPENDIX H: STIMULI FOR THE EVALUATION OF ALARYNGEAL SPEECH

EVALUATION OF THE INJECTION METHOD FOR OBSTRUENTS IN ESOPHAGEAL SPEECH (continued)

Client Name _____   Date _____

X. Five- to six-syllable phrases Voiced and unvoiced obstruents in the releasing and arresting positions	Voicing							Intelligibility				Nonverbal behaviors
	Consistency		Quality		Latency			Articulation		Rate		Describe
	Yes	No	Esoph-ageal	Pharyn-geal	OK	Not OK		OK	Not OK	OK	Not OK	
1. back in the saddle												
2. decent cup of coffee												
3. face down position												
4. vision for the future												
5. Put the car top down.												
6. Schedule time to rest.												
7. Table for two, please.												
8. That is a good show.												
9. Gail's blind as a bat.												
10. fifty-fifty chance												
Total												
Percentage												

APPENDIX H: STIMULI FOR THE EVALUATION OF ALARYNGEAL SPEECH

EVALUATION OF THE INJECTION METHOD FOR SONORANTS AND VOWELS AND FOR THE EVALUATION OF THE INHALATION METHOD IN ESOPHAGEAL SPEECH

Client Name _____   Date _____

| I. One-syllable words beginning with mid and low vowels | Voicing | | | | Intelligibility | | | | | | Nonverbal behaviors |
| | Consistency | | Quality | | Latency | | Articulation | | Rate | | Describe |
	Yes	No	Esoph-ageal	Pharyn-geal	OK	Not OK	OK	Not OK	OK	Not OK	
1. a											
2. oaf											
3. all											
4. of											
5. act											
6. Abe											
7. air											
8. arch											
9. oak											
10. awl											
Total											
Percentage											

APPENDIX H: STIMULI FOR THE EVALUATION OF ALARYNGEAL SPEECH

EVALUATION OF THE INJECTION METHOD FOR SONORANTS AND VOWELS AND FOR THE EVALUATION OF THE INHALATION METHOD IN ESOPHAGEAL SPEECH (continued)

Client Name _____   Date _____

II. One-syllable words beginning with other vowels	Voicing						Intelligibility						Nonverbal behaviors
	Consistency		Quality		Latency		Articulation		Rate				Describe
	Yes	No	Esoph-ageal	Pharyn-geal	OK	Not OK	OK	Not OK	OK	Not OK			
1. ooze													
2. oops													
3. earl													
4. each													
5. ear													
6. aisle													
7. ouch													
8. oil													
9. oozed													
10. oomph													
Total													
Percentage													

APPENDIX H: STIMULI FOR THE EVALUATION OF ALARYNGEAL SPEECH

EVALUATION OF THE INJECTION METHOD FOR SONORANTS AND VOWELS AND FOR THE EVALUATION OF THE INHALATION METHOD IN ESOPHAGEAL SPEECH (continued)

Client Name _____   Date _____

III. One-syllable words	Voicing								Intelligibility						Nonverbal behaviors
	Consistency		Quality		Latency		Articulation		Rate			
Sonorants plus mid and low vowels	Yes	No	Esoph-ageal	Pharyn-geal	OK	Not OK	OK	Not OK	OK	Not OK	Describe
1. wad											
2. lone											
3. raw											
4. young											
5. mask											
6. nail											
7. war											
8. lunch											
9. rack											
10. may											
Total											
Percentage											

APPENDIX H: STIMULI FOR THE EVALUATION OF ALARYNGEAL SPEECH

EVALUATION OF THE INJECTION METHOD FOR SONORANTS AND VOWELS AND FOR THE EVALUATION OF THE INHALATION METHOD IN ESOPHAGEAL SPEECH (continued)

Client Name _____   Date _____

| IV. One-syllable words | Voicing | | | | | | Intelligibility | | | | | | Nonverbal behaviors |
| Sonorants plus other vowels | Consistency | | Quality | | Latency | | Articulation | | Rate | | Describe |
	Yes	No	Esoph-ageal	Pharyn-geal	OK	Not OK	OK	Not OK	OK	Not OK	
1. wounds											
2. look											
3. rhyme											
4. yeast											
5. mill											
6. knife											
7. wow											
8. Lloyd											
9. room											
10. meet											
Total											
Percentage											

APPENDIX H: STIMULI FOR THE EVALUATION OF ALARYNGEAL SPEECH

EVALUATION OF THE INJECTION METHOD FOR SONORANTS AND VOWELS AND FOR THE EVALUATION OF THE INHALATION METHOD IN ESOPHAGEAL SPEECH (continued)

Client Name _____   Date _____

V. Two-syllable words beginning with sonorants and vowels	Voicing								Intelligibility						Nonverbal behaviors
	Consistency		Quality		Latency		Articulation		Rate						Describe
	Yes	No	Esoph-ageal	Pharyn-geal	OK	Not OK	OK	Not OK	OK	Not OK					
1. way out															
2. arrow															
3. lawyer															
4. oolong															
5. really															
6. omit															
7. manner															
8. earn it															
9. eyelash															
10. alert															
Total															
Percentage															

APPENDIX H: STIMULI FOR THE EVALUATION OF ALARYNGEAL SPEECH

EVALUATION OF THE INJECTION METHOD FOR SONORANTS AND VOWELS AND FOR THE EVALUATION OF THE INHALATION METHOD IN ESOPHAGEAL SPEECH (continued)

Client Name _____   Date _____

VI. Three- to four-syllable phrases	Voicing						Intelligibility				Nonverbal behaviors
	Consistency		Quality		Latency		Articulation		Rate		Describe
Sonorants and vowels in releasing positions	Yes	No	Esoph-ageal	Pharyn-geal	OK	Not OK	OK	Not OK	OK	Not OK	
1. wrong yacht launched											
2. unaware											
3. lanolin											
4. I'm all out.											
5. roll away											
6. Earn more money.											
7. You were right.											
8. enormous											
9. Many are nice.											
10. nine new menus											
Total											
Percentage											

APPENDIX H: STIMULI FOR THE EVALUATION OF ALARYNGEAL SPEECH

EVALUATION OF THE INJECTION METHOD FOR SONORANTS AND VOWELS AND FOR THE EVALUATION OF THE INHALATION METHOD IN ESOPHAGEAL SPEECH (continued)

Client Name _____ Date _____

VII. Five- to six-syllable phrases	Voicing						Intelligibility						Nonverbal behaviors
	Consistency		Quality		Latency		Articulation		Rate			Describe
Sonorants and vowels in releasing positions	Yes	No	Esoph-ageal	Pharyn-geal	OK	Not OK	OK	Not OK	OK	Not OK		
1. a lenient nun												
2. early morning noise												
3. Know your enemies.												
4. on area rugs												
5. really low on money												
6. way out maniac												
7. You are in an army.												
8. Illinois laws												
9. lemon marinade												
10. minor error in math												
Total												
Percentage												

APPENDIX H: STIMULI FOR THE EVALUATION OF ALARYNGEAL SPEECH

EVALUATION OF COMBINED METHODS OF ESOPHAGEAL SPEECH

Client Name _____   Date _____

I. Two- to four-syllable phrases and sentences Unrestricted phonetic context	Articulation		Rate		Phrasing		Intonation		Loudness		Nonverbal behaviors
	OK	Not OK	OK	Not OK	OK	Not OK	OK	Not OK	OK	Not OK	Describe
1. Stop the paper.											
2. last to be served											
3. choice garage space											
4. mashed potatoes											
5. Close the door.											
6. all together											
7. Judge for yourself.											
8. What's new with you?											
9. vitamin B											
10. Empty the trash.											
Total											
Percentage											

APPENDIX H: STIMULI FOR THE EVALUATION OF ALARYNGEAL SPEECH

EVALUATION OF COMBINED METHODS OF ESOPHAGEAL SPEECH (continued)

Client Name _____ Date _____

II. Five- to seven-syllable phrases and sentences	Articulation		Rate		Phrasing		Intonation		Loudness		Nonverbal behaviors
Unrestricted phonetic context	OK	Not OK	OK	Not OK	OK	Not OK	OK	Not OK	OK	Not OK	Describe
1. age before beauty											
2. time off for good behavior											
3. How long will we have to wait?											
4. That's what friends are for.											
5. Mail the letter to Boston.											
6. Paul is taller than Jim.											
7. Read the instructions.											
8. Don't talk with your mouth full.											
9. I'll pick you up at eight.											
10. She had a good cry.											
Total											
Percentage											

APPENDIX H: STIMULI FOR THE EVALUATION OF ALARYNGEAL SPEECH

EVALUATION OF COMBINED METHODS OF ESOPHAGEAL SPEECH (continued)

Client Name _____   Date _____

III. Eight-syllable or more phrases and sentences — Unrestricted phonetic context	Articulation		Rate		Phrasing		Intonation		Loudness		Nonverbal behaviors
	OK	Not OK	OK	Not OK	OK	Not OK	OK	Not OK	OK	Not OK	Describe
1. A good start is an early morning walk.											
2. He is on a low salt, fat-free diet.											
3. Just the person I wanted to see!											
4. One for the money and two for the show.											
5. Take off your coat and have some tea.											
6. You can go, or you can stay right here.											
7. more than anything else in the world											
8. Give credit where credit is due.											
9. Take as many as you want.											
10. I told you a hundred times.											
Total											
Percentage											

APPENDIX H: STIMULI FOR THE EVALUATION OF ALARYNGEAL SPEECH

EVALUATION OF COMBINED METHODS OF ESOPHAGEAL SPEECH (continued)

Client Name _____ Date _____

IV. Oral reading of paragraphs Unrestricted phonetic context	Articulation		Rate		Phrasing		Intonation		Loudness		Nonverbal behaviors
	OK	Not OK	OK	Not OK	OK	Not OK	OK	Not OK	OK	Not OK	Describe
1. Headlights have been a standard feature on automobiles for many years.											
2. The accepted rules for use of headlights include turning your lights on between the hours of dusk and dawn.											
3. Special weather conditions, such as fog and rain, may also require use of the vehicle's headlights.											
4. Generally, the use of high beams is reserved for night driving on dark roads when there are no other cars around.											
5. Recently, you may have noticed more cars than usual with their headlights on during the daytime.											

IV. Oral reading of paragraphs Unrestricted phonetic context	Articulation		Rate		Phrasing		Intonation		Loudness		Nonverbal behaviors
	OK	Not OK	OK	Not OK	OK	Not OK	OK	Not OK	OK	Not OK	Describe
6. The reason is that, as of 1995, General Motors has made daytime headlights a standard feature on several of their new models.											
7. These "running lights" do not have as much glare as regular headlights and are designed to come on automatically when the car is started.											
8. The idea is to alert oncoming drivers of the car's presence.											
9. Running lights have already been in use in Canada and Scandinavian countries for a number of years.											

Form continued on next page.

APPENDIX H: STIMULI FOR THE EVALUATION OF ALARYNGEAL SPEECH

EVALUATION OF COMBINED METHODS OF ESOPHAGEAL SPEECH (continued)

Client Name _____ Date _____

IV. Oral reading of paragraphs	Articulation		Rate		Phrasing		Intonation		Loudness		Nonverbal behaviors
	OK	Not OK	OK	Not OK	OK	Not OK	OK	Not OK	OK	Not OK	Describe
Unrestricted phonetic context											
10. Only time will tell whether the use of running lights will reduce traffic accidents in the daylight hours.											
Total											
Percentage											

Note: These stimuli appear in paragraph form in Appendix D, "Oral Reading of Paragraphs," Paragraph 1.

APPENDIX H: STIMULI FOR THE EVALUATION OF ALARYNGEAL SPEECH

EVALUATION OF COMBINED METHODS OF ESOPHAGEAL SPEECH *(continued)*

Client Name _____   Date _____

V. Structured conversation (Respond in 2–3 sentences) Unrestricted phonetic context	Articulation		Rate		Phrasing		Intonation		Loudness		Nonverbal behaviors
	OK	Not OK	OK	Not OK	OK	Not OK	OK	Not OK	OK	Not OK	Describe
1. Describe how to change the batteries in the artificial larynx.											
2. Think of four tourist spots to visit with out-of-town guests in a weekend.											
3. Would it be a good idea to be able to "see" the future?											
4. If you could have dinner with a famous person, what would you talk about?											
5. What television show do you enjoy and why?											
6. How do you use a mail order catalogue?											
7. True or false: Large doses of vitamin C are worthless against the common cold.											
8. How would winning a $1 million lottery change your life?											

Form continued on next page.

APPENDIX H: STIMULI FOR THE EVALUATION OF ALARYNGEAL SPEECH

EVALUATION OF COMBINED METHODS OF ESOPHAGEAL SPEECH (continued)

Client Name _____ Date _____

V. Structured conversation	Articulation		Rate		Phrasing		Intonation		Loudness		Nonverbal behaviors
	OK	Not OK	OK	Not OK	OK	Not OK	OK	Not OK	OK	Not OK	Describe
(Respond in 2–3 sentences) Unrestricted phonetic context											
9. What is the difference between a letter and a postcard?											
10. "A woman's place is in the home." Is this a valid statement today?											
Total											
Percentage											

APPENDIX H: STIMULI FOR THE EVALUATION OF ALARYNGEAL SPEECH

EVALUATION OF COMBINED METHODS OF ESOPHAGEAL SPEECH (continued)

Client Name _____   Date _____

VI. Spontaneous and extended conversation Unrestricted phonetic context	Articulation		Rate		Phrasing		Intonation		Loudness		Nonverbal behaviors
	OK	Not OK	OK	Not OK	OK	Not OK	OK	Not OK	OK	Not OK	Describe
1. Discuss a recently read book or journal article.											
2. What year of your life would you like to repeat? Why?											
3. Describe the most exotic vacation you've ever taken.											
4. Debate political issues surrounding an upcoming election.											
5. Tell about your first car: make and model, cost, performance, "fun" value.											
6. Describe the teacher who had the most influence on you during your school years.											
7. Go through your wallet or purse and talk about some of the items.											

Form continued on next page.

APPENDIX H: STIMULI FOR THE EVALUATION OF ALARYNGEAL SPEECH

EVALUATION OF COMBINED METHODS OF ESOPHAGEAL SPEECH (continued)

Client Name _____   Date _____

VI. Spontaneous and extended conversation	Articulation		Rate		Phrasing		Intonation		Loudness		Nonverbal behaviors
Unrestricted phonetic context	OK	Not OK	OK	Not OK	OK	Not OK	OK	Not OK	OK	Not OK	Describe
8. Teach stoma hygiene care to a new laryngectomee in the group.											
9. Make a phone call to a local airline to inquire about rates to a certain city.											
10. Recommend a good pet and tell about the care and feeding involved.											
Total											
Percentage											

APPENDIX H: STIMULI FOR THE EVALUATION OF ALARYNGEAL SPEECH

EVALUATION OF TRACHEOESOPHAGEAL SPEECH

Client Name _____   Date _____

I. Two- to four-syllable phrases and sentences	Valving		Articulation		Phrasing		Rate		Nonverbal behaviors
Unrestricted phonetic context	OK	Not OK	OK	Not OK	OK	Not OK	OK	Not OK	Describe
1. Stop the paper.									
2. last to be served									
3. choice garage space									
4. mashed potatoes									
5. Close the door.									
6. all together									
7. Judge for yourself.									
8. What's new with you?									
9. vitamin B									
10. Empty the trash.									
Total									
Percentage									

APPENDIX H: STIMULI FOR THE EVALUATION OF ALARYNGEAL SPEECH

EVALUATION OF TRACHEOESOPHAGEAL SPEECH (continued)

Client Name _____ Date _____

II. Five- to seven-syllable phrases and sentences	Valving		Articulation		Phrasing		Rate		Nonverbal behaviors
Unrestricted phonetic context	OK	Not OK	OK	Not OK	OK	Not OK	OK	Not OK	Describe
1. age before beauty									
2. time off for good behavior									
3. How long will we have to wait?									
4. That's what friends are for.									
5. Mail the letter to Boston.									
6. Paul is taller than Jim.									
7. Read the instructions.									
8. Don't talk with your mouth full.									
9. I'll pick you up at eight.									
10. She had a good cry.									
Total									
Percentage									

APPENDIX H: STIMULI FOR THE EVALUATION OF ALARYNGEAL SPEECH

EVALUATION OF TRACHEOESOPHAGEAL SPEECH (continued)

Client Name _____   Date _____

III. Eight-syllable or more phrases and sentences

Unrestricted phonetic context	Valving		Articulation		Phrasing		Rate		Nonverbal behaviors
	OK	Not OK	OK	Not OK	OK	Not OK	OK	Not OK	Describe
1. A good start is an early morning walk.									
2. He is on a low salt, fat-free diet.									
3. Just the person I wanted to see!									
4. One for the money and two for the show.									
5. Take off your coat and have some tea.									
6. You can go, or you can stay right here.									
7. more than anything else in the world									
8. Give credit where credit is due.									
9. Take as many as you want.									
10. I told you a hundred times.									
Total									
Percentage									

APPENDIX H: STIMULI FOR THE EVALUATION OF ALARYNGEAL SPEECH

EVALUATION OF TRACHEOESOPHAGEAL SPEECH (continued)

Client Name _____   Date _____

	Valving		Articulation		Phrasing		Rate		Nonverbal behaviors
IV. Oral reading of paragraphs Unrestricted phonetic context	OK	Not OK	OK	Not OK	OK	Not OK	OK	Not OK	Describe
1. Headlights have been a standard feature on automobiles for many years.									
2. The accepted rules for use of headlights include turning your lights on between the hours of dusk and dawn.									
3. Special weather conditions, such as fog and rain may also require use of the vehicle's headlights.									
4. Generally, the use of high beams is reserved for night driving on dark roads when there are no other cars around.									
5. Recently, you may have noticed more cars than usual with their headlights on during the daytime.									
6. The reason is that, as of 1995, General Motors has made daytime headlights a standard feature on several of their new models.									

	Valving		Articulation		Phrasing		Rate		Nonverbal behaviors
IV. Oral reading of paragraphs Unrestricted phonetic context	OK	Not OK	OK	Not OK	OK	Not OK	OK	Not OK	Describe
7. These "running lights" do not have as much glare as regular headlights and are designed to come on automatically when the car is started.									
8. The idea is to alert oncoming drivers of the car's presence.									
9. Running lights have already been in use in Canada and Scandinavian countries for a number of years.									
10. Only time will tell whether the use of running lights will reduce traffic accidents in the daylight hours.									
Total									
Percentage									

Note: These stimuli appear in paragraph form in Appendix D, "Oral Reading of Paragraphs," Paragraph 1.

APPENDIX H: STIMULI FOR THE EVALUATION OF ALARYNGEAL SPEECH

EVALUATION OF TRACHEOESOPHAGEAL SPEECH (continued)

Client Name _____ Date _____

V. Structured conversation (Respond in 2–3 sentences.) Unrestricted phonetic context	Valving OK	Not OK	Articulation OK	Not OK	Phrasing OK	Not OK	Rate OK	Not OK	Nonverbal behaviors Describe
1. Describe how to change the batteries in the artificial larynx.									
2. Think of four tourist spots to visit with out-of-town guests in a weekend.									
3. Would it be a good idea to be able to "see" the future?									
4. If you could have dinner with a famous person, what would you talk about?									
5. What television show do you enjoy and why?									
6. How do you use a mail order catalogue?									
7. True or false: Large doses of vitamin C are worthless against the common cold.									
8. How would winning a $1 million lottery change your life?									

V. Structured conversation (Respond in 2–3 sentences.) Unrestricted phonetic context	Valving		Articulation		Phrasing		Rate		Nonverbal behaviors
	OK	Not OK	OK	Not OK	OK	Not OK	OK	Not OK	Describe
9. What is the difference between a letter and a postcard?									
10. "A woman's place is in the home." Is this a valid statement today?									
Total									
Percentage									

APPENDIX H: STIMULI FOR THE EVALUATION OF ALARYNGEAL SPEECH

EVALUATION OF TRACHEOESOPHAGEAL SPEECH (continued)

Client Name _____ Date _____

	Valving		Articulation		Phrasing		Rate		Nonverbal behaviors
	OK	Not OK	OK	Not OK	OK	Not OK	OK	Not OK	Describe
V. Spontaneous and extended conversation Unrestricted phonetic context									
1. Discuss a recently read book or journal article.									
2. What year of your life would you like to repeat? Why?									
3. Describe the most exotic vacation you've ever taken.									
4. Debate political issues surrounding an upcoming election.									
5. Tell about your first car: make and model, cost, performance, "fun" value.									
6. Describe the teacher who had the most influence on you during your school years.									
7. Go through your wallet or purse and talk about some of the items.									
8. Teach stoma hygiene care to a new laryngectomee in the group.									

	Valving		Articulation		Phrasing		Rate		Nonverbal behaviors
V. Spontaneous and extended conversation Unrestricted phonetic context	OK	Not OK	OK	Not OK	OK	Not OK	OK	Not OK	Describe
9. Make a phone call to a local airline to inquire about rates to a certain city.									
10. Recommend a good pet and tell about the care and feeding involved.									
Total									
Percentage									

Index